BICTON
COLLEGE
of Agriculture

CULTUS EX MENTIS CULTU

Education
Ce

D1345832

HANDBOOK OF
Small Animal
Toxicology
&
Poisonings

HANDBOOK OF

Small Amimal Toxicology *&* Poisonings

Roger W. Gfeller, DVM

Practitioner, Diplomate American College of
Veterinary Emergency and Critical Care,
Veterinary Emergency Service,
Fresno, California

Shawn P. Messonnier, DVM

Practitioner,
Paws and Claws Veterinary Hospital,
Plano, Texas

 Mosby

St. Louis Baltimore Boston Carlsbad Chicago Minneapolis New York Philadelphia Portland
London Milan Sydney Tokyo Toronto

Publisher: John A. Schrefer
Executive Editor: Linda L. Duncan
Senior Developmental Editor: Teri Merchant
Project Manager: Dana Peick
Manuscript Editor: Carl Masthay
Designer: Elizabeth Rohne Rudder
Manufacturing Manager: Betty Mueller

A NOTE TO THE READER
The authors and publisher have made every attempt to check dosages
and nursing content for accuracy. Because the science of pharmacology
is continually advancing, our knowledge base continues to expand.
Therefore we recommend that the reader always check product information for changes in dosage or administration before administering any
medication. This is particularly important with new or rarely used drugs.

Printed in the United States of America
Composition by Accu-Color, Inc.
Printing/binding by R. R. Donnelley

Mosby, Inc.
11830 Westline Industrial Drive
St. Louis, Missouri 63146

Library of Congress Cataloging-in-Publication Data

Gfeller. Roger W.
     Handbook of small animal toxicology and poisonings / Roger W.
Gfeller, Shawn P. Messonnier.
         p.   cm.
     Includes bibliographical references (p.   ) and index.
     ISBN 0-8151-6454-8
     1. Dogs--Diseases--Treatment--Handbooks, manuals, etc. 2. Cats-
-Diseases--Treatment--Handbooks, manuals, etc. 3. Veterinary
toxicology--Handbooks, manuals, etc. I. Messonnier. Shawn.
II. Title.
SF991.G494   1997   97-42301
636.089'59--DC21   CIP

97 98 99 00 01 / 9 8 7 6 5 4 3 2 1

To our wives (Sandy Messonnier and Margie Gfeller) and our kids (Erica Messonnier, Hayley Gfeller, Heath Gfeller, and Scott Gfeller), whose love and support have allowed us the strength and resolve to complete this worthy project

And

To the many patients who will be helped by caring professionals utilizing the information contained within these pages

Preface

Several years ago I (Shawn Messonnier) recognized that there was literally no one reference for the veterinarian treating the poisoned pet. When I proposed the idea for the book to our editor, Dr. Paul Pratt, he agreed that there was a definite void in the veterinary literature in the area of treating small animal intoxications. With his guidance, our team was formed to address this shortcoming. Now with the completion of this text, veterinarians will have at their disposal a handy reference to use when the need arises to treat the poisoned pet. We truly believe our book, Handbook of Small Animal Toxicology and Poisonings, fills this void in our profession.

We have spent a great deal of time and energy completing this book, doing our best to make sure it contains the latest and most accurate information to help you in your practice. During the course of this research, we discovered how little is truly known about treating poisonings in dogs and cats. Much of the literature is based on case reports and extrapolations from human literature. It is obvious that more research needs to be done in the field of veterinary toxicology.

This book is organized to help the practitioner quickly get the information needed to optimize problem recognition and treatment of the poisoned or intoxicated patient. Section One, Rapid Patient Evaluation and Symptomatic Treatment of the Poisoned Pet, is written to cover those nebulous instructions, "Give symptomatic support." Using this section to identify and treat "problems" rather than a "diagnosis" will allow the practicing veterinarian to handle most poisoned patients, even though the causative agent is unknown.

In Section Two, Toxic Drugs and Chemicals, we have taken the most commonly identified poisons and condensed the information that is known about each. Just underneath each agent, you will find four icons. These icons are designed to provide the reader important information at a glance. (See page viii.)

	EMESIS recommended		EMESIS NOT recommended		Value of EMESIS unknown
L	Gastric LAVAGE recommended		Gastric LAVAGE NOT recommended		Value of gastric LAVAGE unknown
C	Activated CHARCOAL recommended		Activated CHARCOAL NOT recommended		Value of activated CHARCOAL unknown
A	ANTIDOTE exists		NO known ANTIDOTE		Value of ANTIDOTE unknown

The text continues following a format that identifies the most common sources of the poison and a brief description of its mechanism of action. Next, the clinical signs are described in text form followed by a section on treatment. A list of signs is followed by a quick guide to emergency treatment. In this area you will find emergency procedures, instructions for decontamination, antidotal and supportive care information, enhancement of elimination procedures, and any precautions that are known.

Section Three, Toxic Plants, provides an extensive index of common names of plants known to be toxic to small animals. After the index, each plant species is written up with a brief description of the known common names, the toxin or toxins produced by the plant, and the part or parts of the species that are known to be toxic. A paragraph describing clinical signs caused by the plant is followed by known treatment recommendations.

Following Section Three are the appendices. Appendix A is a formulary of drugs often used in treating poisoned patients. We have taken great effort to assure that this section is accurate, but, as with all the research we did, we found great variations in recommended dosage information. We chose the recommendations that we could verify in referenced veterinary literature. Appendix B is the daily fluid requirements for dogs and cats. Appendix C is a series of "recipes" that will allow the veterinarian to accurately formulate and administer drugs by continuous intravenous infusion. Appendix D is a flow chart that may be copied and used in charting the course of treatment of the poisoned pet.

As with all written works, every effort has been made to provide true, factual, and accurate information. We welcome all comments and advice. Although we predict that practitioners will find this book extremely practical and useful, we know that any and all criticism can only make the product better.

Roger W. Gfeller
Shawn P. Messonnier

Acknowledgments

We first would like to say a huge thanks to Brent Ekins, PharmD, ABAT, and his staff at the Central California Regional Poison Control Center in Fresno, California. Their generous assistance and cooperation in making this project a success goes far begond their job descriptions. No matter how busy, they always seemed to manage to find a way to get us the information we needed.

Next, our colleagues at Custer Parkway Animal, Plano, Texas, deserve recognition and our thanks for providing additional reference materials.

Finally, we acknowledge the editorial and production staff of Mosby, Inc. We particularly wish to say thanks to Dr. Paul Pratt, Terri Merchant, and Dr. Carl Masthay, with whom we have had numerous communications in getting this text done.

Roger W. Gfeller
Shawn P. Messonnier

Contents

ABC's of emergency care (Inside front cover)

■ SECTION ONE

*RAPID PATIENT EVALUATION
AND SYMPTOMATIC TREATMENT
OF THE POISONED PET*

The initial contact with the owner of a pet that has been poisoned is frequently by telephone. The advice offered to the caller may have a significant influence on the outcome. Failure to supply the owner with appropriate information may also affect the case and usually not in a positive way (Box 1-1).

The "poisoned" veterinary patient remains a significant challenge to the practicing veterinarian. Not all acutely ill patients are poisoned, and not all poisoned patients are acutely ill. A patient presented with the history of exposure to a toxin or poison should be considered to have a potentially life-threatening problem. The veterinarian faced with a critical patient must immediately evaluate the need for lifesaving procedures and support. As always, the emergent patient is examined and treated using the ABC's.

The chart on the inside front cover includes a quick review of emergency procedures recommended for support of the patient presented with the possibility of being poisoned. Although written in a sequential order, several items may be performed simultaneously as needed by members of the resuscitation team (for example, one member establishes an airway while another gains IV access).

AIRWAY

Lifesaving interventions begin with the airway. Many poisons directly or indirectly cause fluid or secretions to build up in the airway. These may occlude the airway leading to hypoxic complications and possibly even death.

GENERAL

One of the greatest contributors to patient death from poisoning is loss of airway-protective reflexes with subsequent airway obstruction by a flaccid tongue or aspiration of gastric contents.

Evaluate the airway by direct examination if possible. Patients who are awake and alert are not likely to need airway intervention, but the veterinary team must be alert for signs of deterioration that can result in rapid loss of airway control. Loud upper airway sounds such as gurgling, stertor, or stridor are indications that the patient is in danger of losing

BOX 1-1

INSTRUCTIONS TO OWNERS

FIRST AID
Attempt to identify the offending substance and route of poisoning.
Advise the owner as follows:
Bring the package (or what is left of it) to the hospital.

INGESTED TOXINS
Induce emesis only if:
- Ingestion was within the last 30 to 60 minutes.
- The substance ingested was *not* a strong acid or alkali.
- The substance ingested was *not* a petroleum distillate
  (such as kerosene, gasoline, lighter fluid).
- The pet is alert, conscious, and cooperative.

Induce emesis using:
- Syrup of ipecac may be administered at $\frac{1}{2}$ to 1 teaspoon
  per 10 lb PO in the dog or 1 teaspoon PO for an
  average-sized cat.
- Hydrogen peroxide (3%) may be given PO at 1 tablespoon per 20 lb.
- Salt, mustard, and many other substances have been
  advocated but have proved ineffective and possibly even
  dangerous.

If the substance was a strong acid, a strong alkali, or a petroleum
distillate, advise the owner to administer milk or egg and rush the
patient to a treatment facility. Immediate administration of activated charcoal (read label for dose) by the owner should be recommended. Numerous over-the-counter products are available,
but few pet owners have one of them at hand.

INHALED TOXINS
- Move the patient to fresh air or an area with adequate
  ventilation.
- Provide artificial respiration if required.
- Transport to the hospital as soon as possible.

SKIN CONTAMINATION
- If the patient has been contaminated with a dry powder,
  carefully brush the powder away using a firm-bristled

(Continued)

BOX 1-1

INSTRUCTIONS TO OWNERS—cont'd

SKIN CONTAMINATION—cont'd
brush. It is extremely important to protect the patient's and the caregiver's eyes, nose, and mouth to avoid inhalation or ingestion of the powder during this procedure.
- Thoroughly rinse the contaminated area with running water.
- Once the area has been thoroughly rinsed, wash the area with soap and water and rinse well.
- Continue bathing and rinsing for at least 15 minutes.
- Do *not* attempt to neutralize the poison.

TOXIN IN THE EYE
- Promptly flush the eye with water or saline and continue to flush for at least 10 minutes.
- Saline is more comfortable to the ocular tissues and can be made at home by adding 2 teaspoons of table salt to a quart of warm water.

Repeat the need to bring any information about the poison to the hospital (the package, bottle, or anything else that may help identify the active toxic ingredient).

the airway. It is considerably better to secure the airway (perhaps) prematurely than to make the patient "prove" that the airway is in jeopardy.

Test the gag/cough reflex by putting a tongue depressor or other object in the pharyngeal area. Conscious patients usually have an intact gag/cough reflex and can be expected to protect their airway. Obtunded or comatose patients may lack this protection. These patients are in grave danger because they may rapidly lose their airway. If any doubt exists regarding the patient's ability to protect his or her airway, endotracheal or tracheal intubation should be performed.

TREATMENT

Patients should be positioned in left lateral recumbency with the head in a slightly extended position to maximize the airway. Patients with mild risk for vomiting or aspiration should be positioned with the head down so that secretions or vomitus can drain out of the mouth by gravity flow.

If the airway is still not patent, it should be cleared using a suction machine (preferable), bulb syringe, or other suction device. It is wise to have a "ready area" of the hospital where a suction device is set up in advance to anticipate these complications. Foreign bodies are removed using a Heimlich-like maneuver, finger sweep, or forceps.

Endotracheal intubation is necessary when the patient cannot protect his or her own airway (such as coma, obtundation, anesthesia), when there is obstruction, or when the patient suffers ventilatory failure (see below). Endotracheal intubation provides the most reliable protection of the airway. It prevents aspiration and obstruction by swelling of oropharyngeal tissues. Endotracheal intubation also allows for mechanical ventilation.

Tracheal intubation (tracheostomy, tracheotomy) is necessary when endotracheal intubation is not possible because of a physical obstruction of the rostral trachea. Even though this would be an uncommon finding in cases of poisoning, the "ready area" should have a tracheotomy-tracheostomy tray to anticipate such needs.

BREATHING

Once the airway is determined to be open and secure, an evaluation of breathing must be performed. Respiratory complications fall into the categories of ventilatory failure, hypoxia, or bronchospasm and remain one of the major causes of patient morbidity and mortality in the poisoned or intoxicated patient.

Ventilatory failure

GENERAL

Ventilatory failure may occur as a result of failure of the respiratory muscles or central depression of the respiratory drive. Hypoxia from ventilatory failure may result in brain damage, cardiac dysrhythmias, and cardiac arrest. Hypercapnia results in acidosis, which may contribute to dysrhythmias that are often resistant to antidysrhythmic drugs. Examples of drugs and toxins that cause ventilatory failure are listed in Box 1-2.

Arterial blood gases.   If the $Paco_2$ is between 45 and 50 torr or the Pao_2 is 60 to 80 torr, supply supplemental oxygen and obtain serial blood gases to evaluate response. If the patient has a $Paco_2$ of >50 torr or a Pao_2 of <60 torr, begin immediate assisted ventilation (p. 9). Do not wait for more pronounced evidence for the need to provide assisted ventilation (Table 1-1).

Pulse oximetry.   Use a pulse oximeter to obtain hemoglobin saturation (SpO_2, the oxygen saturation in a pulsating vessel). Although there is no consistent relationship that will allow prediction of arterial oxygenation using pulse oximetry, coarse generalizations have been made and are reported in Table 1-2.

Using these generalizations, one can make the following recommendations. If the SpO_2 is >91% but <96%, provide

---

BOX 1-2

SELECT DRUGS OR TOXINS THAT CAUSE VENTILATORY FAILURE

Botulism toxin
Organocarbamates
Tetanus
Strychnine
Organophosphates
Barbiturates
Metaldehyde
Ethanol
Penitrem A (mold toxin)
Human antidepressant drugs or sedatives
Paraquat
Smoke inhalation

supplemental oxygen (see below) and observe response. If the SpO_2 fails to respond appropriately, begin assisted ventilation. If SpO_2 is <90%, provide immediate assisted ventilation (see p. 9).

TREATMENT

Supplemental oxygen.   Provide an enriched source of oxygen to a spontaneously breathing patient using one of the following techniques.

Reservoir bag-mask.   Face masks may be used with the anesthesia machine as an oxygen source. The mask must fit tightly to the face to avoid dilution of the oxygen with room air. This will provide short-term oxygen therapy but is usually not tolerated well by the patient.

TABLE 1-1

Normal blood gas measurements

	Dog		Cat	
	Arterial	**Venous**	**Arterial**	**Venous**
pH	7.4	7.38	7.39	7.34
Pco_2	30.8-36.8	37.4	31.0	38.7
HCO_3^-	22.2	22.5	18.0	20.6
Po_2	92.1	52.1	95.4-118.2	Not reported
SpO_2	97-99.9	Not reported	Not reported	Not reported

TABLE 1-2

Coarse generalizations between Po_2 and SpO_2

Po_2 (mm Hg, or torr)	SpO_2 (%)
90	>95
80	95
60	90
40	75

These are generalizations only. Caution is advised in using SpO_2 monitoring as a detector of life-threatening hypoxemia because there is about a 10% false-negative rate as well as a 14% false-positive rate.

Blow-by oxygen administration. An oxygen line or mask may be held in front of the patient's face and set at a high flow rate. The oxygen flow around the face will need to be near the inspiratory rate of the patient to provide high levels of oxygen supplementation. Large dogs may have inspiratory rates that exceed 50 L/min. This technique is valuable only in emergency settings and is pointed out here to remind the practicing veterinarian that flow rates must be extremely high in the setting described.

Oxygen bag. A clear plastic bag is slipped over the head (and shoulders if size permits), and the oxygen line is placed inside. Initial flow rates of oxygen must be rapid enough to inflate the bag but may be slowed to a maintenance flow of 100 to 200 mL/kg/min. The patient must remain under direct observation at all times during the use of an oxygen bag. "Baggie" oxygen may not be well tolerated by some patients, especially feline patients.

Nasal catheter. Nasal catheterization remains one of the most efficient, economical routes of oxygen supplementation. Inspired oxygen concentrations of >85% are possible. The flow rate required to achieve a desired effect will vary proportionately with the patient's weight and ventilatory pattern. Table 1-3 provides approximate flow rates to achieve target inspired-oxygen concentrations. The technique of catheter insertion and fixation has been described elsewhere (see suggested readings) and is not covered here.

TABLE 1-3

Approximate flow rates (in liters per minute) required to achieve target-inspired oxygen concentrations by nasal catheter

Body weight (kg)	30%-50%	50%-75%	75%-99%
0.1-10	0.5-1	1-2	3-5
10-20	1-2	3-5	>5
20-40	3-5	>5	Not determined

Data from Fitzpatrick RK, Crowe DT: *J Am Anim Hosp Assoc* 22:293-300, 1986.

Oxygen hood. A simple device to administer supplemental oxygen in a small animal patient involves the use of an Elizabethan collar. A collar of sufficient size to extend past the patient's nose is chosen. It is applied routinely, and an oxygen line is inserted between the patient's neck and the collar. The oxygen line is then attached to the collar. The end of the collar is covered with plastic food wrap that is taped in place. A hole is torn in the top (dorsum) of the wrap so that warm exhaled gases can escape. A weight (roll of tape or large metal washer) can be taped to the bottom of the collar to keep the collar positioned properly. Oxygen flow rates of 50 to 200 mL/kg/min are suggested.

Oxygen cage. There are many commercially available cages or cage doors specifically manufactured for the purpose of administering oxygen. Many of these require massive flow rates to increase the inspired oxygen and are no more effective than the above. They also require that the door remain shut; thus the clinician and staff are unable to monitor the patient closely. This "forced neglect" may, however, be a boon to some patients (especially the dyspneic feline) because continued stress from handling may be injurious.

Assisted ventilation. If an endotracheal or tracheal tube has been placed in the patient, ventilation can be assisted.

Volume ventilator. Program the volume ventilator for an appropriate tidal volume (usually 15 to 20 mL/kg) and rate (10 to 12 breaths per minute). Assess patient response and adjust the ventilator as necessary.

Pressure ventilator. Program the pressure-controlled ventilator to an appropriate inspiratory pressure limit (15 to 20 cm H_2O) and rate (10 to 12 breaths per minute). Assess patient response and adjust the ventilator as necessary.

Manual devices. Commercial bag-valve devices (generally referred to as Ambu-Bags) are available and may be used temporarily until the ventilator is readied. The anesthesia machine can be used with the pop-off valve closed down to allow the operator to compress the bag to ventilate the patient.

Hypoxia

GENERAL

Significant or sustained hypoxia may cause brain damage, cardiac dysrhythmias, proximal renal tubular damage, or bowel mucosal necrosis. Selected causes of hypoxia are listed in Box 1-3. Hypoxia can be caused by the following conditions:

- *Insufficient oxygen* in ambient air (such as displacement of oxygen by inert gases).

BOX 1-3 SELECTED CAUSES OF HYPOXIA

INERT GASES
Carbon dioxide
Methane and propane
Nitrogen

CARDIOGENIC PULMONARY EDEMA
Beta-blockers
Quinadine
Procainamide
Verapamil

CELLULAR HYPOXIA
Carbon monoxide
Cyanide
Methemoglobinemia

PNEUMONIA OR NONCARDIOGENIC PULMONARY EDEMA
Aspiration of gastric contents
Aspiration of hydrocarbons
Chlorine and other irritant gases
Cocaine
Ethylene glycol
Metal fumes
Opiates
Paraquat
Salicylates
Sedatives and hypnotic drugs
Smoke inhalation

- *Disruption of oxygen absorption* by the lung (such as that caused by pneumonia or pulmonary edema).

Pneumonia.   A common cause of pneumonia in the poisoned or intoxicated patient is aspiration of gastric contents. Aspiration may occur during vomiting in a conscious or unconscious patient. Often the aspiration takes place "silently" (that is, without any visible signs of retching or vomiting) in the unconscious patient. Irritant gases (smoke, hydrocarbons, and so on) may cause chemical pneumonia. Petroleum distillates often cause pneumonia.

Pulmonary edema.   Irritant gases are also capable of causing direct damage to the lungs, altering capillary membrane permeability. The vessels become "leaky," and the result is noncardiogenic pulmonary edema. In noncardiogenic pulmonary edema, the pulmonary capillary wedge pressure (PCWP) (a reflection of left ventricular filling pressure) is often normal or low. Likewise, central venous pressure (CVP) (a more common monitoring parameter in veterinary medicine) is often normal or low. In contrast, cardiogenic pulmonary edema caused by heart failure or cardiac depressant drugs is characterized by low cardiac output with elevated pulmonary capillary wedge pressure (and often elevated CVP as well.)

Cellular hypoxia may be present, despite a normal arterial blood gas value.

Carbon monoxide poisoning and *methemoglobinemia* may severely limit oxygen binding to hemoglobin (thereby limiting oxygen carrying capacity). These toxins do not alter the Pao_2 because routine blood gas determinations provide a measure of the amount of oxygen dissolved in plasma but do not provide a measure of actual oxygen concentration. Likewise, the SpO_2 will remain normal as pulse oximeters measure hemoglobin saturation, but they cannot distinguish between oxyhemoglobin, carboxyhemoglobin, or methemoglobin. In such cases, a *cooximeter* must by used to reveal true oxyhemoglobin saturation.

Cyanide poisoning and hydrogen sulfide poisoning interfere with cellular oxygen utilization, resulting in decreased oxygen uptake by the tissues. Blood gas determinations will reveal normal to high Pao_2 with a notably high Pvo_2. Venous oxygen saturation levels (in settings where this can be measured) will also be elevated.

TREATMENT

Correct hypoxia. Administer supplemental oxygen as indicated based on arterial blood gases. Intubation and assisted ventilation may be required.

- If carbon monoxide poisoning is suspected, give 100% oxygen.
- See treatment guides for cyanide (p. 120), methemoglobinemia (p. 183), and hydrogen sulfide (p. 153).

Treat pneumonia. Obtain sputum samples or transtracheal wash samples to examine for evidence of bacterial infection.

- Begin appropriate antibiotic therapy only when there is evidence of bacterial infection.
- There is no basis for prophylactic antibiotic treatment of aspiration- or chemical-induced pneumonia.
- Controversy exists regarding the use of corticosteroids in chemical-induced pneumonia. No definitive evidence of their benefit can be found in the literature.
- Nebulization of acetylcysteine (accompanied by coupage) or bronchodilators (terbutaline, albuterol) may be utilized in the patient with pneumonia.

Treat pulmonary edema

- Avoid overzealous fluid administration. At a minimum, central venous pressures should be monitored to guide fluid therapy. (Ideally CVP should be maintained <5 cm H_2O if no signs of shock are noted and urine production remains >0.5 mL/kg/hour). In settings where it is possible, pulmonary artery cannulation with pulmonary wedge pressure determinations provide more accurate guidelines.
- Administer supplemental oxygen to maintain a Pao_2 of at least 60 to 70 torr. Positive-pressure ventilation, ventilation with positive end-expiratory pressure (PEEP) or continuous positive airway pressure (CPAP), may be required to maintain oxygenation.
- It is tempting to recommend the use of colloids, such as plasma, dextran, or hetastarch, instead of crystalloids when there is hypovolemia concurrent with pulmonary edema. Although colloids are more potent volume expanders, studies have failed to show definitive evidence of the advantages of their use. Crystalloids are significantly cheaper. The controversy remains largely unresolved.

- In patients where crystalloids are used to treat hypovolemia or shock, there is no doubt that water moves into the pulmonary interstitium. To minimize this movement and subsequent increase in extravascular lung water (EVLW), the volume of crystalloid should be kept to the minimum required to alleviate the signs of shock or hypovolemia. Diuretic therapy may be initiated to lower CVP (or PAWP) once signs of shock, hypovolemia, or hemodynamic instability are absent. Furosemide (1 to 5 mg/kg IV q1-4h) will lower CVP by inducing a brisk diuresis as well as by a transient vasodilatory effect.
- Inotropic pharmacologic support using dopamine (5 to 20 µg/kg/min IV infusion) or dobutamine (*dogs:* 2 to 40 µg/kg/min IV infusion; *cats:* 2.5 to 15.0 µg/kg/min IV infusion) may be preferable to fluid therapy for hypotension in patients with signs of increased EVLW (radiographic evidence of pulmonary edema, moist lung sounds on auscultation).

Bronchospasm

GENERAL

Animals that are hypoxic, or tachypneic, and demonstrate an increased work of breathing may be suffering bronchospasm. Auscultation often reveals crackles or wheezes. Examination of the breathing pattern will reveal forceful and prolonged inspiratory and expiratory phases of respiration. Prolonged bronchospasm may induce complications associated with hypoxemia including shock, cardiac dysrhythmias, and ventilatory failure. Examples of toxins that cause bronchospasm are listed in Box 1-4. Bronchospasm can result from:

- *Direct bronchial injury* from inhaled gases, liquids, or powders or from pulmonary aspiration of petroleum distillates or stomach contents.
- *Pharmacologic effects* of poisons (such as organophosphates or organocarbamates) or drugs (such as beta-adrenergic blockers).
- *Hypersensitivity* or allergic reactions may cause bronchospasm.

TREATMENT

1. Administer supplemental oxygen sufficient to maintain the Pao_2 >60 torr or the SpO_2 >90%.

> ## BOX 1-4 SELECTED DRUGS AND TOXINS CAUSING BRONCHOSPASM
>
> Beta-blockers
> Chlorine and other irritant gases
> Hydrocarbon aspiration
> Metal fumes
> Organophosphates and other anticholinesterases
> Smoke inhalation

2. Administer bronchodilators.
   a. Administer aerosolized beta$_2$-agonist (such as metaproterenol, albuterol, or terbutaline).
   b. Administer a beta$_2$-agonist by parenteral injection (such as terbutaline—*dogs:* 0.01 mg/kg SC q4h; *cats:* 0.01 mg/kg SC q4h).
3. In cases of organophosphate- or organocarbamate-induced bronchospasm, administer atropine at 0.2 to 2.0 mg/kg *only after oxygen administration* (p. 7).

CARDIOVASCULAR SYSTEM AND CIRCULATORY SYSTEM

Many poisoned or intoxicated patients are presented in a state of cardiovascular collapse that must be recognized and treated early in the course of events after (or concurrent with) airway and breathing assessment and treatment.

General assessment

CHECK PULSE RATE AND RHYTHM
Begin cardiopulmonary-cerebral resuscitation (CPCR) if there is no pulse.

ASSESS THE QUALITY OF THE PULSES
If the patient has an easily palpable pulse in both the femoral artery and anterior metatarsal artery of the same hind

limb, the systolic blood pressure is likely >80 mm Hg. If the femoral pulse is easily palpable but the anterior metatarsal pulse is weak or absent, the systolic pressure is probably 60 to 80 mm Hg. If the femoral pulse is weak or absent, the systolic pressure is likely to be <60 mm Hg. Bounding pulses are often indicative of hypotension. If the patient is believed to be hypotensive, see the discussion of hypotension, p. 16. Pulse character gives no hint of hypertension. *These are generalizations; there are times where reality deviates from these observations.* They will never take the place of actual measurement of blood pressure.

CHECK BLOOD PRESSURE

Blood pressures are readily determined using indirect measurement methods such as the Doppler flow detector (Parks Electronics, Aloha, Oreg.) or the Dinamap (Criticon, Johnson & Johnson, Tampa, Fla.). If experienced personnel and equipment are present, direct measurement of blood pressure is preferred; however, the time it takes to establish a direct line must not delay necessary resuscitation. Hypotension (p. 16) is often seen in the poisoned patient. Hypertension (p. 21) is probably a more frequent problem than currently recognized.

ASSESS MUCOUS MEMBRANE COLOR AND CAPILLARY REFILL TIME

Any color other than pink is not normal.
- Pale pink or white—indicates anemia or vasoconstriction. Evaluate for the need for blood transfusion (PCV, hemoglobin determinations), fluid therapy, or vasodilator therapy.
- Bluish tinge or cyanosis—generally indicates the need for oxygen, though one must remember that for cyanosis to be visible to the human eye, at least 5 g/dL of reduced hemoglobin must be present in the blood. Therefore, not all hypoxic animals will reveal cyanosis, and not all cyanotic animals will be hypoxemic.
- Brown—may indicate the presence of methemoglobinemia (p. 181).
- Red—indicates possible vasodilatation caused by a toxin or cytokines released in response to infection or inflammation. Red mucous membranes may also indicate the presence of cellular toxins such as cyanide (p. 126).

SECURE VENOUS ACCESS

The cephalic vein in the foreleg of the dog and the cat is usually quite easy to catheterize with an over-the-needle catheter. Other sites include the lateral saphenous vein, the femoral vein, and the jugular veins. Cannulation of the jugular vein is technically more difficult but offers the advantage of central vein access, which will allow monitoring of the central venous pressure and will allow multiple samples of blood to be taken for analysis. In settings where it is offered, it also allows the placement of a pulmonary artery catheter or transvenous pacemaker capability. Place the largest-bore catheter possible or place multiple catheters if shock or severe hypovolemia is present. In conditions of severe vascular collapse, placement of an intraosseous catheter provides another option for rapid administration of fluids or drugs. The procedure has been described elsewhere and is not covered here.

DRAW BLOOD SAMPLES FOR AN INITIAL DATA BASE

It is advisable to draw blood samples for routine tests before treatment is begun. Obviously this is not always possible (as in a case of cardiac arrest).

MONITOR ECG

Cardiovascular collapse may be precipitated by a cardiac dysrhythmia.

PLACE A URETHRAL CATHETER

Place a urethral catheter and anchor in place. Empty the bladder and submit urine for a urine analysis and toxicologic testing. Collect and measure hourly urine production. This vastly underutilized monitoring tool can be used to assess the adequacy of fluid therapy (barring renal dysfunction). Normal urine production is 1 to 2 mL/kg/hour in the dog and 0.5 to 1 mL/kg/hour in the cat. Volumes less than or more than this require reevaluation of both the fluid therapy plan and the renal function.

Hypotension

In the poisoned patient, hypotension may be the result of hypovolemia (such as vomiting, diarrhea, blood loss, diuresis), vasodilatation (such as venodilatation or arteriolar dilatation), or decreased cardiac output (such as dysrhythmias, decreased contractility). Severe or prolonged hypotension may result in shock, acute renal failure, brain damage, bowel mucosal necrosis, and death.

ASSESSMENT

Blood pressure.   Direct or indirect measurements of blood pressure are becoming more available in small animal practice. The trend of repeated measurements is more important than a single reading. In general, systolic pressure of less than 80 mm Hg should be considered hypotension and indicates the need for therapy.

Central venous pressure.   Central venous pressure readings of less than 2 cm H_2O most often indicate the need for therapy.

Assess the heart rate.   Hypotension as a result of a loss of volume or vasodilatation is usually associated with a reflex tachycardia. Hypotension accompanied by bradycardia is suggestive of intoxication by sympatholytic agents, membrane-depressant drugs or chemicals, calcium-channel blockers, cardiac glycosides, hypothermia, or anaphylaxis.

Assess the ECG.   Cardiac dysrhythmias may be severe enough to cause hypotension.

TREATMENT

Hypotension usually responds to empirical therapy with intravenous fluids and perhaps low doses of pressor drugs (such as dopamine). When hypotension does not respond, a systematic approach should be followed to determine the cause of hypotension and to select the appropriate treatment.

1.   Maintain the airway and assist ventilation if necessary (p. 9). Administer supplemental oxygen as needed.
2.   Administer crystalloids (LRS, Normosol-R, 0.9% saline) rapidly as a bolus. The dose of crystalloid used for resuscitation has been reported in many references. Too many variables exist to allow one to pick a universal dose that will be adequate for treatment of all hypotensive or shock patients. For example, a dose of 15 mL/kg given rapidly may be too much for an old cat with heart disease who was traumatized, whereas two blood volumes (180 mL/kg

in the first hour) may be "enough" to resuscitate a young, athletic dog who was struck by a car. A more profound example is two similar patients with a PCV of 16%—one having been anemic for 3 months and the other acutely anemic. The patient with chronic anemia will withstand more crystalloid administration than the other because he has compensated to the chronic hypoxemia by producing more 2,3-diphosphoglycerate (DPG).

A more clinical approach to the "dose" of fluids is to give "enough" (if possible) without giving "too much." "Enough" crystalloid is the amount that causes the vital signs to improve. When "enough" is being given:

- The pulses are readily palpable.
- The color is pinker than previously.
- The capillary refill time is between 1 and 2 seconds.
- Urine is being produced at 1 to 2 mL/kg/hour.
- Delta T (ΔT, core temperature minus toe web temperature) is approaching normal (normal is usually thought to be 6 to 8 Fahrenheit degrees less than the core temperature).
- The trend of the central venous pressure (CVP) has been upward and now measures at 4 to 12 cm H_2O.
- Mean arterial blood pressure is at least 80 mm Hg. "Too much" crystalloid is the amount that causes problems rather than correcting problems.
- The packed cell volume is diluted to <25% ±5%.
- The hemoglobin concentration is diluted to 8.0 ±1.0 g/dL.
- (These numbers are inaccurate in patients with pre-existing anemia, where compensation has occurred).
- The total plasma proteins are reduced to <4.0 ±0.5 g/dL.
- Increases in respiratory rate, effort, or moist crackles, or all three, are auscultated.
- The CVP measures higher than 15 to 18 cm H_2O.

To determine the amount of crystalloids to be administered, the attending veterinarian must take into account the variables of the case and estimate (based on blood volume) a safe amount. Dogs have a blood volume of 80 to 90 mL/kg of body weight, whereas cats are estimated to have a blood volume of 45 to 60 mL/kg of body weight. Administer that "safe" amount as rapidly as possible while monitoring the patient closely for signs of having had too much. If the full amount is administered without stabilization taking place and there is still no evidence of "too much," the clinician must decide what additional amount (if any) is appropriate. If the patient's vital signs improve adequately before the safe amount is administered, the flow rate can be reduced and the patient monitored for stability.

A time *will* come when the attending veterinarian is uncomfortable with administering more crystalloids. This time will be different for different clinicians with different patients with different presentations. When the "crystalloid comfort zone" has been exceeded, the clinician is obliged to continue resuscitation using an alternative therapy.

When the "crystalloid comfort zone" is exceeded, resuscitation may be continued with the use of colloids. Colloids mediate against the loss of intravascular water associated with movement of sodium into the interstitium. These products use the oncotic pull of their larger molecules to pull and hold fluid (as well as sodium) in the intravascular fluid compartment. Smaller volumes are required to achieve the same volume expansion achieved by crystalloids. The smaller volume can be administered more rapidly. Fluid products such as plasma, hetastarch, or dextran 70 are commonly used. A volume of 10 to 20 mL/kg is recommended. Colloid therapy is not used first in most cases of shock because colloids are significantly more costly than crystalloid solutions are. When indicated, they are an indispensable part of shock resuscitation.

The use of hypertonic solutions has gained popularity. Hypertonic saline is also a crystalloid, but it has the advantage of restoring vascular volume rapidly by osmotically drawing water from the interstitium to the intravascular compartment. Small volumes are required (4 mL of 7% to 7.5% saline per kilogram of body weight) to achieve volume expansion. The effect is short lived because the sodium quickly (within 15 to 30 minutes) disperses into the interstitium or is eliminated through the kidneys. Adding a colloid to the hypertonic solution has given this form of therapy a longer duration of action than without the colloid. Hypertonic saline is not used in the dehydrated patient. Newer work is looking at the use of hypertonic (2%) sodium lactate solutions as a resuscitation fluid.

3. Treat bradycardias (heart rates <30 to 70 bpm) or tachycardias >150 to 220 bpm (depending on the size and normal heart rate of the individual). These cardiac dysrhythmias may contribute to hypotension.

4. Hypotension associated with hypothermia often will not respond to routine fluid therapy but will rapidly normalize with rewarming. Rewarming efforts include IV or intraperitoneal (IP) administration of warmed fluids, warming of the air the patient breathes, and wrapping of the patient in blankets to prevent further heat loss. Warming measures such as heating pads, hot water bottles, or heat lamps are dangerous because they may contribute to hypotension by dilating vessels in the skin. These measures are also known to cause thermal burns and should be avoided.

5. Administer dopamine at 5 to 20 μg/kg/min. See Appendix C, p. 380, for continuous infusion guidelines. Assess the response and adjust the drip accordingly. Monitor response in blood pressure or pulse quality. Be observant for cardiac dysrhythmias, which may dictate the need to slow the rate of administration or discontinue the drug altogether.

6. In hospital settings where it is possible, the following can be performed and will provide a great deal of information to guide therapy for the cardiovascular system (Box 1-5). Insert a pulmonary artery catheter to measure CVP or pulmonary artery wedge pressure (PAWP) and to measure cardiac output (CO). Cardiac output is usually converted to cardiac index (CI) using the formula:

$$CI = CO/Body\ surface\ area$$

Systemic vascular resistance index (SVRI) is calculated using the formula:

$$SVRI = (MAP - CVP)/CI \times 80$$

Select further therapy based on the results:
a. If the CVP is low or the PAWP is low, give more intravenous fluids.
b. If the CI is low and the SVRI is high, give dobutamine.
c. If the CI is low and the SVRI is low, give dopamine.
d. If the CI is normal and the SVRI is low, give norepinephrine.

BOX 1-5

NORMAL HEMODYNAMIC PARAMETERS

DOGS:

CVP	−1 to 7 cm H_2O
PAWP	3 to 7 mm Hg
CO	130 to 200 mL/kg/min
CI	3.5 to 5.8 L/M²/min
SVRI	1700 to 2600 dynes·sec/cm⁵·m²

CATS:
Data not available

Data from unpublished study by S Haskins et al, personal communication, 1995.

Hypertension

Hypertension is rarely diagnosed in small animal medicine and therefore often goes untreated. Numerous chemicals and drugs are capable of inducing hypertensive states (Box 1-6). If hypertension is present and goes untreated, it may cause severe complications including hypertensive encephalopathy, intracranial hemorrhage, renal failure, retinal hemorrhage or detachment, and congestive heart failure.

GENERAL INFORMATION
Blood pressure.　　Direct measurement of blood pressure is the only reliable way to diagnose hypertension. Indirect measurement of blood pressure is not so reliable as direct measurements. Although firm difinitions of normal ranges of blood pressures have not been established, most recent reports regard sustained systolic pressures in excess of 160 mm Hg or diastolic pressures over 95 mm Hg compatible with hypertension in dogs. Published data for cats with reported pressures exceeding 190 systolic and 140 diastolic are compatible with hypertension.

Fundic examination.　　Retinal detachments, acute blindness, reduced pupillary reflexes, hyphema, and retinal hemorrhages should alert the veterinarian that hypertension may exist.

BOX 1-6

SELECTED POISONS AND DRUGS THAT CAUSE HYPERTENSION

Amphetamines
Antihistamines
Atropine
Cocaine
Ephedrine/pseudoephedrine
Ethanol
Marijuana
Nicotine
Organophosphates (early stages)

HYPERTENSION ASSOCIATED WITH BRADYCARDIA OR ATRIOVENTRICULAR BLOCK
Clonidine
Ergot derivatives
Methoxamine
Phenylephrine

HYPERTENSION ASSOCIATED WITH TACHYCARDIA
Ephedrine
Phenylephrine
Phenylpropanolamine
Pseudoephedrine

TREATMENT
Life-threatening hypertension
1. In a hypertensive crisis *not* associated with hypovolemia, furosemide may lower blood pressure by both eliminating fluid volume as well as by inducing vasodilatation. Administer furosemide IV at 1 to 5 mg/kg IV. This dosage may be repeated hourly as needed.
2. Administer sodium nitroprusside in a continuous infusion at 0.5 to 10 µg/kg/min. Use lower doses initially and administer to effect. Blood pressure must be continuously monitored.
3. Consider alpha-adrenergic receptor blockade if tachycardia is not associated with the hypertension. (Acepromazine 0.05 to 0.1 mg/kg IV PRN; phenoxyben-

zamine and prazosin may be used but are available only in forms for oral administration.)

4. If tachycardia is associated with hypertension, use propranolol with alpha-adrenergic blockade (see above). Administer propranolol 0.02 to 0.06 mg/kg IV over several minutes. CAUTION: Furosemide may potentiate the effects of propranolol. Propranolol should not be used alone to treat hypertensive crisis; this may paradoxically worsen hypertension if the primary cause of hypertension is alpha-adrenergic receptor stimulation.

Moderate hypertension

1. Furosemide or thiazide-derivative diuretics may be administered orally to treat moderate or nonemergency hypertension.
2. Angiotensin-converting enzyme (ACE) inhibitors such as captopril or enalapril have met with much favor in human medicine. Enacard (enalapril) is an ACE inhibitor approved for use in dogs. The dose of enalapril for dogs is 0.25 to 1 mg/kg PO q12-24h and for cats is 0.25 to 0.5 mg/kg PO q12-24h.
3. Calcium-channel blockers such as diltiazem may be used. These drugs are especially indicated where hypertension is accompanied by tachycardia. The dose published for dogs is 0.75 to 1.5 mg/kg PO q8h and for cats is 3.5 to 7.0 mg PO q8h. Amlodipine, another calcium-channel blocker, has recently been shown to lower blood pressure in cats. It is given once daily at a dose of 0.625 mg PO.
4. Beta-blockers (such as propranolol) may be used. The oral dose for dogs is 0.125 to 0.250 mg/kg q8-12h. Cats may be given 2.5 to 5.0 mg PO q8-12h. CAUTION: Propranolol should be used concurrently only with diuretics. Use of propranolol alone may cause sodium and water retention.

CONSCIOUSNESS

Poisonings and intoxications often affect the mental status of the patient. Affected patients may show alterations of consciousness that range from seizures to coma.

Seizures

GENERAL

Seizures remain one of the most common complications resulting from poisoning or intoxication. They may be mild, single episodes or may be severe and continuous resembling status epilepticus. Sustained muscle activity associated with generalized seizures may cause hyperthermia, metabolic acidosis (lactic acidosis) or rhabdomyolysis, or all three. Seizures may cause apnea or hypoventilation resulting in hypoxemia or respiratory acidosis. Pulmonary aspiration is all too often a complication of seizures associated with poisonings.

TREATMENT

1. Maintain an open, secure airway. Endotracheal intubation may be necessary.
2. Assist ventilation if necessary.
3. Administer anticonvulsants.
   a. Diazepam is most commonly administered intravenously at 0.5 to 1.0 mg/kg IV in increments of 5 to 20 mg to effect. It may also be administered rectally at a dose of 1 to 4 mg/kg in increments of 5 to 20 mg to effect for a rapid response. CAUTION: Diazepam has recently been implicated as a possible cause of severe hepatopathy in cats.
   b. Pentobarbital may be given IV 2 to 30 mg/kg to effect if diazepam is ineffective in stopping the seizure. General anesthesia warrants endotracheal intubation, preferably with a cuffed endotracheal tube, because aspiration remains a critical problem in anesthetized patients. *Decontamination by gastric lavage requires that a cuffed endotracheal tube be in place.*
4. Obtain stat. blood chemistry analysis.
   a. Check for hypoglycemia (blood glucose <60 mg/dL). If hypoglycemia is suspected or confirmed, administer 50% dextrose at 0.25 to 2.0 mL/kg IV slowly. Fifty-percent dextrose is extremely hyperosmolar and may cause vasculitis or phlebitis if administered directly. It should be diluted at least 1:1 with a saline solution or with sterile water before administration.
   b. Check serum calcium. If hypocalcemia is confirmed, administer calcium (2 to 15 mg/kg IV over 3 to 15

minutes) while observing response to therapy. Monitoring the electrocardiogram during administration is advisable. If bradycardia or shortening of the Q-T interval is noted, the administration of calcium is slowed or temporarily discontinued.

Calcium gluconate contains 9 mg/mL elemental calcium; calcium chloride contains 27 mg/mL elemental calcium.

5. Check the body temperature. See the discussion of hyperthermia or hypothermia below.
6. Consider the need for thiamine supplementation. Thiamine may be deficient in patients who are anorexic without supplementation, especially if the patient has undergone extensive diuresis. Thiamine deficiency has been reported in cats who are fed all-fish diets (which contain thiaminase) and in dogs fed meat that had been cooked, a process that destroys thiamine.

Hyperthermia

GENERAL

Elevated body temperatures may be the result of continuous muscle activity (seizures), malignant hyperthermia, a reduced ability to dissipate heat (rigidity or weakness of respiratory muscles), a hypothalamic disorder ("resetting of the thermostat"), or increased metabolic rate (uncoupled oxidative phosphorylation).

Untreated, hyperthermia may result in dehydration, rhabdomyolysis, heatstroke, shock, vasculitis, disseminated intravascular coagulation, brain injury, and death. Patients who survive may have permanent brain dysfunction.

TREATMENT

Immediate treatment is necessary when the body temperature exceeds a range of 106° to 107° F to reduce the risk of heat-induced injury and death.

1. Secure the airway and ventilate if necessary. Administer supplemental oxygen.
2. Administer intravenous fluids to support blood pressure or prevent or treat dehydration.
3. Control seizures (see above).
4. Begin external cooling. Dousing the patient with tepid, running water with or without fanning is quite effective in reducing body temperature. Once the

patient is thoroughly wetted, a fine mist of water may be applied. Application of isopropyl alcohol to the foot pads and abdomen may help lower temperature by evaporation. Cold or ice water immersion is no longer considered appropriate because this will cause intense peripheral vasoconstriction resulting in reduced ability to dissipate heat from the core. Cooling efforts should be discontinued when the body temperature reaches 103° to 104° F to prevent complications of hypothermia.

5. If hyperthermia is pronounced (>107° F), consider internal cooling techniques. Tepid or cool water gastric lavage or colonic irrigation may be necessary when external cooling measures are not showing rapid effect at lowering the body temperature to <103° F.

6. Although not widely available or practical in veterinary medicine, neuromuscular paralysis with paralyzing agents (such as pancuronium 0.03 to 0.06 mg/kg IV or vecuronium 10 to 20 µg/kg IV in the dog or 20 to 40 µg/kg IV in the cat) remains the single most rapidly effective means of lowering body temperature. These patients will not be able to breathe and will require ventilation. General anesthesia is required for patient comfort during paralysis.

7. The use of drugs to lower body temperature is not advisable, at least not initially. If the above do not resolve the hyperthermia, administration of steroids or nonsteroidal antiinflammatory drugs (NSAIDs) will block formation of mediators that cause the body's "thermostat" to maintain a higher temperature. If hyperthermia is attributable to formation of these mediators, use of steroids or NSAIDs will lower body temperature. Antipyretic drugs are generally not indicated for toxin-induced hyperthermia.

8. If the above do not resolve the body temperature, think about the presence of malignant hyperthermia and, though dosage and safety have not been established, consider administration of dantrolene.

Rhabdomyolysis

GENERAL

Rhabdomyolysis occurs in poisoned patients as a result of prolonged seizures, prolonged muscular hyperactivity, hyperthermia, or direct effects of the toxin (such as carbon monoxide). Circulating myoglobin released from the damaged muscle cells will be filtered by the kidneys where it may cause acute renal tubular necrosis and acute renal failure. Hyperkalemia, hyperphosphatemia, and hypocalcemia may accompany severe rhabdomyolysis.

1. Urine that contains few or no intact red blood cells but tests positive for blood on a urine dipstick test is suggestive of rhabdomyolysis. Hemolysis may cause similar findings. Affected urine is usually red to brown (color of tea or coffee) in color.
2. Elevated serum creatine phosphokinase levels are suggestive of rhabdomyolysis.

TREATMENT
1. Administer maintenance fluids at a rate to promote a flow of urine of 2 to 3 mL/kg/hour in dogs or 1 to 2 mL/kg/hour in cats. Be observant for signs of fluid overload, preferably by monitoring central venous pressure.
2. If rhabdomyolysis is attributable to excessive muscle activity, use sedation such as diazepam (0.5 to 1.0 mg/kg IV in increments of 5 to 20 mg to effect or 1 to 4 mg/kg per rectum in increments of 5 to 20 mg), acepromazine (0.05 to 0.1 mg/kg IV; CAUTION: phenothiazine-derivative tranquilizers may lower the seizure threshold), muscle relaxants (methocarbamol 50 to 222.2 mg/kg IV), or muscle-paralyzing agents (pancuronium 0.03 to 0.06 mg/kg IV or vecuronium 10 to 20 µg/kg IV in the dog or 20 to 40 µg/kg in the cat).
3. For severe rhabdomyolysis or oliguria, administer IV mannitol (0.1 to 0.5 g/kg). Consider loop diuretics (furosemide 2 to 5 mg/kg IV q1h) or a low-dose dopamine drip (1 to 3 µg/kg/min) for unrelenting oliguria. Consider dialysis (hemodialysis or peritoneal dialysis; see p. 61) for acute renal failure. Kidney function will likely be regained within 3 weeks if renal failure was initiated by rhabdomyolysis.
4. Acid urine promotes precipitation of myoglobin in the renal tubules. Induce and maintain an alkaline urine by administration of sodium bicarbonate (1 to 2 mEq/kg IV every 3 to 4 hours) or potassium citrate (5 to 7 mg/kg/hour) in the IV fluids. *Caution is advised when using potassium citrate. Destruction of muscle cells may release potassium resulting in hyperkalemia. Potassium citrate may*

worsen hyperkalemia. The appropriate dose is added to the quantity of fluids to be administered over an 8-hour period. Monitor and adjust dosage to maintain urine pH >7.0. Monitor blood gases to avoid inducing alkalemia.

Agitation, hyperactivity

GENERAL

Numerous drugs and chemicals (Box 1-7) may result in hyperactivity that is not under the control of the patient. Restlessness, pacing, struggling, and apparent hallucinations (observed as quick head movements as if the patient is watching something move quickly, referred to as "tracers" by some) may be seen. Severe prolonged hyperactivity may result in hyperthermia and exhaustion.

TREATMENT

1. Hypoxemia may cause delirium and restlessness. Maintain an open airway and administer supplemental oxygen, as needed. Ventilate the patient if necessary.
2. Move the patient to a quiet, darkened area with minimal external stimulation and observe. This may allow the patient to relax adequately.
3. Administer diazepam IV or per rectum.

BOX 1-7

SELECTED CAUSES OF UNCONTROLLED HYPEREXCITABILITY

Amphetamines
Antihistamines
Atropine
Carbon monoxide (hypoxemia)
Cocaine
Fluoroacetates (Compound 1080, Compound 1081)
Lead
LSD
Marijuana
PCP
Phenylpropanolamine
Pseudoephedrine

4. Gain IV access.
    a. Check for and treat hypoglycemia as needed (p. 46).
    b. Check for hyperthermia and treat as needed (p. 25).
    c. Check for dehydration or hemoconcentration (PCV >60%). Administer crystalloid fluids to reduce PCV rapidly to ≤55%.
    d. Check for rhabdomyolysis and treat as needed (p. 26).

Stupor and coma

GENERAL

Numerous toxins reduce the level of consciousness directly or indirectly by depressing the brain's reticular activating system. Stupor or coma may also be a postictal sign after a toxin-induced seizure. Toxins may result in seizure-induced (as with strychnine) or direct cellular hypoxia (as with carbon monoxide, cyanide), which may manifest as stupor or coma. Anticoagulant poisons or head trauma experienced during a toxin-induced seizure may induce intracranial bleeding. Respiratory depression may result in hypoxemia and hypercapnia resulting in reduced cerebral blood flow, which may induce cerebral edema and ischemia. Hypoglycemia may result in a reduced level of consciousness.

TREATMENT

1. Establish or maintain the airway. Ventilate as necessary. Administer supplemental oxygen.
2. Administer fluids to treat hypotension or prevent dehydration, or both. Maintain CVP ≥8 cm H_2O, mean arterial pressure ≥80 mm Hg.
3. Check blood glucose. Administer dextrose if hypoglycemia is present.
4. Rule out other causes of depressed level of consciousness.
5. If the stupor or coma is believed to be related to increased intracranial pressure:
    a. Administer:
        (1.) Furosemide (1 to 5 mg/kg IV) followed by mannitol (0.1 to 0.5 g/kg IV slowly).
        (2.) Methylprednisolone sodium succinate
        (3.) Dexamethasone sodium phosphate
    b. Consider ventilating the patient to maintain a P_{CO_2} of 30 to 35 mm Hg.

c. Do not put any compression on jugular veins, which could possibly interfere with venous drainage of the head, which is kept level or elevated.

d. Do not perform procedures that would likely result in sneezing or coughing (nasal oxygen, intubation) without appropriate measures.

6. Check body temperature and treat for hypothermia (see below) or hyperthermia (p. 25) as needed.

Hypothermia

GENERAL

Hypothermia (body temperature ≤100.5° F) is a common sequela to poisoning, especially in patients with reduced levels of consciousness. Toxins may induce hypothermia by interfering with the patient's ability to shiver, causing vasodilatation or hypotension, decreasing metabolic activity, or inducing a coma state. Toxins may also act directly on the hypothalamus to "reset the thermostat." Hypothermia may result in severe hypotension and bradycardia. Ventricular fibrillation may occur spontaneously.

TREATMENT

1. Establish and maintain an airway. Ventilate as necessary. Administer supplemental oxygen.

2. Cautiously administer warm (100° to 102° F) IV fluids. Hypothermic patients are easily volume overloaded. Do not attempt to raise blood pressure to normal until the body temperature has been raised.

3. *Slowly* rewarm the patient using blankets and circulating water pads. Increase the ambient temperature to near normal body temperature if possible. Electric heating pads or heat lamps are known to cause thermal burns and are not recommended. *Rapid external rewarming may cause peripheral vasodilatation resulting in profound hypotension.*

4. Internal rewarming measures include gastric or peritoneal lavage with warmed fluids and warm water enemas. Warmed mist or warmed air inhalation will add heat to the core circulation.

5. Cardiopulmonary-cerebral resuscitation (CPCR) is futile during profound hypothermia. Antidysrhythmic agents and defibrillation countershocks are ineffective until the

core temperature is elevated. Open-chest CPCR and direct irrigation of the ventricle with warm saline may improve chances of successful resuscitation.

DIAGNOSIS

Although literature implores veterinarians to "treat the patient, not the toxicant," a correct diagnosis may have tremendous effect on the outcome. Proper identification of the offending substance may afford the use of specific antidotes or therapies that may be lifesaving, prevent complications, or speed recovery. An accurate diagnosis will be invaluable in medicolegal cases. If the offending substance goes unrecognized, further human and animal exposure is possible. Accurate diagnosis also improves the probability that the veterinarian will recognize subsequent cases of poisoning by the same substance.

A proper diagnosis of poisoning is made using a thorough history, clinical signs, and submission of samples for analysis.

History

The owner may be able to provide insight into what intoxicants may be in the animal's environment. It is, of course, ideal when the owner can provide information that leads to a diagnosis. This may occur when they witness the poisoning (ingesting the snail bait as the owner put it out) or are a part of it (dipped the pet and the signs started within minutes). It is more difficult when the exposure is not witnessed. All members of the family must be interviewed to ascertain what drugs or chemicals might be within the pet's environment. Many times owners will be unaware of potential intoxicants. The authors have found the following questions to be helpful.

- Have you fed your roses (other plants)? This often reveals the use of fertilizers that contain insecticides or other toxins.
- Is anyone at home taking any medication for illness or allergies? If so, what products are being used? Ingestion of human over-the-counter (OTC) medications has often been revealed with this line of questioning, even though the owners may arduously deny the possibility of exposure.

- Are you presently working on your house or automobile? Information regarding exposure to paints, solvents, linoleum, or antifreeze may be determined.

Clinical signs

It is unwise to say that physical examination of a patient can accurately diagnose the exact cause of poisoning. There are, however, many chemicals and toxins that cause signs that may allow the veterinarian to suspect a specific agent or group. Often this identification will allow more specific empirical treatment to proceed.

MUSCULOSKELETAL AND NERVOUS SYSTEM FINDINGS

The appearance of muscle activity may be specific enough to cause suspicion of a specific etiologic agent. This may allow more specific questions to be asked of the client and direct more specific diagnostics and treatment.

Strychnine. Ingestion of compounds containing strychnine will result in typical signs. The victim shows a muscular rigidity characterized by the so-called sawhorse stance. The activity may progress to seizures with violent tonic-clonic muscular contractions. These seizures may be spontaneous or may be *consistently* induced by visual, tactile, or auditory stimulation.

Metaldehyde. Snail bait or similar molluscicidal poisons cause the patient to be anxious and have fine muscle tremors. The muscular activity will progress to tonic-clonic spasms, which may be mildly inducible with tactile stimulation; auditory and visual stimulation rarely induce spasms. This muscle activity cannot be consistently induced as it is with strychnine and therefore should not be confused with strychnine ingestion.

Fluoroacetates (Compound 1080 and Compound 1081). These patients will vomit, urinate, or defecate, but such behavior does not give any hint toward a specific diagnosis. These nonspecific signs will be followed by bursts of wild activity mostly characterized as "running fits," which are characteristic for poisoning by Compound 1080 and Compound 1081. Any patient with this type of activity should alert the clinician to look for a source of these compounds and may prompt specific diagnostic tests. Compound 1080 is the sodium salt, and Compound 1081 is fluoroacetamide.

Penitrem A.   The neurotoxin is produced by a mold that grows in rich moist mediums such as fallen walnuts or almonds or even in garbage. The mold may be more widespread than previously believed because the source was traced to mold growing on tree bark in a patient seen by one of the authors. Ingestion of the mold releases the toxin, which causes muscular activity similar to that by strychnine and metaldehyde. The spasms are often induced by tactile stimulation, not so consistently as with strychnine but perhaps more consistently than that with metaldehyde. It should be suspect when no source of metaldehyde can be identified.

AUTONOMIC FINDINGS

The physical examination may reveal changes in parameters that are under the control of the autonomic nervous system (ANS). Several syndromes have been described. Each is characterized by signs that are attributable to a specific receptor or receptors of the ANS.

Alpha-adrenergic syndrome.   Drugs such as phenylpropanolamine or phenylephrine will stimulate alpha-adrenergic receptors resulting in findings of hypertension and tachycardia. The mucous membranes may be pale because of peripheral vasoconstriction. The pupils are usually dilated, and there are fewer bowel sounds than usual. These patients are often hyperactive and will pace incessantly. They are often noted to snap their head about as if they are seeing flies or "tracers." Other examples include ephedrine and pseudoephedrine, which are common ingredients in cold or allergy preparations.

Beta-adrenergic syndrome.   Drugs that stimulate the beta$_2$-receptors cause weakness and tachycardia. Activation of beta$_2$-receptors induces vasodilatation resulting in hypotension. Hypokalemia is common because of beta$_2$-receptor mediated activation of the Na$^+$/K$^+$-ATPase pump, which results in increased intracellular potassium. Examples include exposure to drugs used by asthmatics such as albuterol or salbutamol.

Mixed alpha- and beta-adrenergic syndrome.   Simultaneous activation of alpha- and beta- adrenergic receptors results in hypertension and tachycardia. The pupils are commonly dilated. Mucous membranes are usually dry. Examples of chemicals that cause this syndrome include cocaine and amphetamines.

Sympatholytic syndrome.   Hypotension with bradycardia or tachycardia may be seen. The pupils are often constricted. Bowel sounds are often decreased or absent. Examples causing the sympatholytic syndrome include opiates, hydralazine, and alpha-adrenergic blockers.

Nicotinic cholinergic syndrome.   Nicotinic receptors are located in both the sympathetic and parasympathetic systems. Stimulation of these receptors by toxins or drugs results in a variety of signs. Early signs are usually associated with stimulation of the CNS. Signs such as vomiting, diarrhea, muscle fasciculations, salivation, and tachycardia are seen early. Later, the signs are more consistent with depression of the CNS. Late signs include paresis or paralysis, convulsions, collapse, loss of reflexes, bradycardia, weak pulses, respiratory muscle weakness with resultant respiratory failure, and death. Examples include tobacco, insecticides, and some drugs including succinylcholine.

Muscarinic cholinergic syndrome.   Stimulation of the muscarinic receptors results in bradycardia, salivation, miosis, urination, and defecation. Wheezing and excess lung secretions are seen. Pure muscarinic cholinergic stimulation is rare. We could find no examples of toxins that stimulate muscarinic receptors only.

Mixed cholinergic syndrome.   Drugs or chemicals that stimulate both nicotinic and muscarinic receptors result in a mixture of the signs listed above. Most often, the patient is found to have miosis (muscarinic), muscle fasciculations or tremors (nicotinic), urination (muscarinic), and diarrhea (both). Examples of this intoxication are common in veterinary medicine. Causative agents include the organophosphates and organocarbamates.

Anticholinergic syndrome.   Signs associated with anticholinergic agents include rapid pulse, hypertension, mydriasis, tonic-clonic muscle activity, hyperthermia, and decreased bowel sounds. Examples include atropine and scopolamine (which may be found in motion sickness preparations), antihistamines, and some antidepressants.

ODORS

Some poisons (such as bleach) have characteristic odors, which may be identified so as to direct diagnostics and therapy. These odors may be quite strong or may be so mild as to be missed. If an odor is noted, it may be helpful in diagnosis.

Garlic odor. A garlic-like odor has been discribed in cases of poisoning with several compounds, such as arsenic, organophosphates, thallium, and zinc phosphide (also said to smell like acetylene).

Acetone-like odor. Aspirin or other salicylates, acetone, benzene, toluene, phenols, xylene, creosote, pine tar, isopropanol.

Bitter almonds. Cyanide.

Formaldehyde. Metaldehyde (having an odor that quickly dissipates from stomach contents).

LABORATORY TESTS

Laboratory testing can be useful in identifying the cause of poisoning or may be useful in defining parameters that may be addressed to improve symptomatic therapy. Specific testing is ideal but not practical unless the attending clinician is able to narrow the field of potential agents causing the syndrome.

SPECIFIC IN-HOUSE TESTING

There are two in-house tests that are extremely valuable in small animal medicine. These tests can be performed by most technicians and veterinarians and may be lifesaving.

PIVKA test. The Thrombotest (Nycomed Pharma AS, Oslo, Norway) is a test sensitive to coagulation factors II, VII, and X and to proteins induced by vitamin K absence (PIVKA). Prolongation of coagulation time of the test reveals a deficiency of one of the above factors or the presence of PIVKA (inactive forms of factors II, VII, IX, and X) and indicates a very high index of suspicion of poisoning by the vitamin K–antagonist rat poisons, such as warfarin or brodifacoum. This test is said to be more sensitive than other coagulation tests (such as PT, PTT) used to detect bleeding abnormalities attributable to vitamin K–antagonist poisons. The test kit is available from Accurate Chemical and Scientific Corp., Westbury, NY 11590.

Ethylene glycol test.   Ethylene glycol is relatively nontoxic until it is degraded into its metabolites by the body. These metabolites are quite toxic. Treatment of ethylene glycol poisoning is aimed at preventing degradation of ethylene glycol. Clearly, early diagnosis is essential to success of treatment. A kit available from PRN Pharmacal, Inc. (PRN Pharmacal, Inc., Pensacola, Fla.) is designed to detect levels of ethylene glycol (but not its metabolites) 1 to 4 hours after ingestion. A blood sample is drawn from the patient and put through the series of steps in the kit. A positive test result is indicated by developement of a reddish violet color in the final tube. If the color intensity in the sample tube is greater than that in the positive control, the dog has ingested ethylene glycol. Cats are much more sensitive to ethylene glycol. *This test kit is not sensitive enough for use in cats.* Although a positive result in cats indicates lethal ingestion of ethylene glycol, a negative result does not indicate that a cat has not ingested enough ethylene glycol to cause severe poisoning or even death.

OUTSIDE LABORATORY TESTING

Identification of a toxin by an outside laboratory is not likely to be helpful in the initial handling of a patient who has potentially been poisoned. The time to submit the test and receive results is usually too long to make much difference. There are cases where identification or quantification of the level of poisoning may make a difference, especially in medicolegal cases.

Specific tests.   Commercial laboratories have the capability to either test for specific compounds or screen for the more common causes of poisoning. Because there are more than 6 million potential causes (drugs, toxins, and chemicals) of poisoning, specific testing is not commonly undertaken unless the clinician has good reason to suspect a particular compound and wishes to confirm or refute that suspicion.

Toxicology screening. Toxiologic screens are performed by most commercial laboratories. These screens include 40 to 50 of the most common toxicants found and therefore are not really very sensitive or specific. A positive finding on a toxicologic screen is a fairly reliable finding; however, a negative screen does not rule out the possibility of poisoning.

Submission of samples for toxicologic screening should be preceded by a consultation with the laboratory staff to determine the content of the screen and the samples necessary for testing. They will also be able to provide any tips on handling the samples, which may make a difference in testing.

MINIMUM DATA BASE

Although routine blood tests are not likely to provide a specific diagnosis in the case of poisoning, the results may provide important clues that may direct treatment and stimulate additional, more specific diagnostic efforts. Although some of these tests are not routinely available in the majority of small-animal veterinary hospitals, they are included in the interest of completeness.

1. Hemogram.
2. Electrolyte determination with calculation of anion gap.
3. Blood or serum glucose.
4. Blood urea nitrogen and creatinine.
5. Liver enzymes including serum alanine transaminase (SALT) and alkaline phosphatase (SAP).
6. Electrocardiogram.
7. Urine analysis.
8. Blood gases (venous or arterial) for acid-base status.
9. Activated clotting time or other means of evaluating coagulation.
10. Radiographs.

Hemogram. The finding of hemoconcentration is helpful in identifying the need for increased fluid administration (for example, when toxins cause fluid losses such as salivation, urination, diarrhea). A finding of anemia in a potentially poisoned pet may stimulate the thought of zinc or lead ingestion, prompting the need for radiographs.

Electrolyte and anion gap determination

High anion gap. The anion gap (AG) is calculated by subtracting the measured anions (Cl^- and HCO_3^-) from the measured cations (Na^+ and K^+). The normal anion gap (12 to 25 mEq/L) is made up of unmeasured anions such as sulfates or phosphates. Accumulation of unmeasured anions will cause an increase in the AG (high AG). Most often a high AG is associated with a metabolic acidosis. High anion gap acidosis is caused by lactic acidosis (shock, liver failure, methanol), toxins (aspirin, ethanol, methanol, ethylene glycol, toluene) or organ dysfunction or failure (diabetic ketoacidosis, heart failure, renal failure, liver failure). *In small-animal medicine, ethylene glycol ingestion should be included in the differential diagnosis in patients with unexplained signs and high AG.*

Hypernatremia. Hypernatremia is a level of plasma or serum sodium greater than normal. This value is different for different laboratories and for different technologies. It is important that each practitioner know the normals for his or her laboratory. In general, plasma sodium levels greater than approximately 155 mmol/L in dogs or 165 mmol/L in cats are considered to indicate hypernatremia.

Hypernatremia may result as a loss of pure water (rare), loss of water greater than sodium (most common), or a gain of a salt (as in sodium phosphate enema toxicity, salt ingestion, overzealous replacement fluid administration). Hypernatremia may be present with hypovolemia, euvolemia, or even hypervolemia.

The body responds to increased plasma sodium levels by rapidly moving fluid from the intracellular fluid (ICF) to the extracellular fluid (ECF) and by moving sodium from the ECF into the ICF. The latter process is much slower than the fluid shift; thus cellular dehydration (and therefore cellular shrinkage) is the more dramatic result. This effect is most devastating to the brain. As the brain shrinks away from the calvarium, fine meningeal vessels are torn. Subarachnoid and subcortical hemorrhages, subdural hematomas, and activation of the coagulation system lead to further ischemic injury.

The brain has a unique response to *chronic* hypernatremia (as it does with any hypertonic extracellular fluid compartment condition). To defend itself against dehydration caused by fluid shifts, the brain has the capability of producing nondiffusible intracellular solutes. These are known as "idiogenic osmoles." These idiogenic osmoles increase intracellular osmolality, which prevents water loss and resultant shrinkage of the brain. The production of these osmoles begins rapidly with the onset of any hypertonic condition but takes several days to complete a state of osmotic equilibration.

TREATMENT OF HYPERNATREMIA

1. Evaluate for perfusion deficits first (capillary refill time, tachycardia, pallor, weak pulses, and so on). If evidence of hypovolemia or perfusion deficits exists, it must be treated first. This *volume deficit* must be treated with a crystalloid solution such as normal saline, lactated Ringer's solution, or other replacement solution. Although it may seem inappropriate to treat a hypernatremic patient with a salt-rich solution, it is important to realize that volume must be restored rapidly, and this cannot be done effectively with a salt-poor solution. Rapidly infuse enough crystalloid to improve the signs of hypoperfusion and hypovolemia.

2. Estimate the water deficit. Such estimation may be done by several methods. We prefer to estimate the water deficit using the magnitude of the sodium elevation above normal. It can be estimated that there is a deficit of 4 mL of water per kilogram of body weight per milliequivalent elevation of sodium above normal. For example, if a 20 kg dog presents with a sodium level of 176 mEq/L (lab normal = 155), the water deficit is:

$$176 - 155 = 21 \text{ mEq Na}^+ \text{ elevation over normal}$$

$$4 \text{ mL} \times 20 \text{ kg} \times 21 \text{ mEq} = 1680 \text{ mL water deficit}$$

This water deficit should be replaced slowly. It is recommended that the sodium level be lowered no faster than 0.5 to 1.0 mEq/hour. Using the above example, the water deficit would be replaced over 21 to 30 hours or approximately 60 to 80 mL/hour. The water deficit is best replaced using the oral route. If the oral route is inappropriate (as when vomiting is present), the water may be administered intravenously by use of 5% dextrose in water. Sodium levels should be monitored frequently.

3. If signs of hypervolemia are present (especially pulmonary edema), the patient should be treated with loop diuretics such as furosemide. If neurologic signs of hypernatremia are present, judicious use of salt-poor solutions may be required to treat brain dehydration, but continuous monitoring must be employed to prevent this addi-

tional fluid from worsening the pulmonary edema (see discussion of treating pulmonary edema, p. 12).
4.   It should be noted that many of these hypernatremic patients may have a concurrent metabolic acidosis. Sodium bicarbonate is contraindicated in these patients unless the blood pH is less than 7.05. Administration of sodium bicarbonate will worsen the hypernatremia.

Hyponatremia.   Hyponatremia is not a common finding in patients suspected of being poisoned. Acute hyponatremia will result in a shift of water into the brain. The resulting cerebral edema and ischemia may result in overt signs of neurologic impairment and even death. The majority of animals suffering acute hyponatremia will die of neurologic complications if untreated. Overzealous treatment of severe *chronic* hyponatremia, however, may result in central pontine myelinolysis and irreversible brain impairment.

Hyponatremia most commonly exists with decreased plasma osmolality but may occur with normal or increased plasma osmolality. It may also occur with hypovolemia, euvolemia, or even hypervolemia.

TREATMENT OF HYPONATREMIA
1.   Mild hyponatremia with no neurologic signs may be treated with mild water restriction and monitoring of serum sodium levels.
2.   Patients suffering hyponatremia with hypovolemia will require treatment of the volume deficit with an infusion of saline or other replacement crystalloid solution. Enough crystalloid should be given rapidly to improve the signs of hypovolemia or hypoperfusion. The sodium deficit can then be calculated and replaced over time. Sodium deficit can be calculated using the formula:

$$\text{Na}^+ \text{ deficit (in mEq)} = 0.6 \times \text{Body weight in kg} \times (\text{Normal Na}^+ - \text{Patient Na}^+)$$

Thus the sodium deficit in a 20 kg patient with a serum sodium of 130 (lab normal 150) would be:

$$0.6 \times 20 \times (150 - 130) = 240 \text{ mEq sodium}$$

This sodium can be replaced slowly using replacement crystalloid solutions such as normal saline (154 mEq/L), lactated Ringer's solution (130 mEq/L) or Normosol-R (140 mEq/L).

3. Patients with neurologic signs suffering severe (<120 mEq/L) or chronic (2 to 3 days in duration) hyponatremia must be treated aggressively to correct the edema, but care must be taken to prevent myelinolysis. Literature recommends that enough saline be given to raise the serum sodium approximately 5% to improve the cerebral edema without undue risk of myelinolysis. The remainder should be replaced at a rate not to exceed an elevation in serum sodium of 0.5 mmol/hour. An example:

A 20 kg patient has a serum sodium of 120 mEq/L (laboratory normal = 155 mEq/L). *Note that the laboratory normal is not the same as the example above to reinforce the point that each laboratory establishes its own normal reference range.* A 5% increase in serum sodium would require adding 6 mEq/L (120 × 5% = 6). In this patient, this translates to 72 mEq of sodium (0.6 × 20 × 6), which is administered rapidly to minimize the effects of cerebral edema. If normal saline were used, this would require an infusion of 467 mL (72 mEq/154 mEq per L × 1000 mL per liter). In theory, this would raise the sodium concentration to 126 mEq/L in this patient. The sodium deficit can then be calculated as above (0.6 × 20 × [155 − 126] = 348) and replaced slowly. These calculations will provide guidelines for treatment, but frequent measurements of serum sodium are required to assure that treatment is adequate but not too aggressive.

Hyperkalemia. The finding of hyperkalemia in a patient should direct emergency therapy first, followed by diagnostics to find the cause. Endogenous causes of hyperkalemia are more likely; however ingestion of some agents can cause hyperkalemia. Agents such as beta-blockers (propranolol) will cause a shift of potassium out of the cell. This is usually not severe enough to cause clinical problems. Potassium levels >6.5 mEq/L should be considered a medical emergency.

TREATMENT OF HYPERKALEMIA

1. Rapid infusion of potassium-free crystalloid fluids (such as 0.9% saline, D_5W) will have dilutional effects. Crystalloid administration may also treat existing acidemia, which will raise the pH toward normal. As pH rises, H^+ shifts out of the cell following its concentration gradient. Plasma potassium will move intracellularly to retain intracellular electroneutrality.

2. Intravenous calcium will antagonize the effects of hyperkalemia on cell membranes. Calcium gluconate 10% should be administered IV at a dose of 0.25 to 1.5 mL/kg. It must be given slowly while the ECG is being monitored. If bradycardia is noted, the infusion should be discontinued. Calcium chloride may also be used but may cause tissue damage if given perivascularly. CAUTION: If the hyperkalemia is caused by digitalis toxicity, do not use calcium preparations because refractory dysrhythmia may result.

3. Glucose infusion will stimulate insulin release in normal patients. Insulin and glucose will drive potassium from the plasma into the cells. Administration of 50% dextrose at a dose of 1 to 2 mL/kg (or rapid administration of a 5% to 10% dextrose solution) will usually result in potassium shifts in normal animals. Some clinicians prefer to administer insulin as well. Regular insulin (0.5 to 1 unit/kg) with dextrose (2 g of dextrose per unit of insulin) is given intravenously over 30 minutes. CAUTION: Observe closely for signs of hypoglycemia.

4. Sodium bicarbonate administration promotes movement of potassium from the plasma into the cell. The dose of bicarbonate should be calculated from blood gas analysis. Bicarbonate required = 0.3 (BW_{kg} × Base deficit). If blood gas anlysis is unavailable, one may administer 0.25 to 1 mEq/kg IV over 30 minutes. CAUTION: Administration of sodium bicarbonate may result in alkalinization of the patient, especially the patient suffering diabetic ketoacidosis.

5. Sodium polystyrene sulfonate, a cation-exchange resin, administered orally or as an enema at a dose of 0.25 to 0.5 g/kg/day may extract excess potassium from the gastrointestinal tract.

6. If all other methods fail, dialysis may be the patient's only hope. Hemodialysis will rapidly lower serum potassium but is likely only available in large referral institutions. Ambulatory peritoneal dialysis using potassium-free dialysate may be a more widely available option (p. 61).

Hypokalemia. Hypokalemia has been reported in dogs in cases of poisoning from beta$_2$-agonists. Drugs such as albuterol, metaproterenol, and terbutaline are packaged in pressurized containers and are used extensively by asthma patients. Typically the poisoning occurs when the dog punctures the cannister discharging the contents. Beta$_2$-agonists cause a rapid and profound shift of potassium from the plasma into the cell. Hypokalemia may also be caused by other drugs or toxins that induce renal or gastrointestinal losses.

TREATMENT OF HYPOKALEMIA

1. Hypokalemia is usually mild and not life threatening. Oral supplementation with potassium chloride (0.1 to 0.25 mL/kg PO q8h) or potassium gluconate (5 to 8 mEq PO q12-24h) is usually sufficient.

2. Life-threatening hypokalemia is manifested more by signs than by measured levels. Signs of life-threatetning hypokalemia include profound weakness, ileus, and tachycardia. Electrocardiographic findings with hypokalemia are found in Table 1-4. Severe hypokalemia may cause rhabdomyolysis and should be treated with intravenous administration of potassium chloride (Table 1-5). Intravenous potassium should be given at a rate not to exceed 0.5 mEq/kg/hour. The volume of the infusion should be kept to a minimum because rapid volume administration of fluids may treat an existing acidemia resulting in a shift of K^+ into the cell, further lowering plasma potassium levels. The ECG should be monitored continuously during IV potassium supplementation. Hypokalemia that is refractory to supplementation should alert the clinician to supplement magnesium as well. The mechanism between refractory hypokalemia and hypomagnesemia is believed to involve the inhibition of the Na^+/K^+-ATPase pump, which maintains intracellular potassium levels. Supplementation of magnesium ranges from simply using magnesium-containing solutions (such as Normosol-R, which contains 3 mEq/L) to administering magnesium chloride or magnesium sulfate at a rate of 1 mEq/kg/day in intravenous fluids. Life-threatenting hypomagnesemia has reportedly been treated with magnesium sulfate at a dose of 0.15 to 0.3 mEq/kg given IV over 5 to 15 minutes.

Blood or serum glucose.   Numerous drugs and toxins (as well as disease states) can cause alterations in blood glucose. Rapid

TABLE 1-4

Possible electrocardiographic abnormalities seen with electrolyte disturbances

Hyperkalemia
Spiked T-waves, increased P-R interval, decreased P-wave amplitude, atrial standstill, sinoventricular rhythm, and bradycardia. These changes are magnified by hyponatremia, acidosis, hypocalcemia, and hypermagnesemia.

Hypokalemia
Inversion of the T-wave, flattening of the T-wave, development of U-waves, sinus bradycardia, ST-segment depression, first- and second-degree heart block, atrial flutter, paroxysmal atrial tachycardia, atrioventricular dissociation, cardiac arrest.

Hypercalcemia
Tachycardia, possibly prolongation of the Q-T interval, increased P-R interval, several dysrhythmias including ventricular fibrillation.

Hypocalcemia
Tachycardia, possibly prolongation of the Q-T interval, T-wave alternans.

Hypernatremia
Usually no changes are evident.

Hyponatremia
Usually no changes are evident. May magnify the changes seen with concurrent hyperkalemia.

TABLE 1-5

Potassium supplementation guidelines

Serum K$^+$	mEq of potassium required
<2.0	80
2.0-2.49	60
2.5-3.0	40
3.0-3.5	28
>3.5	13-20

determination of glucose levels can be accomplished by the use of relatively inexpensive glucometers available from many sources. These glucometers are widely used by human diabetics and use whole blood as the sample. They are rapid (2 minutes or less) and reasonably accurate for use in dogs and cats. They are known to be inaccurate in birds or in animals that have increased PCV (>60%).

Hyperglycemia. Hyperglycemia (serum glucose >200 mg/dL) caused by drugs or toxins is usually mild and transient requiring no treatment. In cases of sustained hyperglycemia or levels above 500 mg/dL, fluid may shift from the brain to the plasma. If this occurs rapidly, the brain will dehydrate resulting in CNS depression or coma. Central pontine myelinolysis has been reported from rapid dehydration of brain tissue caused by fluid shifts.

To prevent this shift, the brain will manufacture "idiogenic osmoles." These osmotically active molecules attract water and balance the effects of sustained hyperglycemia. Danger arises when glucose levels are normalized rapidly. When this occurs, the active idiogenic osmoles attract water, and the brain becomes edematous resulting in decreased cerebral perfusion pressure and coma. Sustained hyperosmolar states should be treated slowly to allow the brain to rid itself of the idiogenic osmoles.

TREATMENT OF SUSTAINED HYPERGLYCEMIA. Hyperglycemia should be treated if it is not resolving spontaneously or if the patient is symptomatic. Correct fluid deficits with isotonic crystalloid solutions. Often, once the patient is rehydrated, the osmotic diuresis lowers the glucose levels though renal losses. If the glucose levels remain elevated despite adequate fluid therapy, insulin therapy may be necessary. The goal of therapy is to reduce glucose levels slowly; reduction of 100 to 150 mg/dL/hour are appropriate. Administer regular insulin (0.25 units/kg) intramuscularly followed by 0.1 unit/kg IM every hour. Monitor blood glucose levels every 1 to 2 hours. When glucose levels reach 200 to 250 mg/dL, discontinue insulin. Continue to monitor glucose. If glucose levels begin to rise, consider a diagnosis of diabetes mellitus and begin therapy with intermediate or long-acting insulins. CAUTION: As the patient responds to insulin therapy, potassium levels may fall to low levels. Monitor potassium frequently and supplement if necessary.

Hypoglycemia. Hypoglycemia (measured levels <60 mg/dL) may manifest as weakness, alterations of consciousness, or even seizures. If the patient's mental status is profoundly affected, the first priority is to protect the airway (p. 2) and administer supplemental oxygen. Ventilate the patient if necessary. If hypoglycemia is suspected or confirmed, administer 50% dextrose at 0.25 to 1.0 mL/kg. Fifty-percent dextrose is extremely hyperosmolar and may cause vasculitis or phlebitis if administered directly. It should be diluted at least 1:1 with a sterile saline solution or sterile water before administration.

Blood urea nitrogen and creatinine. Kidney function should be evaluated initially and monitored serially. The finding of impaired renal function on initial evaluation should alert the astute clinician that toxins that are eliminated via the kidneys will remain in the body for a prolonged period. Acute renal failure may be caused by many poisons; by direct or indirect action of the poison; or by reduced renal perfusion brought on by shock, hypovolemia, or cardiovascular collapse. Serial measurements of BUN and creatinine will disclose damage to the kidneys, allowing prompt therapy.

Liver enzymes including serum alanine transaminase (SALT) and alkaline phosphatase (SAP). The liver is responsible for metabolism and elimination of many poisons from the body. It is also sensitive to damage from many toxins and thus should be monitored for damage. Rising or high levels of liver enzymes may indicate a prolonged course of recovery from poisons requiring degradation by the liver. The discovery of hepatic damage will alert the clinician to watch the patient closely for signs of hepatic encephalopathy, coagulation deficits, or other complications.

Electrocardiogram. The electrocardiogram may be useful in detecting electrolyte abnormalities when laboratory support is not available. Abnormal ECG findings for electrolyte disturbances are found in Table 1-4. The ECG is also useful in diagnosing dysrhythmias caused directly or indirectly by toxins. Ingestion of oleander, for example, will result in cardiotoxicity and ECG abnormalities. Shock or hypoxemia may result in ECG abnormalities.

Urine analysis. The bladder should be emptied and a urine analysis performed. A sample should be saved for possible toxicologic testing; especially if there may be legal implications. Urine production should be monitored to detect oliguria or anuria. If urine production drops below 1 mL/kg/hour (0.5 mL/kg/hour in the cat) in a patient at risk for acute renal failure, aggressive therapy is indicated.

The urine should be monitored for the presence of crystals, which could indicate a specific cause (such as hippuric acid or calcium oxalate crystals being indicative of ethylene glycol toxicity).

The appearance of granular casts in the urine may herald proximal tubular cell damage or death and is *one of the earliest findings in acute renal failure.* These casts often appear before a rise in BUN or creatinine is seen. Aggressive therapy for acute renal failure should be initiated upon the discovery of granular or renal tubular cell casts.

Blood gases (venous or arterial) for acid-base status. Arterial blood gas analysis is important in cases of poisoning that result in damage to the respiratory system or when aspiration may have occurred (see the discussion of ventilatory failure, p. 6). More commonly, arterial or venous blood gas analysis will reveal acid-base abnormalities associated with poison cases.

Activated clotting time or other coagulation tests. Abnormal coagulation may be a direct or indirect consequence of a toxicosis. The advent of the more potent second-generation vitamin K–antagonist poisons has made this much more important in the diagnostic profile of the patient. Small animal patients may be secondarily poisoned by ingesting an animal that died after eating the poison. This means that the owners will have no idea that the pet could possibly be exposed.

Clinical signs associated with internal bleeding are quite variable; many times the bleeding is not grossly evident and is uncovered only after finding an abnormal laboratory parameter. Activated clotting tests that demonstrate prolonged clotting should alert the clinician that a coagulation system defect exists and a more thorough work-up of the coagulation system is necessary. An activated clotting time that is shorter than reference range may indicate a hypercoagulable state and prompt the clinician to look for a cause (such as DIC).

The PIVKA test is preferred for diagnosis of intoxication with a vitamin K antagonist (see above). Other tests that may indicate a problem in the coagulation cascade include prothrombin time, activated partial thromboplastin time, fibrinogen levels, fibrin/fibrinogen degradation product levels, platelet counts, analysis of a complete blood cell count, and antithrombin III levels.

Radiographs. Occasionally radiographs may provide hints as to the cause of toxicosis. Radiographs can be useful in diagnosing zinc toxicosis (recent pennies, metal from transportation cages, game pieces), ingestion of iron tablets, or ingestion of drugs such as lithium salts. Illicit drug trafficking using condoms filled with cocaine of other drugs have resulted in poisoning of animal patients. These packets can be seen radiographically.

DECONTAMINATION

Decontamination procedures are necessary to remove the poison so that a patient does not have repeated or ongoing absorption of the toxin. Poisons may gain access to the systemic circulation from topical application, inhalation, injection, or ingestion.

Skin decontamination

Poisons or toxins applied to the skin may cause physical injury. Topically applied toxins may also be absorbed through intact skin resulting in systemic effects. To prevent injury and systemic absorption, the toxin should be removed as rapidly as possible.

Prevent exposure to yourself or anyone else during decontamination. Wear protective gloves, aprons, and splash shields. During decontamination, be aware that an animal may attempt to shake off powders or liquids that may cause injury to bystanders.

Protect the patient from injury during decontamination. If the patient is moribund, protect the airway to prevent aspiration. If the patient is active, make certain that he or she does not ingest the contaminant while it is brushed or bathed off. Watch for hypothermia if bathing is necessary. Prevent exposure of sensitive occular tissues by using a petrolatum oph-thalmic ointment in the eyes.

If the patient has received exposure from a dry or powdered toxin or poison, gently brush it away with a stiff-bristled brush or piece of cardboard. Take care to prevent the powder gaining access to the patient's or caregiver's eyes or respira-tory tract.

Bathe the patient thoroughly in tepid, running water. Use an unmedicated pet shampoo or mild dishwashing liquid and work thoroughly through the hair. Rinse with copious amounts of running water. Continue rinsing for a minimum of 15 minutes. Repeat bathing if the odor of the toxin remains. Actively dry the patient to prevent hypothermia.

Do not use neutralizing agents on the skin. The heat generated by these chemical reactions is likely to cause more harm than good.

Eye decontamination

Corneal tissues are very sensitive and are quickly injured by exposure to toxins. If the toxin is not removed quickly, the eye may be permanently damaged.

The owner should be told to flush the eye with water for 10 minutes before attempting to bring the pet to the hospital. Tap water is uncomfortable to the sensitive tissues of the eye. Saline is a better option. The client may be instructed to make saline by dissolving 2 teaspoons of table salt per quart of water. This solution can be used to flush the eye with less dis-comfort. Saline in squirt bottles may be purchased commer-cially to have on hand for these emergencies.

Upon arrival at the hospital, continue irrigating the eye with sterile saline for a total of at least 30 minutes. For com-fort, the saline solution should be warmed to body tempera-ture. Topical ophthalmic anesthetic drops may be instilled to make the procedure more comfortable for the pet. Stain eyes after flushing and treat appropriately.

Inhalation decontamination

Most toxins that gain access to the systemic circulation through the respiratory system are inhaled as a gas. The patient must be removed from the source of the noxious sub-stance. Protect the airway. Administer humidified oxygen. Intubate the patient and ventilate if necessary.

Injection decontamination

The most common exposure to toxins through injection is from bee or wasp stings or snakebite. Injection of toxins through intact skin have occurred in farm or industrial accidents using high-pressure spraying equipment.

Some stinging insects, such as bees, embed the stinger into the victim's skin. When these bees fly away, the stinger and a venom sac remain. The venom sac continues to contract slowly until the contents are fully emptied into the victim. Immediate removal of the venom sac will prevent further injection of venom. If a stinger is found, one should remove it by grasping the stinger near the victim's skin or by scraping across the stinger with a credit card. The venom sac should not be compressed while the stinger is being removed because this injects more venom into the victim.

Snakebites are a type of injected toxin. See Coral snakes, p. 115, and Pit vipers, p. 223.

High-pressure injection accidents are rare. High-pressure spray equipment may be used to apply insecticides or other chemicals high into the trees of orchards. It is also used in some painting equipment. Should a pet run close to the spray nozzle, the product being applied may be forcefully injected through intact skin. Liquids that are generally nontoxic may "tattoo" an animal, resulting in toxic signs if not decontaminated. Decontamination of areas that have been subjected to injection injury usually requires surgical drainage or débridement.

Gastrointestinal decontamination

Ingestion is the most common route of significant poisoning in small animal patients. There is much controversy over the advisability and effectiveness of various procedures used to decontaminate gastrointestinal tract. If the exposure was >2 hours previously, there is little reason to decontaminate the stomach unless examination (physical examination or radiographs) reveals that the stomach contains ingesta.

EMESIS

Induction of emesis may be a rapid and convenient way to empty some ingested poison from the stomach. Studies have shown that some patients fail to empty even half of the stomach's contents during emesis. Still, the procedure is useful in the home setting to eliminate some of the toxin from the chance of absorption. The earlier emesis can be induced, the better.

1. Induce emesis *only* if:
   a. Ingestion occurred within the last 60 minutes.
   b. The patient is fully conscious and alert.
   c. The toxin is known and is not a strong corrosive agent (acid or alkali) or a petroleum distillate. Corrosive substances will cause further damage to the esophagus if they are put in contact again through the act of vomiting. Petroleum distillates (hydrocarbons) carry a great risk of aspiration if emesis is induced.

2. *Do not* induce emesis if:
   a. The toxin was ingested over 60 minutes previously.
   b. The patient is weakened or severely ill.
   c. The patient is suffering an alteration of consciousness. Pets suffering toxin-induced central nervous system hyperexcitability have increased risk of seizures. Aspiration of gastric contents is a common mishap in obtunded or comatose patients who vomit.
   d. The toxin is a strong corrosive agent (acid or alkali) or a petroleum distillate. Corrosive substances will cause further damage to the esophagus if they are put in contact again through the act of vomiting. Petroleum distillates (hydrocarbons) carry a great risk of aspiration if emesis is induced.
   e. The toxin is unknown. The risk of aspiration or repeat exposure of the esophageal tissues to the toxin is too great when compared to the effectiveness of emesis to warrant induction of emesis in the case of an unknown intoxicant.

3. Induce emesis with:
   a. *Syrup of ipecac.* Syrup of ipecac is usually sold commercially as a 7% solution. Administer 1 to 2.5 mL/kg PO in dogs or 3.3 mL/kg PO in cats. Onset of vomiting should occur in 10 to 15 minutes. The dose may be repeated once if the patient does not vomit within 20 to 30 minutes. The patient may be given a small amount of water (4 to 5 mL/kg) and made to move about to speed the onset of nausea and vomiting. CAUTION: *Syrup of ipecac should not be confused with the fluid extract of ipecac, which is the concentrated form and may cause cardiotoxicities.*

b. *Hydrogen peroxide* (3%). Onset of vomiting is seen within 10 to 15 minutes after administration of hydrogen peroxide at a dose of 1 to 2 mL/kg PO. This may be repeated once if vomiting has not occurred within 20 minutes after first administration.

c. *Apomorphine.* Apomorphine remains the most useful emetic in dogs. A dose of 0.04 to 0.08 mg/kg IV will produce rapid emesis. It is also effective to place a portion of the apomorphine tablet in the conjunctival sac. When the dog begins to vomit, any remaining tablet is flushed from the eye with saline. The use of apomorphine in cats is controversial. Some experts state that it should not be used in this type of animal because it is much less effective than either xylazine or ipecac syrup and possibly less safe.

d. *Xylazine.* Xylazine injected at a dose of 1.1 to 2.2 mg/kg IM may induce vomiting in 5 to 10 minutes. In cats 0.44 mg/kg IM or SC is quite effective. Xylazine causes bradycardia, sedation, and respiratory depression. It can be reversed with yohimbine if these effects become excessive.

GASTRIC LAVAGE

Gastric lavage remains an effective means of removing gastric contents. Controversy exists regarding whether gastric lavage is superior to emesis for recently ingested toxins. If more than 1 or 2 hours have passed since ingestion, the stomach may be empty and there is little reason to perform lavage. For this reason, we recommend getting a scout radiograph to assess the presence or absence of ingesta in the stomach. If nothing can be seen in the stomach, there is little reason to assume the risks of gastric lavage.

Advantages of gastric lavage
1. *Rapid* removal of gastric contents.
2. *Caustic* or corrosive substances are diluted and retrieved through a tube, avoiding reexposure of the esophagus to the toxin.
3. *Allows* introduction of activated charcoal into the stomach of uncooperative patients.

Disadvantages of gastric lavage
1. *Requires* general anesthesia.
2. *Carries* the risk of trauma to the esophagus or stomach.

3. *Carries* the risk of aspiration of charcoal or lavage of fluids or stomach contents, even though the patient is intubated.
4. *Is often* not effective in removing undissolved or undigested tablets, large amounts of ingesta, or large pieces of food.

Procedure

1. The patient must be lightly anesthetized.
    a. Induce with tiletamine-zolazepam, ketamine-diazepam, oxymorphone, propofol, or short-acting barbiturates.
    b. If the patient has been seizuring or may have increased intracranial pressure, do not use ketamine, tiletamine, or opioids. These anesthetics may cause further increases in intracranial pressure and, even though the effect may be minimized by concurrent use of benzodiazepines, are not worth the risk.
    c. Intubate the patient with a cuffed endotracheal tube. Inflate the cuff just enough to effect a seal between the tube and the trachea.
    d. Maintain on oxygen and an appropriate anesthetic (gas, injectable).
2. Two tubes will be passed into the stomach, if possible. If not, one tube may be used. The patient is secured in lateral recumbency, and the table is tipped so that the head is lower than the stomach.
    a. The distance from the tip of the nose to the last rib is measured and marked on a stomach tube. This stomach tube should be at least as large as the endotracheal tube (preferably larger) and is the egress tube.
    b. A smaller tube is also marked with this distance. This is the ingress tube.
    c. Both tubes are passed gently into the stomach (as indicated by the mark on the tube or by the return of stomach contents through the tube). Do not pass the tubes farther than the marked distance.
3. Perform lavage of the stomach thoroughly with warm (body-temperature) water or saline infused through the small tube. Do not use excessive amounts of infusate, which may distend the stomach unnecessarily. A volume of 5 to 10 mL/kg is appropriate. The infused fluid should leave the stomach via the large-bore tube,

carrying stomach contents. If the egress tube does not allow free flow of fluid from the stomach, it may extend too far into the stomach or may be plugged. Withdraw the tube slowly. If flow begins, continue the lavage. If no flow can be established, infuse a small amount of water or air through the large-bore tube to dislodge material. If no flow is established, remove the tube and check for a plug. Gently reinsert to establish flow.

Continue the lavage until the effluent is clear. In cases where the stomach is filled with food, this may take large volumes of lavage solution and a great deal of time. The patient should be lavaged in both left and right lateral recumbency to ensure that the stomach is thoroughly emptied. In some cases, it is helpful to move the egress tube gently to and fro to help mix and dislodge stomach contents. If this is necessary, it must be done gently to avoid trauma to the pharynx, esophagus, and stomach.

4. When the effluent is clean, crimp one of the tubes and remove. Ensure that the endotracheal tube is still properly placed and the cuff remains inflated. Instill activated charcoal through the remaining tube. Crimp or clamp the tube and remove.

5. To minimize the chances of aspiration, recover the patient with the endotracheal tube in place and the cuff inflated until the swallowing reflex returns. Carefully check the oropharynx for fluid, activated charcoal, or stomach contents and suction clean before removing the endotracheal tube.

ACTIVATED CHARCOAL, KAOLIN, BENTONITE

Recent human studies have found that administration of activated charcoal alone is more effective in decontamination of the gastrointestinal tract than emesis or gastric lavage. Although current human literature recommends that repeated doses of activated charcoal should replace the practice of inducing emesis or gastric lavage, we recommend emesis or lavage followed by repeated doses of activated charcoal. Repeated doses of activated charcoal may be beneficial in managing toxicoses by interrupting the enterohepatic recycling of some poisons.

Not all substances will be adsorbed by activated charcoal. A list of selected poisons that are poorly adsorbed by activated charcoal is included in Box 1-8. The clays kaolin and bentonite have also been recommended for use as adsorbents. They are, in general, less effective than activated charcoal with one exception: they are reported to be more effective in adsorbing paraquat.

Activated charcoal is administered by nasoesophageal, nasogastric, or orogastric tube. Some patients will allow administration by gavage.

WHOLE BOWEL IRRIGATION

Whole bowel irrigation is a newer technique useful in removal of toxins from the gut. It is especially useful to remove toxins that are poorly adsorbed by activated charcoal (see Box 1-8) or that are slowly digested (such as iron, lithium, or sustained-release preparations).

The technique uses polyethylene glycol (PEG) electrolyte preparations such as GoLYTELY (Braintree Laboratories, Braintree, MA 02185). These preparations are given in large quantities and pass through the gastrointestinal tract without being absorbed. Intestinal contents are forced through the intestines by sheer volume.

A nasoesophageal or nasogastric tube may be used for continuous administration of PEG solutions. If the patient is unconscious or anesthetized, the airway must be protected by endotracheal intubation. An initial dose of 25 to 40 mL/kg followed by continuous infusion of 0.5 mL/kg/hour. Orogastric intubation is satisfactory in an anesthetized patient; however, the procedure usually requires infusion for

BOX 1-8

POISONS THAT ARE POORLY ADSORBED BY ACTIVATED CHARCOAL.

Acids	Fluoride
Alkalis	Iron
Chlorate	Isopropanol
Chloride	Methanol
Cyanide	Mineral acids
Detergents	Nitrate
Ethanol	Paraquat
Ethylene glycol	Potassium
Ferrous sulfate	Sodium

more than a range of 1.5 to 2 hours. Alternatively, PEG solution may be given by gavage at a dose of 30 to 40 mL/kg given every 2 hours.

Expect large volumes of stool within 2 hours. Reported side effects include apparent abdominal cramping and discomfort. Vomiting has also been reported. Vomiting and regurgitation carry the risk of pulmonary aspiration. Reports indicate that administration of PEG solutions may interfere with the effectiveness of activated charcoal. Studies of this treatment are ongoing. The role of whole bowel irrigation is unclear.

ENEMAS

Enemas may be useful in decontamination of the lower gastrointestinal tract (GIT). Commercial phosphate enemas may cause hyperphosphatemia, hypocalcemia, and hypomagnesemia and are not recommended; this is especially true for the feline patient. Mineral oil enemas are messy and are not proved to be more effective than water. Mineral oil enemas are never to be used with dioctyl sodium sulfosuccinate (DSS) because emulsification and subsequent absorption of mineral oil will result. *The best enema solution is lukewarm water.*

Lukewarm water is infused into the rectum of a patient. The patient may be unmedicated or may require sedation or even light anesthesia for treatment. Conscious patients and lightly anesthetized patients will expel the contents when the colon becomes distended. Water is infused into the rectum until the return is clear. If difficulty is encountered in cleaning the lower GIT, it is better to repeat the enema in 2 hours than to be overzealous on the initial attempt.

The effectiveness of enemas is not clear. Certainly, in some cases they help to decontaminate the lower GIT, but most toxins have been absorbed before they reach the lower GIT. Disadvantages of enemas include patient discomfort, cramping, and nausea.

CATHARTICS

Little data exist to confirm or deny the effectiveness of cathartics in removing toxins from the GIT; however, most literature still advocates their use. It does seem logical that decreased transit time of gastrointestinal contents would limit

TABLE 1-6

Commonly used cathartics with dosage recommendations

	Dogs	**Cats**
Magnesium sulfate (Should be mixed with 5 to 10 mL/kg water and administered orally)	250 to 500 mg/kg	200 mg/kg
Magnesium hydroxide (milk of magnesia) (Dosage may be repeated q6-12h PRN)	10 to 150 mL PO	15 to 50 mL PO
Sodium sulfate (Should be mixed with 5 to 10 times as much water and administered orally)	250 to 500 mg/kg	200 mg/kg
Sorbitol	4 g/kg PO	4 g/kg PO

absorption time and therefore would be beneficial. Common cathartics include sodium sulfate (Glauber's salts), magnesium sulfate (Epsom salt), and sorbitol (Table 1-6).

Cathartics would seem to be indicated to help passage of activated charcoal compounds, which have adsorbed toxins, or to help pass toxins that are poorly adsorbed by activated charcoal. They would not be indicated if ileus is present or there is evidence of intestinal obstruction. Caution must be taken not to worsen the clinical picture with the use of cathartics. Hypermagnesemia has been seen in patients with renal insufficiency when magnesium-containing cathartics were used. Absorption of magnesium may worsen CNS depression caused by toxins. *Therefore magnesium-based cathartics are not indicated for use with poisons that have caused CNS depression.*

Sorbitol is widely used as an additive in activated charcoal preparations. It is normally administered by gavage or by orogastric tube. It is too thick to administer through tubes that will pass through the nose of most small animal patients. The dose is repeated in 2 to 4 hours. Nausea, cramping, and vomiting have been reported after administration.

Oil-based cathartics (such as mineral oil) are not indicated. They decrease effectiveness of activated charcoal and may actually enhance absorption of some toxins such as insecticides (such as chlorinated hydrocarbons).

ENHANCED REMOVAL AND ELIMINATION

There are methods of enhancing elimination of drugs, chemicals, or other toxins from the body. Although this is a worthy goal, it must be understood that these techniques are not necessary in most cases and in some cases may be deleterious. Some of these techniques are impractical or economically unfeasible for some pet owners. Techniques discussed in the following section include urinary manipulation, hemodialysis, hemoperfusion, peritoneal dialysis, ion-exchange resins, precipitating, or chelation therapy. Before any of these therapies are incorporated in the treatment of a poisoned patient, the clinician must be familiar with the technique and its limitations and side effects. Check each poison in Section 2 of this text. If the poison is not listed, consultation with a poison control center is strongly advised.

Urinary manipulation

DIURESIS

Toxins or poisons that are eliminated from the body largely through the kidneys (such as cholecalciferol, ethylene glycol) may be cleared from circulation more quickly if the glomerular filtration rate (GFR) is increased. Administration of crystalloid fluids or diuretics may enhance GFR. Fluid, such as saline, lactated Ringer's solution or other crystalloid solution, is administered at a rate to promote urine production >2 mL/kg/hour. Central venous pressure must be monitored to avoid volume overload or overhydration. Diuretics may be added to enhance GFR. Osmotic diuresis may be initiated with mannitol at a dose of 0.25 to 0.5 g/kg IV given over a 30-minute period. Furosemide given at 2 to 5 mg/kg IV may enhance urine production. Dopamine at 1 to 3 μg/kg/min will dilate afferent renal arterioles, so that the renal blood flow and GFR may be enhanced.

The drawbacks to forced diuresis is that aggressive fluid therapy is not very effective for removal of most toxins and carries the risk of iatrogenic complications. The use of diuretics carries the risks of dehydration, electrolyte and acid-base imbalances, and hypotension and subsequent perfusion deficits. Osmotic diuretics like mannitol are hyperosmolar and may aggravate any hyperosmolar condition. If the patient is anuric, mannitol should not be used. Before initiating forced diuresis, the clinician should consult Section 2 of this text or a poison control center to see if the target poison is suitable for enhanced elimination using the technique.

ION TRAPPING

Weak acids and weak bases are present as ionized and non-ionized forms in the body. Equilibrium between the forms is established by conditions within the body. Substances in the ionized form do not diffuse easily across cellular membranes; of particular interest is the inability of these ions to diffuse across luminal membranes of the renal tubules. This phenomenon may be used to "trap" ionized molecules in urine. The balance of equilibrium may be shifted when the pH of the urine is adjusted.

Urine acidification.   Administration of ammonium chloride will acidify the urine. Acid urine favors a shift of equilibrium of certain toxins (weak bases) to the ionized form. Examples of toxins that may be eliminated using this technique are amphetamines, PCP, and strychnine.

Urinary acidification is not very effective and may aggravate kidney damage in patients with rhabdomyolysis, myoglobinuria, or hemoglobinuria. (Strychnine is known to cause exertional rhabdomyolysis.)

Urine acidification is accomplished by use of ammonium chloride to maintain a urine pH of 5.5 to 6.5. Ammonium chloride is administered at a dose of 100 to 200 mg/kg in the dog or 20 mg/kg in the cat. It is given twice a day in an oral preparation. The patient must be monitored closely for development of metabolic acidosis. Use of ammonium chloride is contraindicated in patients who have renal or hepatic insufficiency. Ammonia toxicity, manifested by CNS depression or coma, may develop in patients with impaired renal or hepatic function.

Urine alkalinization. Urinary alkalinization has been used in the treatment of animals poisoned with salicylates, ethylene glycol, 2,4-D, and phenobarbital. Urinary alkalinization requires that the renal threshold for bicarbonate (24 mEq/L) be exceeded. Administration of sodium bicarbonate at 1 to 2 mEq/kg IV every 3 to 4 hours may accomplish this excess. It should be given by slow, continuous intravenous administration for best results. The goal is to induce a urine pH >7; however, carnivores have acidic urine and administration of bicarbonate sufficient to induce urinary alkalinization may induce metabolic alkalemia. Metabolic alkalemia, hypokalemia, and hypochloremia (systemic alkalinization results in chloride and potassium wasting) are common complications of attempts to alkalinize urine in small animal patients.

Hemodialysis

Drugs or toxins that are small (<500 daltons), are water soluble, and experience low protein binding are suitable for clearance using hemodialysis. The procedure is performed by use of a venovenous (double-lumen) or arteriovenous catheter through which blood is extracted, circulated through a hemodialysis system, and returned to the body. Inside the hemodialysis system, drugs and toxins flow passively through semipermeable membranes down concentration gradients into a dialysate solution. Systemic anticoagulation is required. Hemodialysis systems are not widely available in the small animal practice.

Hemoperfusion

Blood is extracted through a double-lumen catheter and pumped through a column that contains an adsorbent material (charcoal or Amberlite resin) and returned to the body. Because the drug or toxin is in direct contact with the adsorbent, molecular size, water solubility, or plasma protein binding does not play an important role. Drug or toxin clearance rates can be greatly enhanced by this technique.

Hemoperfusion requires systemic anticoagulation, often requiring higher doses than hemodialysis. Thrombocytopenia following the procedure is common. The equipment including the perfusion column is relatively expensive. These systems must be primed before use; that is, they must be filled with an appropriate fluid that will be pumped into the body to replace blood that is being extracted and pumped through the column. If crystalloids are used as priming liquid, the volume required may cause excessive hemodilution of the patient. If blood products are used to prime the column, blood should be typed and cross-matched.

Peritoneal dialysis

Peritoneal dialysis is widely available to veterinarians and within economical reach for many more pet owners than hemodialysis is. It does not require systemic anticoagulation. Although peritoneal dialysis is not so effective as hemodialysis or hemoperfusion, it can be continued 24 hours a day. The procedure utilizes the gut wall and peritoneum as the semipermeable membrane.

TECHNIQUE FOR PERITONEAL DIALYSIS

The patient is placed in dorsal or lateral recumbency. The abdomen is shaved and surgically prepared. The bladder is emptied. Local anesthesia is used to facilitate implantation of the catheter. Commercial peritoneal dialysis sets are available. The catheter is implanted according to instructions for the catheter used. In lieu of a commercial catheter, silicone elastomer tubing (Silastic brand medical-grade tubing, Dow Corning Corp., Midland, MI 48686) with multiple fenestrations or a large-bore intravenous (14-gauge) catheter with added fenestrations can be used. The placement site depends somewhat on the catheter used. If Silastic tubing or a modified IV catheter is used, it should enter the abdomen just to the right of the midline a few centimeters caudally to the umbilicus.

The Column Disc Peritoneal Dialysis Catheter (VetCath-Physio-Control, Redmond, WA 98052) is recommended when the need for continuous ambulatory peritoneal dialysis is likely to exceed 1 or 2 days. The catheter is implanted through a surgical incision in the caudoventral abdomen near the urinary bladder. The disk should be pulled firmly against the abdominal wall and the peritoneum closed over the base. The abdominal muscles should be sutured tightly around the first Dacron velour cuff. The free end of the catheter is tunneled subcutaneously and exits through a stab incision at a point beyond the second Dacron velour cuff.

Commercial dialysate (Dianeal 137, Peridial, or Inpersol) or lactated Ringer's solution with glucose added to form a 1.5% to 4.5% solution (see p. 378 in Appendix C) is warmed to body temperature and infused into the abdomen through the catheter. Strict aseptic technique is observed. Masks, caps, and sterile gloves are worn. The dialysate is infused until the abdomen distends slightly but does not interfere with normal respiration. The dose required is variable but is usually 30 to 40 mL/kg. The dialysate is allowed to remain in the abdomen for 45 minutes (dwell time) and then allowed to drain off by gravity flow. The recovered volume is recorded. It is common to find that less dialysate is recovered than is infused. This is attributable to absorption of the water from the dialysate and is minimized with adequate fluid therapy. The process is repeated each hour until no longer necessary. As the patient improves, the dwell time may be extended to 3 or 4 hours, and exchanges are done less frequently.

Frequently the catheter becomes plugged with fibrin (or tissue) after several hours of use. Addition of 1000 units of heparin to each liter of dilaysate may help prevent this complication. The Column Disc Peritoneal Dialysis Catheter is reported to become less frequently plugged than other catheters (unfortunately this catheter may not be manufactured any longer). Electrolyte imbalances are also a complication of peritoneal dialysis, particularly when the dialysate is not a commercially prepared solution made specifically for the purpose of peritoneal dialysis. Serum electrolyte levels should be checked frequently, especially during the initial exchanges. Protein loss is also seen with this technique. Serum protein should be monitored at least twice daily. Hypoproteinemia, if present, may warrant treatment with plasma or other colloid.

Peritonitis is a dangerous complication of peritoneal dialysis. The collected fluid should be examined carefully after each collection. If the fluid is grossly clear, there is probably little reason to perform microscopic examination. If, however, the fluid collected is turbid or bloody, a sample should be examined directly under the microscope. If no evidence of peritonitis can be seen on a direct examination, a sample should be centrifuged and the sediment examined microscopically for evidence of bacterial infection. Returned dialysate samples should also be added to culture media for culture, identification, and antibiotic sensitivity testing. It has been reported that addition of 1 g of ampicillin to 2 liters of dialysate may be used to prevent bacterial contamination of the dialysis catheter and tubing during continuous peritoneal dialysis.

Ion-exchange resins

Ion-exchange resins can ionically bind certain drugs or toxins. Cholestyramine and sodium polystyrene sulfonate are examples of ion-exchange resins. These resins delay absorption from the gut lumen. Cholestyramine is especially effective in delaying absorption of fat-soluble toxins. Ion-exchange resins have been used to delay absorption of warfarin, phenylbutazone, phenobarbital, tetracycline, digitalis glycosides, and organochlorine compounds. These resins have limited indication and have largely been replaced by activated charcoal as the treatment of choice.

Chelation therapy

Administration of a drug or compound that combines with a toxin or toxin metabolite to form an insoluble salt resulting in poor absorption is the principle behind chelation therapy. Chelation therapy is most useful in heavy-metal poisoning but may also provide an additional avenue of treatment of certain alkaloids or oxalates. Examples of compounds administered in chelation therapy include BAL, calcium salts, desferoxamine, succimer, EDTA, and D-penicillamine.

Surgical removal

On occasion, the toxin will not be removed by any other means than surgical removal. Iron tablets may adhere tenaciously to the stomach or intestine wall. Drug-filled condoms may rupture, spilling their contents if attempts are made to remove them through gastric lavage or whole bowel irrigation.

Multiple-dose activated charcoal

Repeated administration of activated charcoal may enhance the elimination of certain toxins. Two mechanisms are believed to be responsible for this. First, if the toxin enters the enterohepatic circulation, it will come into contact with the charcoal and be removed from recirculation. The second mechanism is sometimes referred to as "gut dialysis." Certain toxins, while following equilibrium gradients, will cross from the bloodstream into the bowel lumen where they are "trapped" by repeat doses of activated charcoal. For suitable toxins, activated charcoal may be administered every 2 to 4 hours.

Suggested Reading

Crowe DT: Managing respiration in the critical patient, *Vet Med* 84:55-76, 1989.

Fitzpatrick RK, Crowe DT: Nasal oxygen administration in dogs and cats: experimental and clinical investigations, *J Am Anim Hosp Assoc* 22:293-300, 1986.

Mann FH, Wagner-Mann C, Allertt JA, et al: Comparison of intranasal and intratracheal oxygen administration in healthy, awake dogs, *Am J Vet Res* 53(5):856, 1992.

■ SECTION TWO

TOXIC DRUGS AND CHEMICALS

ACETAMINOPHEN AND PHENACETIN

E L C A

Sources Many prescription and over-the-counter brands of analgesic and antipyretic drugs contain acetaminophen or its ethyl ether, phenacetin. Examples are Tylenol, SineAid, Sine-Off, Anacin-3, Comtrex, Daytril, Nyquil, Allerest, and Vanquish.

Mechanism of action Phenacetin is metabolized to acetaminophen. Acetaminophen is metabolized by enzymes of the cytochrome P-450 series to intermediate products: nonreactive glucuronides and sulfates (which are conjugated and eliminated in the urine), and reactive metabolites, which are metabolized with glutathione to nontoxic mercapturic acid (which is eliminated). If the toxic metabolites accumulate as a result of insufficient glucuronide or sulfate metabolism or insufficient glutathione, they are converted to toxic macromolecules that directly cause cellular death. Cats lack glucuronyl transferase and inefficiently form glucuronic acid and sulfate conjugates, leaving more acetaminophen or phenacetin to be metabolized to toxic metabolites. The glutathione stores are rapidly depleted in cats, leaving a large amount of toxic metabolites. Methemoglobinemia occurs.

Clinical signs Acute signs in cats are related to methemoglobin formation, whereas acute signs in the dog are related to hepatic damage. Toxicity is mainly seen in cats when even a small amount of acetaminophen is ingested (half of a 325 mg tablet for a 3.5 kg cat); dogs can usually tolerate dosages up to 100 mg/kg. Signs include cyanosis (which is caused by methemoglobinemia), dyspnea, facial edema (a hallmark of acetaminophen poisoning—mechanism unknown), depression, hypothermia, vomiting. Signs may progress to weakness, coma, and subsequently death. Increased ALT from hepatic damage may be seen.

Treatment Since the toxic metabolites bind preferentially with glutathione rather than cell macromolecules, supplying a glutathione precursor is an important part of treatment. *N*-Acetylcysteine provides the cysteine needed for glutathione synthesis and also increases serum sulfate levels, which supplies sulfate for conjugation. Ascorbic acid is used to change methemoglobin to reduced hemoglobin. Acetaminophen is rapidly absorbed and reaches peak blood levels within 30 to 60 minutes; emesis is performed immediately after ingestion (if possible), and a saline cathartic is given. Steroids should not be given because they have been reported to cause a dose-dependent increase in mortality. Antihistamines have been reported to be contraindicated.

Signs

Cyanosis
Dyspnea
Facial edema
Depression
Hypothermia
Vomiting
Increased ALT
Weakness
Coma
Death

EMERGENCY TREATMENT

Procedures

1. Secure the airway and ventilate as necessary (pp. 5, 9).
2. Administer supplemental oxygen (p. 7).
3. Secure venous access. Collect blood for laboratory testing. Administer fluids as needed to support blood pressure and perfusion. See p. 17.
4. Control seizures (p. 24).

Decontaminate

1. Induce emesis if safe to do so (p. 50) or perform gastric lavage (p. 52).
2. Administer activated charcoal. Repeat dose every 3 to 4 hours. *If N-acetylcysteine is to be given orally, activated charcoal administration should be delayed for 30 to 60 minutes.*
3. Administer saline or osmotic cathartics (p. 56).

Administer antidotes or other indicated supportive care

1. *N*-Acetylcysteine (Mucomyst) 280 mg/kg PO loading dose (dogs) or 140 to 240 mg/kg PO loading dose (cats), followed by 140 mg/kg PO q4h for 3 days (dogs) or 70 mg/kg q6h for 3 days of treatments (cats). Mucomyst, although not labeled for IV use, can be administered intravenously (either directly from the bottle or diluted in D_5W) by infusion through a 0.2 µm filter. The oral route is preferred because Mucomyst is rapidly absorbed from the GI tract where it enters the portal circulation. This is believed to increase the amount of drug presented to the liver, the site of utilization.
2. Administer fluids to maintain hydration and urine output.
3. Treat increased intracranial pressure if suspected (p. 29).
4. Ascorbic acid at 30 mg/kg PO, SC, or 20 mg/kg IV may be given as an attempt to convert methemoglobin to oxyhemoglobin.
5. If severe acidosis (pH <7.1, rare), sodium bicarbonate can be used (pp. 139, 372).
6. Cimetidine reduces metabolism of acetaminophen by the cytochrome P-450 system. Metabolism of acetaminophen by this system results in the production of a hepatotoxic metabolite. Therefore the administration of cimetidine is warranted.

Enhancement of elimination

Hemoperfusion has been shown to enhance elimination of acetaminophen.

Avoid

Excessive handling and stress.

Suggested Reading

Aronson LR, Drobatz KJ: Acetaminophen toxicosis in 17 cats, *J Vet Emerg Crit Care* 6(2):65-69, 1996.

Cullison R: Acetaminophen toxicosis in small animals: clinical signs, mode of action, and treatment, *Compend Cont Ed Pract Vet* 6(4):315-320, 1984.

Hjelle J: Acetaminophen-induced toxicosis in dogs and cats, *J Am Vet Med Assoc* 188(7):742-745, 1986.

Oehme F: Aspirin and acetaminophen. In Kirk RW, editor: *Current veterinary therapy,* Philadelphia, 1986, Saunders.

ACETONE

See *Organic solvents and fuels*

ACIDS AND ALKALIS

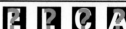

Sources   Household cleaning products, toilet bowl and drain cleaners, dishwasher detergents, cleaners, antirust compounds, alkaline batteries.

Mechanism of action   Acids produce corrosive burns, resulting in coagulation necrosis, which limits their penetration into deeper tissues. Visible lesions (necrotic eschars) are seen on mucous membranes; laryngeal spasm and edema may occur. Alkalis produce liquefaction necrosis, allowing deep tissue penetration that continues until the alkali is neutralized by the tissues.

Clinical signs   Irritation of the oral mucous membranes is prominent; ptyalism is common. Oral ulcers and burns may be present but, when absent, do not indicate a lack of esophageal involvement. Gray, yellow, or black lesions most commonly result from acids. Pain, vocalization, dysphagia, panting, laryngeal edema with upper airway obstruction, abdominal pain, hematemesis, and shock have been reported. In cases of severe injury, perforation of the esophagus or stomach (especially in the region of the pylorus) may be seen. Signs include ptyalism, pain, pneumothorax, peritonitis, pleuritis, sepsis, shock, collapse, and death.

Treatment

GENERAL

Emesis and lavage are contraindicated. Activated charcoal is ineffective. Both acids and alkalis can induce pain upon exposure to mucous membranes; this usually limits the amount of concentrated poison ingested, which minimizes esophageal injury. Diluted agents produce less pain and potentially more severe esophageal burns. Injury to the pharynx, larynx, or glottis may cause loss of airway requiring immediate endotracheal tube placement or tracheostomy tube placement.

In general, caustic substances such as acids or alkalis cause local injury, mostly to the mouth, esophagus, and stomach. The degree of oral injury does not correlate well with deeper injuries. For this reason, endoscopic examination of the esophagus and stomach is indicated in patients who have ingested a caustic substance. The procedure should be performed 12 to 24 hours after the incident based on clinical signs.

Treatment of ingestions usually is limited to administration of diluents such as water or milk. Systemic supportive measures must be instituted on a case-by-case basis. Some patients will require intensive shock therapy, whereas others may require only minimal treatment for oral burns.

Pain control is almost always indicated. Corticosteroids may minimize scar formation and thus limit the degree of stricture in cases of esophageal burns. They should be started within 48 hours of injury. Broad-spectrum antibiotics are indicated when steroid therapy is used.

ALKALI INGESTION

Emesis and lavage are contraindicated in alkali ingestion. Gastric secretions are usually sufficient to neutralize the alkali. Activated charcoal is ineffective in alkali ingestion. Since the clinical signs rarely correlate to the degree of esophageal or gastric injury, endoscopic exam should be performed in patients with alkali burns. The procedure should be delayed until the patient has been evaluated for at least 12 hours, and then the procedure should be performed carefully. The procedure should be halted at the first sign of esophageal necrosis.

Ingested alkaline batteries should be removed from the esophagus endoscopically as soon as possible to prevent perforation. If the battery is in the stomach, the probability of perforation is greatly reduced, but the battery should be retrieved in a timely manner. Consider induction of emesis, whole bowel irrigation (p. 55), or endoscopic retrieval. Serial radiographs to monitor the position of the battery are indicated.

ACID INGESTION

When acids contact mucous membranes, intense pain results. For this reason, most animals will not ingest very much. Emesis is contraindicated. The patient should be given copious quantities of diluents such as water or milk. Activated charcoal is ineffective. Supportive care is advised. With severe esophageal injury, food and water are withheld until endoscopic evidence of healing is available; the animal is maintained on parenteral food and water or with a feeding tube (as with a jejunostomy, gastrostomy).

TOPICAL EXPOSURE

Topical exposure to acids or alkalis should be treated with extensive irrigation with running water. The area should be flushed for at least 30 minutes. If the eye was exposed, it should be flushed with water or saline (strongly advise sterile saline if available) for 30 minutes.

Signs

Irritation of oral mucous membranes
Salivation
Oral ulcers or burns
Oral lesions colored gray, yellow, or black (acids)
Hematemesis
Panting, dyspnea (especially upper airway although pulmonary edema has been reported)
Pain
Vocalization
Dysphagia
Shock
Perforation of the esophagus (stomach or intestines may perforate but are less likely to do so)
Pneumothorax
Peritonitis
Pleuritis
Sepsis
Shock, collapse, and death

EMERGENCY TREATMENT

Procedures

1. Secure the airway and ventilate as necessary (pp. 5, 9).
2. Administer supplemental oxygen (p. 7).
3. Secure venous access. Collect blood and urine for laboratory testing.
4. Administer large volumes of water (preferable) or milk orally.

Decontaminate

1. GI exposure (ingestion). *Emesis and gastric lavage are contraindicated in alkali and acid injuries.* Rarely the use of gastric lavage with aluminum hydroxide at 30 to 90 mg/kg for acid injury *if esophageal injury is minimal* has been recommended.
2. Dermal exposure. Wash thoroughly with warm water (with or without soap) for a minimum of 30 minutes. Wear rubber gloves when bathing the patient; avoid inducing hypothermia.
3. Exposure of the eyes. Flush the eyes with water or sterile saline (preferable) for 30 minutes.
4. Administer crystalloid fluids to maintain blood pressure or hydration and urine output (p. 17).

Enhancement of elimination

There are no known effective techniques

Avoid

Do not give "neutralizing agents." These are usually heat-producing reactions, which may cause additional injury.

ACUTE ORGANOPHOSPHATE AND ORGANOCARBAMATE POISONING

E L C A

Sources Malathion, parathion, Diazinon, carbaryl (Sevin), bendiocarb (Ficam), propoxur (Baygon, Sendran), chlorpyrifos (Dursban), methylcarbamate, chlorfenvinphos (Dermaton Dip), cythioate (Proban), dichlorvos (Vapona), dioxathion, fenthion (ProSpot), ronnel, phosmet, disulfoton (Di-Syston), Golden Malrin (fly bait).

Mechanism of action Acetylcholine is utilized as a neurotransmitter in many nerve junctions. In the normal animal, acetylcholine is quickly inactivated by acetylcholinesterase and pseudocholinesterase. Organophosphates and organocarbamates competitively inhibit acetylcholinesterase and pseudocholinesterase allowing the continued presence of acetylcholine to maintain a constant state of nerve stimulation. Acetylcholinesterase inhibition by organophosphates tends to be irreversible; inhibition by organocarbamates tends to be reversible. Organophosphates and carbamates are readily absorbed from the skin and the GI tract and by inhalation.

Clinical signs Signs may be muscarinic, nicotinic, or generalized CNS signs; usually a combination of signs are seen. Muscarinic signs include dyspnea (caused by bronchorrhea and bronchoconstriction), excessive lacrimation, salivation, miosis, micturition (urination), and defecation. Bradycardia is often seen, but tachycardia resulting from catecholamine release may be seen. Nicotinic signs include twitching of facial muscles, tremors, generalized muscle fasciculations, and then weakness and eventually paralysis. Signs referrable to the CNS include convulsions, seizures, ataxia, and anxiety; centrally mediated respiratory depression may lead to respiratory failure and death. Depression or aggression may be seen.

Diagnosis History, exposure to toxin, and blood cholinesterase depression are useful in the diagnosis of organophosphate or organocarbamate poisoning. Blood (not plasma) cholinesterase depression of 50% of normal (or more) indicates exposure.

Depression of cholinesterase activity to less than 25% of normal are often seen in toxicities. Levels may remain depressed for several days to several weeks; some depression is normal after exposure to routine application of insecticides. Although not a definitive test, an atropine trial may be useful. Administer atropine IV at 0.02 to 0.04 mg/kg. If signs of atropinization occur (tachycardia, dry mouth, mydriasis), there is little likelihood that the pet has been poisoned by a cholinesterase inhibitor.

Treatment Atropine is antidotal for carbamates and organophosphates and relieves muscarinic signs. Nicotinic signs can be controlled with diphenhydramine hydrochloride and sedatives such as diazepam. Pralidoxime (2-PAM) will reactivate cholinesterase by freeing the active part of the alkylphosphorylated enzyme complex. 2-PAM has been reported to be of no benefit in treating carbamate toxicosis and may actually further inhibit cholinesterase; however, this report is now disputed. Most recent literature indicates that, if it is uncertain what the toxin is but signs suggest a cholinesterase inhibitor, the use of 2-PAM is indicated. If no response is seen within 3 or 4 doses, the value of the drug is minimal and it is discontinued. 2-PAM should be given early (within 24 hours) in the course of treatment to prevent "aging" of the enzyme complex. Acidosis is treated with fluid therapy and bicarbonate as needed. Emesis and gastric lavage are indicated if oral ingestion occurred (drinking the toxin or licking the toxin from the coat).

Clinical Signs

MUSCARINIC
SLUD (salivation, lacrimation, urination, defecation), vomiting, dyspnea, bradycardia

NICOTINIC
Muscle fasciculations and then weakness or paralysis, ataxia.

CNS
Convulsions, ataxia, anxiety, respiratory depression or failure, death.

NOTE: Cats that have been poisoned with chlorpyrifos often have lethargy or weakness as the only sign. Blood cholinesterase or plasma pseudocholinesterase levels may be valuable in differentiating intoxication with chlorpyrifos from other causes of lethargy and weakness in cats.

EMERGENCY TREATMENT ∎

Procedures

1. Secure the airway and ventilate as necessary (pp. 5, 9).
2. Administer supplemental oxygen (p. 7).
3. Secure venous access. Collect blood and urine for laboratory testing.
4. Administer isotonic crystalloids as needed to support blood pressure and perfusion.
5. Control seizures (p. 24).
6. Treat hyperthermia if present (p. 25).

Decontaminate

INGESTION

- Induce emesis *only* if the ingestion was within the last 60 minutes and the patient shows no clinical signs.
- Perform gastric lavage if indicated (p. 52).
- Give repeated doses of activated charcoal.
- Administer saline cathartic, if necessary. This is usually not necessary because these patients often have diarrhea already caused by the toxin. Magnesium-containing cathartics should be avoided if CNS signs are present.

DERMAL EXPOSURE

- Wash thoroughly with warm, soapy water. Wear rubber gloves when bathing the patient. Avoid induction of hypothermia.
- Oral administration of activated charcoal is indicated in dermal exposure.

Administer antidotes or other indicated supportive care

1. Atropine sulfate 0.2 to 2.0 mg/kg (give ¼ dose IV, remainder IM or SQ). *In cases of severe dyspnea associated with OP or OC toxicity, it is important to administer oxygen before administration of atropine. Failure to do so may result in tachycardia in a patient who cannot meet the demands of increased myocardial oxygen consumption.* Repeat atropine frequently in decreasing dosages (approximately half the initial dose) as needed. Although the decision to repeat has often been

based on the presence or absence of salivation or miosis, this is not appropriate. The clinical decision to repeat atropine should be based on reappearance or persistence of respiratory signs (wheezing, bronchorrhea, dyspnea). Atropine effects usually last for 4 to 6 hours. *Avoid overdosage.*

2. Pralidoxime chloride (2-PAM) 20 to 50 mg/kg IV slowly or SC q12h. Start with lower dose. If no response after 3 or 4 doses, discontinue 2-PAM therapy.

3. Diphenhydramine 1 to 4 mg/kg IM, PO q8h to relieve muscle tremors (nicotinic signs); start with lower dose when giving IM.

4. Treat acidosis as needed, preferably based on blood gases.

Enhancement of elimination

There are no known effective techniques.

Avoid

Morphine, succinylcholine, phenothiazine tranquilizers, and any drugs that decrease the respiratory drive are contraindicated. Other drugs that are contraindicated include procaine, anything with magnesium, inhaled anesthetics, depolarizing neuromuscular-blocking agents, aminoglycoside antibiotics, clindamycin, lincomycin, polymixin A and B, colistin, cimetadine, theophylline, and theophylline-ethylenediamine.

Suggested Reading

Carson T: Organophosphate and carbamate poisoning, In Kirk RW, editor: *Current veterinary therapy*, ed 9, Philadelphia, 1986, Saunders.

Fikes JD: Toxicology of selected pesticides, drugs and chemicals: organophosphorus and carbamate insecticides, *Vet Clin North Am Small Anim Pract* 20(2):353-367, 1990.

Jaggy A, Oliver JE: Chlorpyrifos toxicosis in two cats, *J Vet Intern Med* 4(3):135-139, 1990.

Miller E: Organophosphate toxicity in domestic animals—1: acute toxicity, *Vet Med Small Anim Clin* 78:482-488, 1983.

Murphy MJ: Toxin exposures in dogs and cats: pesticides and biotoxins, *J Am Vet Med Assoc* 205(3):414-421, 1994.

AMITRAZ

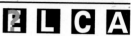

Sources   Amitraz is found in external lotions and dip used in treatment of demodectic mange. Products known to contain amitraz include Mitaban (Upjohn) and Preventic flea and tick collars. (Mitaban also contains xylene [see Organic solvents and fuels, p. 199]). Dogs and cats have been poisoned by dermal absorption after application of amitraz. Ingestion of the dip or accidental ingestion of a portion of a collar are most commonly reported as the source of poisoning.

Mechanism of action   Amitraz acts at $alpha_2$-adrenergic receptor sites in the CNS and at both $alpha_1$- and $alpha_2$-adrenergic receptor sites in the periphery.

Clinical signs   Vomiting, ataxia, staggering, and CNS depression or sedation are noted. This may progress to coma. Central $alpha_2$-stimulation results in bradycardia and hypotension. Peripheral vasoconstriction (and possibly hypotension) contribute to pallor of the mucous membranes. Gastrointestinal hypomotility, hypothermia, and hyperglycemia are often noted. Polyuria is noted within 2 to 3 hours of poisoning.   Seizures have been reported as a sign of amitraz intoxication. (It has been suggested that sedation, ataxia, and even coma may additionally be signs of xylene toxicosis if intoxication was caused by Mitaban [see Organic solvents and fuels, p. 199]).

Treatment   Treatment of amitraz poisoning is best accomplished by decontamination of the patient and administration of antidotes (yohimbine or atipamizole).

Signs

Vomiting
Ataxia, incoordination, staggering
Sedation
Gastrointestinal hypomotility
Hyperglycemia

Pallor of mucous membranes
Hypotension
Bradycardia
Polyuria
Sedation or coma
Seizures(?)

EMERGENCY TREATMENT

Procedures

1. Secure the airway and ventilate as necessary (pp. 5, 9).
2. Administer supplemental oxygen (p. 7).
3. Secure venous access. Collect blood for laboratory testing. Administer fluids as needed to support blood pressure and perfusion. (See p. 17.)
4. Control seizures if necessary (p. 24).

Decontaminate

1. Induce emesis if safe to do so (p. 50) or perform gastric lavage (p. 52). *In cases of Mitaban intoxication, induction of emesis is not advisable because of the presence of xylene, an organic solvent that is known to cause aspiration pneumonia.*
2. Administer activated charcoal. Repeat dose every 3 to 4 hours.
3. Administer saline or osmotic cathartics (p. 56).

DERMAL EXPOSURE
Wash thoroughly with warm, soapy water. Wear rubber gloves when bathing the patient; avoid chilling the patient.

Administer antidotes or other indicated supportive care

1. Alpha-adrenergic receptor antagonists are antidotal.
    *   Atipamizole administered at 50 µg/kg IM reverses signs within 10 minutes. Doses may be repeated every 3 to 4 hours if necessary.
    *   Yohimbine
        Dogs   0.11 mg/kg IV slowly
        Cats   0.5 mg/kg IV slowly

Or 50 µg/kg atipamezole given IM followed by 0.1 mg/kg yohimbine IM q6h.

2. Administer fluids to maintain hydration and urine output.

Enhancement of elimination

Because of the effective nature of the antidotes, there is no reason to consider enhanced elimination techniques.

Avoid

Avoid treating bradycardia with anticholinergic drugs such as atropine.

Suggested Reading

Duncan KL: Treatment of amitraz toxicosis, *J Am Vet Med Assoc* 203(8):1115-1116, 1993.

Hugnet C, Buronfosse F, Pineau X, et al: Toxicity and kinetics of amitraz in dogs, *Am J Vet Res* 57(10):1506-1510, 1996.

AMPHETAMINES

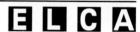

Sources   Diet pills, drugs used in the treatment of narcolepsy and hyperactivity, illegal drugs ("uppers," "speed," and "bennies"). Sustained-release preparations are available.

Mechanism of action   Amphetamines are CNS stimulants with some adrenergic properties. They are believed to stimulate the release of norepinephrine and act directly on both alpha$_1$- and beta$_1$-adrenergic receptor sites as well as inhibiting monoamine oxidase. Amphetamines are rapidly absorbed from the GI tract; high concentrations develop in the brain and CNS.

Clinical signs   Signs in amphetamine poisoning include flushing or pallor followed by restlessness, hyperactivity, tachypnea, tachycardia, tremors, hypertension or hypotension, dysrhythmias, heart block, circulatory collapse, mydriasis, hyperthermia, ptyalism, hypoglycemia, and lactic acidosis. Life-threatening toxicosis is rare because of the large margin of safety between therapeutic and lethal doses (in people) though deaths have been reported after ingestion of low dosages (1.3 mg/kg) of methamphetamine.

Treatment   Sedatives are used, and external stimuli are minimized. Fluids and perhaps steroids are used if shock develops. Urinary acidification with oral ammonium chloride will enhance renal elimination (but use only if the pet is not acidemic). Repeated doses of charcoal and cathartics are needed if sustained-release products were ingested. Chlorpromazine or haloperidol are used to combat drug-induced hyperthermia, convulsions, and hypertension. Diazepam is used for seizures; increased intracranial pressure (ICP) should be treated with furosemide and mannitol or corticosteroids (though no scientific data could be found to prove that corticosteroids improve morbidity and mortality in treatment of increased ICP). The electrocardiogram should be monitored for dysrhythmias.

Clinical findings

Flushing or pallor
Restlessness
Hyperactivity
Tachypnea
Tremors
Hypertension or hypotension
Dysrhythmias or heart block
Circulatory collapse
Mydriasis
Hyperthermia

EMERGENCY TREATMENT

Procedures

1.   Secure the airway and ventilate as necessary (pp. 5, 9).
2.   Administer supplemental oxygen (p. 7).

3. Secure venous access. Collect blood and urine for laboratory testing.
4. Control seizures (p. 24).
5. Treat hyperthermia if present (p. 25).

Decontaminate

1. Remove toxins by induction of emesis or gastric lavage if ingestion was within the last 60 minutes.
2. Administer activated charcoal. Repeat dose every 3 to 4 hours.
3. Administer saline cathartics (p. 56).

Administer antidotes or other indicated supportive care

1. Chlorpromazine at 1 to 2 mg/kg IV, IM q12h PRN or haloperidol at 1 mg/kg IV. Chlorpromazine in higher doses (10 to 18 mg/kg IV) have been reported to be beneficial in dogs that have consumed large quantities of an amphetamine.
2. Furosemide, mannitol, and corticosteroids may be indicated for treatment of increased intracranial pressure (p. 29).
3. Administer fluids to maintain hydration and urine output.

Enhancement of elimination

Amphetamines are suitable for ion trapping by urinary acidification (p. 59).

Ammonium chloride 100 to 200 mg/kg/day PO divided dose q8-12h (dog) or 20 mg/kg PO q12h (cat).

Contraindicated if rhabdomyolysis (myoglobinuria), renal failure, or acidemia is present.

Suggested Reading

Dumonceaux GA, Beasley VR: Emergency treatments for police dogs used for illicit drug detection, *J Am Vet Med Assoc* 197(2):185-187, 1990.

Kisseberth WC, Trammel HL: Illicit and abused drugs, *Vet Clin North Am Small Anim Pract* 20(2):405-418, 1990.

ANTIHISTAMINES

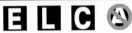

Sources Many brands of antihistamines are available as over-the-counter products, including diphenhydramine (Benadryl, Sominex, Nytol, Sleep-Eze, various cough preparations), clemastine (Tavist), brompheniramine and chlorpheniramine (Chlor-Trimeton and various cough preparations), dimenhydrinate (Dramamine), meclizine (Bonine), and cyclizine (Marezine). Prescription antihistamines include terfenadine (Seldane), hydroxyzine (Atarax, Vistaril), and loratidine (Claritin).

Mechanism of action Antihistamines block the binding of histamine to H_1-receptors of effector cells.

Clinical signs Signs of intoxication in people can include drowsiness, fatigue, nervousness, restlessness, nausea, vomiting, dry mucous membranes, epistaxis, skin eruptions, and cardiac dysrhythmias. Classic antihistamine intoxication in children causes CNS excitement; in adults, classic signs more commonly include drowsiness or possibly coma.

Antihistamines may potentiate the depressant effects of alcohol and benzodiazepines (such as diazepam). Ketaconazole, itraconazole, erythromycin, and hepatic dysfunction interfere with the metabolism of certain antihistamines, which may potentiate the toxic effects. Most cases of antihistamine intoxication in pets are mild and result in sedation and ataxia.

A case report on terfenadine toxicosis in dogs reported hyperthermia, agitation, ataxia, vomiting, premature ventricular contractions, mydriasis, and convulsions as clinical signs. Signs have been reported in dogs ingesting doses of terfenadine from 6.6 to 557 mg/kg; signs were noted within 10 minutes to 24 hours with no correlation between time of onset and dosage ingested. Even though terfenadine does not cross the blood-brain barrier at therapeutic doses (making it an ideal antihistamine), it may overwhelm the blood-brain barrier at high dosages and cause CNS signs.

Treatment Treatment is supportive and includes emesis or lavage, charcoal and cathartic administration, maximizing excretion with fluid therapy, monitoring cardiac rhythm and treating conduction disturbances as needed, and controlling seizures as needed.

Signs

Drowsiness
Fatigue
Nervousness
Ataxia
Restlessness
Nausea
Vomiting
Dry mucous membranes
Epistaxis
Skin eruptions
Cardiac dysrhythmias
Hyperthermia
Premature ventricular contractions
Mydriasis
Convulsions

EMERGENCY TREATMENT

Procedures

1. Secure the airway and ventilate as necessary (pp. 5, 9).
2. Administer supplemental oxygen (p. 7).
3. Secure venous access. Collect blood for laboratory testing. Administer fluids as needed to support blood pressure and perfusion. See p. 17.
4. Control seizures (p. 24). CAUTION: Some antihistamines potentiate the depressant effects of diazepam. Administer diazepam slowly to effect.
5. Treat hyperthermia if present (p. 25).

Decontaminate

1. Induce emesis (p. 50) or perform gastric lavage (p. 52) if exposure was by recent ingestion.
2. Administer activated charcoal. Repeat dosages are not necessary because such practice will not remove additional antihistamine.
3. Administer saline or osmotic cathartics (p. 56).

Administer antidotes or other indicated supportive care

1. There are no known effective antidotes.
2. Administer fluids to maintain hydration and urine output. Antihistamines are eliminated via the kidney; therefore urine production is imperative.
3. Treat increased intracranial pressure if suspected (from hypoventilation, hypoxemia, or hyperthermia) (p. 29).
4. Treat cardiac dysrhythmias as indicated by electrocardiographic diagnosis.
   Atropine
   Beta-blockers (such as propranolol, metoprolol)
   Lidocaine

Enhancement of elimination

There are no known effective techniques.

Suggested Reading

Merchant SR, Taboada J: Antihistaminic drugs: H_1-receptor antagonists in dogs and cats, *J Am Vet Med Assoc* 195(5):647-649, 1989.

Otto CM, Greentree WF: Terfenadine toxicosis in dogs, *J Am Vet Med Assoc* 205(7):1004-1006, 1994.

Owens JG, Dorman DC: Drug poisoning in small animals, *Vet Med* 92(2):149-156, 1997.

Papich M: Toxicoses from over-the-counter human drugs, *Vet Clin North Am Small Anim Pract* 20(2): 431-451, 1990.

ANTITUSSIVES

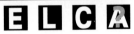

Sources   The most common antitussive available in over-the-counter preparations (in the United States) is dextromethorphan. Codeine may be found in OTC preparations sold in Canada and other countries.

Mechanism of action   Dextromethorphan has a structure similar to the opioids. Its antitussive action is mediated by receptors in the medullary cough center, which are distinct from the mu and kappa opioid receptors.

Signs   Sedation is probably the only sign of dextromethorphan ingestion. Poisoning by overdosing dextromethorphan is unlikely. Codeine may cause sedation, miosis, and respiratory depression.

EMERGENCY TREATMENT

Treatment is usually not necessary for ingestion of dextromethorphan or codeine. In the case of profound signs after ingestion of an OTC cold or allergy preparation, it is much more likely that the signs are related to one or more of the other compounds in the product.

- Activated charcoal may be useful in speeding elimination from the body.
- Codeine may be antagonized by administration of naloxone.

Suggested Reading

Owens JG, Dorman DC: Drug poisoning in small animals, *Vet Med* 92(2):149-156, 1997.

Papich MG: Toxicoses from over-the-counter human drugs, *Vet Clin North Am Small Anim Pract* 20(2):431-451, 1990.

ARSENIC

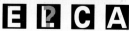

Sources   Arsenic and arsenates are found in nature (pyrites and sulfides) and are common ingredients in herbicides, defoliants, insecticides, ant baits, and rodent baits. They may be found in insulation and some forms of vermiculite or may be a by-product of metal ore refining. Several forms of arsenic are used as wood preservatives. The ashes of treated wood may remain toxic.

Mechanism of action   Soluble forms of arsenic are readily absorbed through skin, mucous membranes, and the respiratory system and from the gastrointestinal tract. Toxicity is influenced by the route of exposure, rate of absorption, metabolic rate and excretion rate, and most important the type of arsenical present. Arsenic may be present as the trivalent form (arsenite) or the pentavalent form (arsenate). Trivalent forms are 4 to 10 times more toxic than the pentavalent form. The mechanism of action of the trivalent form is believed to be its ability to disrupt cellular respiration by binding to sulfhydryl groups on several important enzymes. Vasodilatation and loss of capillary integrity result in fluid losses and hypovolemia. This occurs in all tissues rich in oxidative enzymes (such as lungs, kidney, liver) but is most pronounced in the gastrointestinal tract. The mechanism of action of the pentavalent forms has not been fully elucidated but may involve interference with vitamin B_1 and B_6 metabolism.

Clinical findings

ACUTE
Acute onset of gastroenteritis with severe abdominal pain
Staggering, weakness, and perhaps tremors
Salivation, vomiting
Odontoprisis
Diarrhea, perhaps bloody
Possible hematuria
Shock, thready pulses
Oliguria, dehydration
Death in hours to 2 or 3 days

SUBACUTE
Depression, anorexia
Watery diarrhea, which may contain blood and shreds or
    pieces of intestinal mucosa
Polydipsia with polyuria initially followed by anuria
Dehydration
Possible hematuria
Rear limb weakness, paresis, paralysis
Seizures may occur
Death in 4 or 5 days

CHRONIC

Rarely diagnosed in veterinary medicine

Lackluster appearance with rough, dry hair coat

Skin may become paper thin and crack, secondary pyo-
derma

If respiratory system is affected, the animal may have
tachypnea and dyspnea, especially when excited.

Brick red oral mucous membranes may be seen.

Polydipsia

Laboratory findings

- Results of biochemical profiles will reveal the systems involved, but results are nonspecific.
- Commonly see evidence of dehydration with hemoconcentration.
- Specific tests would be indicated for the diagnosis of arsenic poisoning.
- Liver, kidney, stomach, and intestinal contents may be analyzed for arsenic. Urine may also be analyzed for presence
of arsenicals.

EMERGENCY TREATMENT

Procedures

Stabilize the patient:

1. Secure the airway and ventilate if necessary (pp. 5, 9).
2. Administer crystalloid fluids to treat hypovolemia and
shock and to maintain hydration (p. 17).
3. Monitor and treat electrolyte imbalances caused by diarrhea.
4. Monitor blood gases (venous blood gas determination
will be appropriate if the patient has no respiratory
signs) and treat acidemia with sodium bicarbonate as
needed. See p. 139 or 372.

Decontaminate

1. If ingested within the last 1 to 2 hours and no other contraindications exist, induce vomiting (p. 50).

2. If contraindication to emesis exists and the exposure has been within the last 2 to 4 hours, gastric lavage is indicated. If signs are pronounced, there is a relative contraindication to performing a gastric lavage because of increased likelihood of perforation.

3. Gastric lavage should be followed by administration of activated charcoal. Cathartics are not indicated because diarrhea usually results from poisoning.

4. Dermal exposure may require that the offending substance be brushed or vacuumed off or removed by bathing. Care must be taken to avoid contamination and exposure of the caregivers to the offending substance. (See Cautions on p. 48.) Masks, face shields, and other precautions are advisable.

Administer antidotes or other indicated supportive care

1. Administer dimercaprol (BAL) 3 to 4 mg/kg IM q8h until recovery. In severe exposures, dose may be increased to 6 to 7 mg/kg IM q8h on the first day.

2. A new chelator that is more effective than dimercaprol has recently been used in children. Succimer (*meso*-dimercaptosuccinic acid, also listed as DMSA) is available as Chemet (from McNeil Consumer Products, a division of McNeil-PPC, Inc., Fort Washington, PA 19034). This chelator has shown promise in the treatment of heavy metal toxicosis in children and adults. It is known to have greater specificity for arsenic and lead than calcium EDTA or penicillamine. Studies have shown succimer to be effective in treating lead poisoning in dogs. The dose used in the study was 10 mg/kg PO every 8 hours for 10 days. It has a wide margin of safety.

3. Administer acetylcysteine. A study of the toxicity of sodium arsenite in rats showed that administration of acetylcysteine reduced the toxicity. It has the advantage that it can be administered IV for acute arsenic poisoning.
   DOSE:
Cat	140 to 240 mg/kg PO; then 70 mg/kg PO q6h for 3 days
Dog	280 mg/kg PO loading dose; then 140 mg/kg PO q4h for 3 days

   Acetylcysteine may be given intravenously if the patient is vomiting. It is recommended that the solution be administered at the *lower dose, diluted with D_5W, and given through a 0.2 μm filter over 15 to 30 minutes.*

4. Blood (whole blood, packed red blood cells, plasma) may be necessary.
5. Dopamine may be required to support blood pressure or urine production.
6. B vitamins in the fluids have been recommended.

Suggested Reading

Murphy MJ: Toxin exposures in dogs and cats: pesticides and biotoxins, *J Am Vet Med Assoc* 205(3):414-421, 1994.

Ramsey DT, Casteel SW, Fagella AM, et al: Use of orally administered succimer (*meso*-2,3-dimercaptosuccinic acid) for treatment of lead poisoning in dogs, *J Am Vet Med Assoc* 208(3):371-375, 1996.

ASPIRIN (ACETYLSALICYLIC ACID, SALICYLATE)

E L C A

Sources Many analgesic, antiinflammatory, antipyretic, and antidiarrheal (Pepto-Bismol) agents that contain salicylates are sold as OTC preparations. Some keratolytic products contain salicylates.

Mechanism of action Acetylsalicylic acid inhibits cyclooxygenase, which then inhibits production of certain prostaglandins, including protective prostaglandins of the E series. High levels are known to directly stimulate the respiratory center (early) to cause an initial respiratory alkalosis. High doses are also known to uncouple oxidative phosphorylation and may cause hyperglycemia and glycosuria.

Clinical signs The biologic half-life of aspirin is 7.5 to 8 hours in dogs and 38 to 45 hours in cats at a dose of 25 mg/kg/day. The toxic dose in cats is >25 mg/kg/day in cats and >50 mg/kg/day in dogs. Signs are noted within 4 to 6 hours after ingestion of a toxic dose and include depression, vomiting, anorexia and lethargy, tachypnea (caused by initial respiratory alkalosis), and hyperthermia. The vomitus may be blood-tinged from GI ulceration. CNS depression leads to muscle weakness and ataxia; coma and death can occur within 1 or more days. Gastrointestinal ulceration or perforation may be seen after the administration of repeated doses over several days' duration. Anemia, bone marrow depression, Heinz body formation (cats), and toxic hepatitis may occur.

Toxic signs may be seen at doses of Pepto-Bismol >7 mL/kg/day in dogs and cats. Two tablespoons of Pepto-Bismol contain the salicylate equivalent of one 5-grain aspirin tablet.

Treatment   There is no specific antidote. The stomach should be emptied by induction of emesis or lavage if within <2 hours of ingestion though there are literature reports that gastric evacuation may be of value up to 12 hours after ingestion of enteric-coated aspirin preparations. Multiple-dose activated charcoal is warranted. Acid-base balance is corrected as needed; diuresis is instituted. Alkalinization of the urine with sodium bicarbonate can be done to hasten urinary excretion, though this requires intense monitoring and is difficult to achieve safely. Peritoneal dialysis allows direct removal of salicylic acid from serum. Gastric ulceration or perforation is treated as needed.

Clinical findings

Depression
Vomiting (possibly blood tinged)
Anorexia or lethargy
Tachypnea
Pulmonary edema (infrequent)
Hyperthermia or hypothermia (late)
Anemia
Bone marrow depression
Heinz body formation (cats)
Toxic hepatitis
Muscle weakness
Ataxia

Seizures
Cerebral edema
Coma
Death

Laboratory findings

Hyperglycemia or hypoglycemia are possible.
Respiratory alkalemia with metabolic acidosis early. Metabolic
   acidemia later.
Electrolyte abnormalities are common
   Wide anion gap acidosis
   Hypokalemia
   Hypernatremia
Increased bleeding time
Anemia, possibly with Heinz body formation
Increased liver enzyme levels
   Alkaline phosphatase (ALK-P)
   AST
   ALT
   GGT

EMERGENCY TREATMENT

Procedures

1.   Secure the airway and ventilate as necessary (pp. 5, 9).
2.   Administer supplemental oxygen (p. 7).
3.   Secure venous access. Collect blood for laboratory
     testing. Administer fluids as needed to support blood
     pressure and perfusion. See p. 17.
4.   Control seizures (p. 24).
5.   Treat hyperthermia if present (p. 25).
6.   Treat pulmonary edema (p. 11).

Decontaminate

1.   Induce emesis (p. 50) or perform gastric lavage (p. 52).
2.   Administer activated charcoal. Repeat dose every 3 to 4
     hours.

3. Administer saline or osmotic cathartics (p. 56). Enemas may also be indicated.

Administer antidotes or other indicated supportive care

1. There are no known antidotes.
2. Administer fluids carefully to initiate brisk diuresis. Closely observe for onset of pulmonary edema.
   a. Furosemide
   b. Dopamine drip (1 to 3 µg/kg/min)
   c. Mannitol is not usually recommended.
3. Treat increased intracranial pressure if suspected (p. 29).
4. Correct acid-base and electrolyte imbalances.
   a. Sodium bicarbonate should be administered to combat metabolic acidemia as well as induce renal elimination of salicylates. Blood gases and urine pH should be monitored carefully to guide dosage and avoid complications caused by therapy. When blood gases are not available, sodium bicarbonate may be administered at 1 to 2 mEq/kg IV very slowly.
   b. Hypokalemia must be corrected because potassium depletion inhibits alkalinization of the urine.
5. Optional glucose
6. Protect the GI tract:
   a. Administer sucralfate at 250 to 1000 mg for dog q6-8h PO and 250 mg for cat q6-12h PO.
   b. Administer misoprostol (Cytotec) at 1 to 5 µg/kg q8-12h PO (dog only) for ulcer prophylaxis.
   c. Administer omeprazole at 0.7 mg/kg q24h PO for dog only. H_2-receptor antagonists have *not* been shown to be of benefit as a prophylactic therapy against NSAID-induced GI ulcers. Their use in aspirin intoxication is also questionable.

Enhancement of elimination

1. Urinary alkalinization enhances urinary excretion (p. 60).
2. Hemodialysis is effective.
3. Hemoperfusion.
4. Peritoneal dialysis is effective.

Suggested Reading

Murphy MJ: Toxin exposures in dogs and cats: drugs and household products, *J Am Vet Med Assoc* 205(4):557-560, 1994.

Oehme F: Aspirin and acetaminophen. In Kirk RW, editor: *Current veterinary therapy*, ed 9, Philadelphia, 1986, Saunders.

BARBITURATES

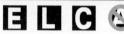

Sources   Sleeping pills, anticonvulsants, tissues of animals that were euthanatized, and illicit drugs.

Mechanism of action   Barbiturates are known to cause global depression of neuronal activity in the brain. These effects are apparently mediated through enhancement of gamma-aminobutyric acid (GABA)–mediated synaptic inhibition (by opening membrane chloride channels). Barbiturates do not act directly on the chloride channel or GABA receptors but affect an allosteric site that prolongs the increase in chloride-channel conductance and facilitates GABA action. Different mechanisms of action may be seen in different areas of the CNS by different doses of different barbiturates.

Clinical findings

SEVERE INTOXICATIONS
- Coma, anesthesia
- Hypothermia
- Miosis or mydriasis
- Respiratory depression, hypoxemia, hypercapnia, respiratory acidosis
- Hypotension, reflex tachycardia
- Depression of cardiac contractility
- Splenomegaly
- Death

MODERATE INTOXICATIONS

- Hypothermia
- Ataxia
- Lethargy
- Sleepiness
- Nystagmus may be seen
- Splenomegaly
- Possible hypotension
- Possible hypothermia

Laboratory findings

Barbiturates are easily detected with routine toxicologic screens.

EMERGENCY TREATMENT

- Support the patient.
- Secure the airway and ventilate the patient if necessary.
- Treat coma (p. 29), hypotension (p. 17), and hypothermia (p. 30) if they exist.

Decontamination

- Induce emesis *only* if the ingestion was within the last 60 minutes and the patient shows no clinical signs.
- Perform gastric lavage if the ingestion was within the last 2 to 4 hours.
- Give repeated doses of activated charcoal.
- Administer saline cathartic. Magnesium-containing solutions should be avoided.
- Consider whole bowel irrigation using CoLyte or GoLYTELY.

Enhanced elimination

- Alkalinization of the urine (p. 60) has been shown to increase the elimination of phenobarbital but none of the other barbiturates. Its value in acute overdose has not been proved, and it may contribute to fluid overload and pulmonary edema.

- Hemoperfusion (p. 60) is indicated for the severely over-dosed patient.

Avoid

- Lactate, glucose, and epinephrine if used improperly (at very high doses) may cause prolonged effects of some of the barbiturates. If these solutions are used properly, there is no clinical significance.
- Chloramphenicol will potentiate the effects of many of the barbiturates and is contraindicated.

Suggested reading

Dayrell-Hart B, Steinberg SA, VanWinkle TJ, Farnbach GC: Hepatotoxicity of phenobarbital in dogs: 18 cases (1985-1989), *J Am Vet Assoc* 199(8):1060-1066, 1991.

Dumonceaux GA, Beasley VR: Emergency treatments for police dogs used for illicit drug detection, *J Am Vet Assoc* 197(2):185-187, 1990.

Owens JG, Dorman DC: Drug poisoning in small animals, *Vet Med* 92(2):149-156, 1997.

BATTERIES

See *Acids and alkalis*

BENZENE

See *Organic solvents and fuels*

BENZOL

See *Organic solvents and fuels*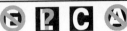

BIRTH CONTROL PILLS

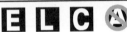

Uses   Birth control, treatment of endometriosis.

Common products   Many brands.

Mechanism of action: Except for high-dose estrogen pills, or pills containing iron, acute ingestion probably is of little consequence.

Clinical signs   Usually none. With iron toxicity, see p. 158.

EMERGENCY TREATMENT

Procedures

Usually none required. If signs are severe, consider other toxicity.

Decontaminate

- Induce emesis if the ingestion was within the last 60 minutes and the patient shows no clinical signs.
- Perform gastric lavage if the ingestion was within the last 2 to 4 hours.
- Give activated charcoal.
- Administer saline cathartic.
- Consider whole bowel irrigation using CoLyte or GoLYTELY.

Administer antidotes or other indicated supportive care

There are no specific antidotes.

BLEACHES

Sources   Household laundry bleaches most commonly contain sodium hypochlorite at concentrations of 3% to 6%. Industrial-strength bleaches and swimming pool supplies may contain 50% sodium hypochlorite. Other common ingredients in (nonchlorine or colorfast) bleaches include trichloroisocyanuric acid and sodium perborate.

Mechanism of action   Sodium hypochlorite is corrosive and usually has local effects on the mucous membranes and esophageal tissues. Animals rarely ingest enough bleach to cause systemic signs. Further, ingestion of a bleach solution usually results in vomiting, limiting the quantity of toxic principal absorbed. The hypochlorite bleaches are alkaline, and tissues exposed to it will suffer alkali burns. Trichloroisocyanuric acid is corrosive but of low toxicity. Sodium perborate degrades to hydrogen peroxide (which may cause gastritis and emesis) and borate (which may cause systemic signs of boric acid poisoning, p. 99).

Clinical signs   Most pets have a "bleach" odor and may show bleaching of the hair. Ptyalism, emesis, and rebound tenderness of the cranial side of the abdomen may occur. Hematemesis and pharyngeal edema may be seen.

Treatment   Although induction of emesis within 3 hours of ingestion has been recommended by at least one reference, we advise against this. Bleaches are alkalis, and the rules of alkali exposure should be followed (pp. 70 to 72). Although most patients will vomit within minutes after ingestion of common bleaches, vomiting should not be the goal of the veterinarian presented with a case of bleach ingestion. Current advice for ingestion of bleaches includes administering large volumes of water or milk.

Past recommendations included administering milk of magnesia, egg whites, or powdered milk slurry. Baking soda (sodium bicarbonate) causes carbon dioxide formation and gastric distension as well as formation of hypochlorous acid and should not be given.

Signs

Bleach odor
Bleaching of hair
Salivation
Emesis, hematemesis
Rebound tenderness of cranial abdomen
Pharyngeal edema

EMERGENCY TREATMENT

Procedures

1. Secure the airway and ventilate as necessary (pp. 5, 9).
2. Administer supplemental oxygen (p. 7).
3. Secure venous access. Collect blood and urine for laboratory testing.
4. Administer large volumes of water or milk.
5. Administer analgesics.
6. Administer antidotes.
   a. There are no known antidotes.
   b. Milk of magnesia has been recommended at 2 to 3 mL/kg PO.

Decontaminate

GI EXPOSURE (INGESTION)
   See step 4 above.

DERMAL EXPOSURE
   Wash thoroughly with warm, soapy water. Wear rubber gloves when bathing the patient. Avoid chilling the patient.

Enhancement of elimination

Administer fluids to maintain blood pressure or hydration and urine output (p. 17).

BORATES/BORON

Sources Borates and boric acid are contained in many products including roach killers, flea products, fertilizers, herbicides, antiseptics, disinfectants, and contact lens solutions. Sodium perborate is found in mouthwashes and denture cleansers. Other boron-containing compounds include sodium borate, sodium biborate, sodium pyroborate, sodium tetraborate, boric anhydride, boron oxide, boron trioxide, boric oxide, boron sesquioxide, borax, sodium metaborate, and magnesium perborate.

Mechanism of action The lethal oral dose for boric acid for small mammals is 0.20 to 0.50 g/kg of body weight. Emesis usually occurs only after substantial amounts of borate have been ingested. Borates are readily absorbed from the GI tract. They are absorbed through abraded skin, but do not easily penetrate intact skin. Borates are excreted in the urine, with 40% to 60% of the dose excreted within 12 to 24 hours. Blood concentrations of borate above 50 µg/mL are diagnostic for borate poisoning. The exact mechanism of action is not understood. Borates are generally cytotoxic to all cells. Because borates are concentrated by the kidney and excreted in the urine, the kidneys are often damaged more than other systems. The brain and liver are also known to be damaged by borates.

Clinical signs Signs include ptyalism, diarrhea, abdominal pain, rebound cranial abdominal tenderness, ataxia, hyperesthesia, tremors, muscle weakness, metabolic acidosis, seizures, coma, and death. Mild hyperthermia, shock, disseminated intravascular coagulation, and Cheyne-Stokes respiration occur.

Treatment Emesis or gastric lavage should be induced if ingestion occurred within 2 hours. Although borates are poorly adsorbed by activated charcoal, it is commonly recommended (in addition to adminstration of a cathartic). To be effective in removing borates from a patient, activated charcoal would have to be administered in dosages 5 to 10 times normal recommendations. The authors find this clinically impractical. The use of activated charcoal in patients known to have ingested borates is therefore not recommended. Persistent vomiting and seizures are controlled as needed. Hemodialysis is known to be effective in humans and should be considered in pets.

Signs

Salivation
Diarrhea, possibly bloody
Abdominal pain
Rebound cranial abdominal tenderness
Ataxia
Hyperesthesia
Tremors
Muscle weakness
Seizures
Coma
Mild hyperthermia
Shock
Disseminated intravascular coagulation
Cheyne-Stokes respiration
Death

EMERGENCY TREATMENT

Procedures

1. Secure the airway and ventilate as necessary (pp. 5, 9).
2. Administer supplemental oxygen (p. 7).
3. Secure venous access. Collect blood and urine for laboratory testing.
4. Control seizures (p. 24).
5. Treat hyperthermia if present (p. 25).
6. Administer crystalloids fluids to maintain perfusion and blood pressure (p. 17).

Decontaminate

GI EXPOSURE (INGESTION)
- Induce emesis if recent ingestion and if signs are not present (p. 50).

- Gastric lavage if signs are present after ingestion (p. 52).
- Administer saline cathartic unless diarrhea already present.

DERMAL EXPOSURE
Wash thoroughly with warm, soapy water. Wear rubber gloves when bathing the patient; avoid chilling the patient.

Administer antidotes and other supportive care

Induce a brisk diuresis
- Administer fluids at 2 or 3 times maintenance dose. Monitor for signs of overhydration.
- Administer furosemide if the patient has normal renal function and is adequately hydrated.

Enhancement of elimination

Hemodialysis is effective. Peritoneal dialysis. Exchange transfusions.

BOTULISM

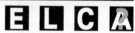

Source   The botulinus toxins are produced by strains of *Clostridium botulinum,* which are often found in garbage, especially decaying animal carcasses. Seven serotypes have been identified. Although these toxins are serotypically different, they act similarly.

Mechanism of action   The toxins bind to receptors in nerve terminals where they inhibit release of acetylcholine resulting in cessation of all cholinergic transmission.

Clinical signs   Signs of botulism are seen 24 to 48 hours after ingestion of food contaminated with botulinus toxin. These signs are usually attributable to type C toxin in the dog. Signs include a generalized weakness followed by ascending paresis progressing to flaccid paralysis (lower motor neuron signs). There is often mydriasis, slow pupillary responses, and decreased palpebral response (often resulting in dry eyes). There is often poor jaw tone and dysphagia. Failure to swallow saliva may give the impression of hypersalivation. Vomiting or regurgitation and generalized weakness (and rarely megaesophagus) may result in aspiration pneumonia. Death as a result of respiratory paralysis is possible.

Differential diagnosis includes tick paralysis, polyradiculoneuritis, coral snake envenomation (p. 115), drug intoxication, rabies, bromethalin poisoning (p. 103), and myasthenia gravis.

EMERGENCY TREATMENT

Procedures

1. Secure the airway and ventilate as necessary (pp. 5, 9).
2. Administer supplemental oxygen (p. 7).
3. Secure venous access. Collect blood and urine for laboratory testing if desired.

Decontamination

If a patient has recently eaten contaminated food, emesis, gastric lavage, and activated charcoal administration may be beneficial.

Administer antidotes or other supportive care

1. Botulism antitoxin is available and has been recommended by various authors. However, since most pets will recover with good nursing care and the use of the antitoxin is controversial, we do not currently recommend its use.
2. Penicillin G (20,000 units/kg IM q12h), metronidazole (10 mg/kg PO q12h), or amoxicillin (10 to 20 mg/kg IM, SC, PO q8-12h). *Avoid aminoglycosides because of possible augmentation of neuromuscular blockade.*
3. Physostigmine may help to increase neuromuscular function by inhibiting acetylcholinesterase. (This treatment regimen is risky and should be used only in cases where death is imminent.) Atropine is indicated as needed to reduce the muscarinic effects caused by administration of physostigmine or neostigmine.
4. Administer fluids by IV or enteral route to support hydration.

5. Nutritional needs must be attended to using the parenteral or enteral (preferred) route.
6. Deep bedding, water beds, physical therapy, and frequent turning of the patient may help to avoid decubitus ulcer formation. *Recovery may take several weeks.*

Sources Rodenticides including brand names such as Vengeance, Assault, and Trounce.

BROMETHALIN

  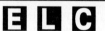

Mechanism of action Bromethalin is a potent diphenylamine neurotoxin that acts by uncoupling oxidative phosphorylation leading to decreased Na^+/K^+-ATPase activity. Without normal Na^+/K^+-ATPase activity, the ability to maintain normal cellular membrane potential and osmotic gradient is lost. Sodium flows into the cell following its electrochemical gradient, and fluid follows resulting in swelling and loss of function. Signs are related to CNS dysfunction. Death is usually caused by respiratory paralysis.

Clinical signs

Clinical signs are extremely variable depending on amount of toxin ingested. High doses may result in onset of signs within hours, whereas lower doses may not have noticeable effects for several days. High doses in dogs have produced signs of hyperexcitability, tremors, hyperreflexia of the hindlimbs, running fits, focal or generalized seizures, and death. Low doses produced depression, anorexia, vomiting, tremors, paresis (of one or more limbs), paralysis, and death. Animals poisoned with bromethalin have been noted to assume Schiff-Sherington posture or to have extensor rigidity. Miosis and anisocoria have been noted. Cats have similar signs including depression, ataxia, progressive motor dysfunction to paralysis, abdominal swelling, convulsions, and death. Death is seen with low doses as well as with high doses.

Bromethalin poisoning should be suspected whenever acute signs of cerebral edema or posterior paresis or paralysis are seen. Differential diagnosis includes alcohol intoxication, ethylene glycol intoxication, salt poisoning, rabies, polyradiculoneuritis, tick paralysis, and botulism.

Treatment   Mainly supportive because no antidote exists. Treatment is aimed at decreasing absorption of the toxin and decreasing cerebral edema. Fluids should be used carefully to prevent aggravation of the cerebral edema. Mannitol and corticosteroids may be ineffective in treating bromethalin toxicity though they are currently recommended in reducing cerebral edema from other causes. Activated charcoal improves survivability when given early.

Signs

ACUTE EXPOSURE
Hyperexcitability
Severe muscle tremors
Running fits
Grand mal seizures
Hindlimb hyperreflexia
Depression
Death

CHRONIC EXPOSURE
Tremors
Depression
Ataxia
Vomiting
Lateral recumbency

EMERGENCY TREATMENT

Procedures

1. Secure the airway and ventilate as necessary (pp. 5, 9).
2. Administer supplemental oxygen (p. 7).
3. Secure venous access. Collect blood and urine for laboratory testing.
4. Administer isotonic crystalloids as needed to support blood pressure and perfusion.
5. Control seizures (p. 24).
6. Treat hyperthermia if present (p. 25).

Decontaminate

- Induce emesis *only* if the ingestion was within the last 60 minutes and the patient shows no clinical signs.
- Perform gastric lavage if the ingestion was within the last 2 to 4 hours.
- Give repeated doses of activated charcoal.
- Administer saline cathartic. Magnesium-containing solutions should be avoided.
- Consider whole bowel irrigation using CoLyte or GoLYTELY.

Administer antidotes or other indicated supportive care

There are no known antidotes.
Treat cerebral edema. (Treatment may not be effective in cases of edema known to be caused by bromethalin.)

1. Furosemide
2. Mannitol administered at 0.1 to 0.5 g/kg IV slowly q1-6h PRN
3. Methylprednisolone sodium succinate at 25 to 30 mg/kg IV initially followed by 12.5 to 15 mg/kg IV at 2 and 6 hours later and then 2.5 mg/kg/hour IV continuous infusion for 8 to 42 hours.
4. Dexamethasone sodium phosphate at 2 to 3 mg/kg IV followed by 1 mg/kg SC q6-8h in doses tapering off.

Enhancement of elimination

There are no reported techniques (other than repeated doses of activated charcoal) that are effective in enhancing the elimination of bromethalin from the body.

Avoid Drugs that might induce hypoventilation (such as high doses of narcotics or tranquilizers).

Suggested Reading

Carson T: Bromethalin poisoning. In Kirk RW, Bonagura JD, editors: *Current veterinary therapy*, ed 10, Philadelphia, 1989, Saunders.

Osweiler GD: *Toxicology*, Philadelphia, 1996, Williams & Wilkins, pp 286-288.

BUILDERS

See also *Detergents, Soaps*

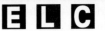

Mechanism of action Builders, which bind elements in detergents and are responsible for water hardness, act by inflicting caustic burns and inducing hypocalcemia by binding calcium (oxalates). Common compounds in descending order of toxicity include metasilicate, sodium carbonate or sesquicarbonate, polyphosphates, silicates, and bicarbonates.

Clinical signs Similar to acids in causing highly corrosive coagulation necrosis. Hypocalcemia may also be seen.

Treatment Treatment is aimed at flushing the mucous membranes and other exposed areas with copious amounts of water. Calcium and diuresis with intravenous fluids and furosemide may be needed in oxalate ingestions.

Signs

Highly corrosive coagulation necrosis
Hypocalcemia

EMERGENCY TREATMENT

Procedures

1. Secure the airway and ventilate as necessary (pp. 5, 9).
2. Administer supplemental oxygen (p. 7).
3. Secure venous access. Collect blood for laboratory testing. Administer fluids as needed to support blood pressure and perfusion. See p. 17.
4. Treat hyperthermia if present (p. 25).

Decontaminate

1. Induce emesis (p. 50) or perform gastric lavage (p. 52) if exposure was by ingestion.

2. Administer activated charcoal. Repeat dose every 3 to 4 hours.
3. Administer saline or osmotic cathartics (p. 56). Enemas may also be indicated.

Administer antidotes or other indicated supportive care

1. Pulverized chalk, slurry of powdered milk (100 mL PO), lime water (150 to 200 mL) may be given orally to precipitate oxalates in the GI tract.
2. If signs of hypocalcemia are present, administer calcium gluconate 0.25 to 1.5 mL/kg IV slowly over 20 to 30 minutes observing for bradycardia to effect if serum calcium decreases.
3. Osmotic diuresis with mannitol 20% at 0.1 to 0.5 g/kg IV q1-6h PRN or furosemide at 1 to 5 mg/kg IV PRN q1-4h. CAUTION: *Furosemide may promote calciuresis, thus enhancing hypocalcemia.*

Enhancement of elimination

There are no known effective techniques.

CARBON MONOXIDE

Sources   Combustion, fires, patients suffering smoke inhalation, vehicles (automobiles, airplanes) with faulty exhaust systems, improperly vented heaters.

Mechanism of action   Carbon monoxide has an affinity for hemoglobin that is 240 times greater than that of oxygen. When carbon monoxide is combined with hemoglobin, it is known as carboxyhemoglobin. Carboxyhemoglobin causes a leftward shift of the oxygen dissociation curve; that is, the oxygen is bound more tightly and is not released to the tissues so readily.

Clinical findings   The most characteristic finding in the patient suffering carbon monoxide poisoning is cherry red blood (similar to cyanide) and red or dark pink mucous membranes, skin, and other tissues. Blood gases may reveal hypoxemia or acidosis; however they do not reveal the presence or absence of carbon monoxide. Blood gas measurements are for the most part unaffected by the presence of carboxyhemoglobin. Oxygen saturation levels are falsely normal when determined by pulse oximetry because carboxyhemoglobin is "invisible" to this technologic method. Carboxyhemoglobin may be detected using direct oximetry or co-oximetry, technologic methods not widely available in veterinary medicine.

Signs

Signs noted depend on the level of carboxyhemoglogin. Carboxyhemoglobin levels of 10% or higher will cause confusion and dyspnea. Additional signs include ataxia, lethargy, deafness, seizures, psychomotor disturbances, and coma. Levels >60% (or sometimes less) are fatal.
- Tachypnea, dyspnea, hyperpnea
- Signs of shock
- Bright red mucous membranes
- Collapse
- Hypoxemia-induced mentation changes including confusion, dizziness (staggering), seizures, and coma.
- Agonal respirations followed by respiratory paralysis. Cyanosis may be noticed soon after onset of hypoventilation.
- Classic finding is the cherry red blood.

EMERGENCY TREATMENT

Procedures

1. Secure the airway and ventilate as necessary (pp. 5, 9).
2. Administer supplemental oxygen (p. 7). Administer 80% to 100% oxygen for at least 30 minutes. The half-life of carboxyhemoglobin approaches 300 minutes in room air but is decreased to about 30 minutes in 100% oxygen.
3. Secure venous access. Collect blood for laboratory testing. Administer fluids as needed to support blood pressure and perfusion. See p. 17.
4. Control seizures (see p. 24).

Decontaminate

Remove the patient from the source of carbon monoxide.

Administer antidotes or other indicated supportive care

There are no known effective antidotes.

Enhancement of elimination

There are no known effective techniques other than administration of high levels of oxygen.

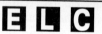

CHOCOLATE (THEOBROMINE) AND CAFFEINE POISONING

Sources Cooking, baking, candy, landscaping (with cacao shells), white chocolate (negligible amounts of theobromine), sweetened milk chocolate ($^1/_{10}$ the amount of theobromine as found in unsweetened chocolate, approximately 45 to 60 mg/oz), semisweet or dark chocolate contains 130 to 185 mg/oz. Unsweetened (baking) chocolate (450 mg/oz), cocoa powder (150 to 600 mg/oz); coffee, tea, soft drinks.

Mechanism of action Theobromine inhibits phosphodiesterase, which results in increased cAMP and release of catecholamines. Caffeine directly stimulates the myocardium and central nervous system. It also causes a competitive antagonism of cellular adenosine receptors. Increased muscle contractility is caused by increased entry of calcium and inhibition of sequestration by the sarcoplasmic reticulum (mechanism unknown). Benzodiazepine receptors in the brain are competitively antagonized.

Clinical signs

THEOBROMINE

A slight increase in blood pressure is seen. Bradycardia or more commonly tachycardia occurs, and myocardial dysrhythmias, especially ventricular premature beats, are possible. Central nervous system excitability, manifested as nervousness, excitement, tremors, seizures, and ultimately coma, are seen. Panting and urinary incontinence are also possible. Death occurs within 6 to 24 hours with acute exposure. With chronic ingestion (over several days), death may result from cardiac failure.

CAFFEINE

Tachycardia, tachypnea, hyperexcitability, tremors, seizures, premature ventricular beats. Dilatation of coronary, pulmonary, and systemic vessels may cause congestion or hemorrhage. The lethal dose for caffeine is 150 mg/kg for dogs, cats, and people.

Treatment No antidote exists; treatment is supportive. Emesis is used and may be effective even after several (4 to 6) hours have passed since ingestion; gastric lavage is useful if emesis is only partially productive or contraindicated. Activated charcoal is useful and can significantly decrease the half-life of theobromine. Diazepam is used to control tremors, anxiety, or seizures. Bradycardia is treated with atropine; tachycardias are treated with lidocaine, metoprolol, or propranolol. The urinary bladder should be catheterized to prevent reabsorption of theobromine through bladder mucosa. Fluids are given as part of supportive treatment.

Signs

THEOBROMINE

Mild hypertension
Bradycardia or tachycardia
Dysrhythmias (especially PVCs)
Nervousness
Excitement
Tremors
Seizures
Panting
Urinary incontinence

Coma
Death

CAFFEINE
Tachycardia
Tachypnea
Hyperexcitability
Tremors
Seizures
Dysrhythmias (especially PVCs)
Generalized congestion or hemorrhage.

EMERGENCY TREATMENT

Procedures

1. Secure the airway and ventilate as necessary (pp. 5, 9).
2. Administer supplemental oxygen (p. 7).
3. Secure venous access. Collect blood and urine for laboratory testing.
4. Control seizures (p. 24). Diazepam is indicated as first choice in controlling seizures but is often ineffective because of the antagonism of the benzodiazepine receptors. If diazepam is ineffective, use phenobarbital followed by pentobarbital if necessary.
5. Treat hyperthermia, if present (p. 25).
6. Monitor ECG for cardiac dysrhythmias. Treat dysrhythmias when noticed with generally accepted treatment options. (See notes below.)

Decontamination

1. Although chocolate is not very effectively removed during vomiting because of its "sticky" composition when melted, it is still most commonly recommended to induce emesis if ingestion was recent. (See p. 50.)
2. Gastric lavage (p. 52) with warm water will help to remove the melted chocolate from the stomach. Cool or cold water may actually worsen retrieval of chocolate.
3. Administer activated charcoal and a saline cathartic; repeat PRN q4-6h (pp. 54 and 56).

Administer antidotes or other supportive care

1. There are no effective antidotes.
2. Atropine (for bradycardia) at 0.02 mg/kg IV PRN.
3. Metoprolol. *Dog:* 0.5 to 1.0 mg/kg PO q8h; *cat:* 12.5 to 25 mg/cat PO q8-12h (*an IV dose has been published as 0.04 to 0.06 mg/kg given slowly IV q8h; we have not used this route of administration and would advise caution*) or propranolol (*acute dysrhythmias:* 0.02 to 0.06 mg/kg IV over several minutes; *nonacute:* dogs: 2.5 to 10 mg/dog PO q8-12h; cats: 2.5 to 5.0 mg/cat PO q8-12h) for atrial or ventricular tachycardias. NOTE: *Metoprolol is the beta-blocker of choice because propranolol is known to slow renal excretion of xanthines (in humans).*
4. Lidocaine (in place of metoprolol or propranolol for ventricular tachycardias) at 1 to 2 mg/kg IV bolus followed by 25 to 75 µg/kg/min IV infusion (dogs) or 0.25 to 1.0 mg/kg IV bolus followed by 5 to 40 µg/kg/min IV infusion (cats).
5. Administer fluids to support blood pressure and to maintain hydration and urine output (p. 17).

Enhancement of elimination

1. Fluid diuresis may enhance excretion.
2. Dialysis and ion trapping are not effective.

Avoid

1. Erythromycin and corticosteroids are known to interfere with excretion of methylxanthines.
2. Hypoventilation

Suggested Reading

Hooser S, Beasley V: Methylxanthine poisoning (chocolate and caffeine toxicosis), In Kirk RW, editor: *Current veterinary therapy*, ed 9, Philadelphia, 1986, Saunders.

Murphy MJ: Toxin exposures in dogs and cats: drugs and household products, *J Am Vet Med Assoc* 205(4):557-560, 1994.

Owens JG, Dorman DC: Drug poisoning in small animals, *Vet Med* 92(2):149-156, 1997.

Vig M, Daldi R, Kufuor-Menfah E, et al: Acute caffeine poisoning in a dog, *Compend Cont Ed Pract Vet* 8(2):82-84, 1986.

COCAINE

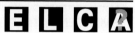

Sources   Commercial preparations include topical and local anesthetics. Free-based cocaine is called "crack," "rock," or "flake." Illicit cocaine may contain impurities including other "caine" anesthetics, caffeine, amphetamine, or quinine.

Mechanism of action   Cocaine is rapidly absorbed from mucous membranes, whereas there is a slight delay of absorption from the GI tract. Cocaine causes an initial sympathetic discharge by interfering with reuptake of endogenous catecholamines. It also is known to interfere with reuptake of dopamine resulting in an increase in dopaminergic neurotransmission. Direct cardiotoxicity is seen with large doses.

Clinical signs   Cocaine causes CNS excitement, peripheral vasoconstriction, increased muscle activity, and secondary hyperthermia. Depression may follow stimulation. Death is caused by the effects of hyperthermia, respiratory arrest, or cardiac arrest.

Treatment   Emesis followed by charcoal and a cathartic. Because cocaine is rapidly absorbed from the GI tract (which may make emesis ineffective), gastric lavage may be preferable. Surgery is needed if bags of cocaine are ingested. If surgery is not an option, consider whole bowel irrigation using polyethylene glycol solutions such as CoLyte or GoLYTELY. Chlorpromazine may antagonize many of cocaine's effects and may control hyperthermia, though it should not be used if seizures are present because phenothiazines are known to aggravate seizures. Seizures are controlled with diazepam or barbiturates; hyperthermia is treated as needed (see Hyperthermia, p. 30). Respiratory support should be assisted as needed.

Signs

Shock
Tachycardia, cardiac dysrhythmias
Pulmonary edema, tachypnea, dyspnea
CNS excitement, hyperactivity, seizures, hyperthermia, acidosis
Depression, coma
Death after respiratory or cardiac arrest or hyperthermia

EMERGENCY TREATMENT ◼

Procedures

1. Secure the airway and ventilate as necessary (pp. 5, 9).
2. Administer supplemental oxygen (p. 7).
3. Secure venous access. Collect blood for laboratory testing. Administer fluids as needed to support blood pressure and perfusion. See p. 17.
4. Control seizures (p. 24).
5. Treat hyperthermia if present (p. 25).

Decontaminate

1. Remove toxins by induction of emesis (p. 50) or gastric lavage (p. 52) if appropriate.
2. Administer activated charcoal. Repeat dose every 3 to 4 hours.
3. Administer saline or osmotic cathartics (p. 56). Enemas may also be indicated.
4. Surgical retrieval of balloons or condoms should be considered if necessary. Consider whole bowel irrigation with polyethylene glycol solutions such as GoLYTELY or CoLyte. (See p. 55.)

Administer antidotes or other indicated supportive care

1. There are no known antidotes. Chlorpromazine at very high doses (up to 15 mg/kg) have reduced signs of cocaine toxicosis. This drug may lower the seizure threshold; therefore it should be used with caution.
   (Butylcholinesterase, known to be present in human

plasma, metabolizes cocaine to inactive metabolites. Potential exists for more rapid inactivation of cocaine if this compound can be isolated or manufactured and safely administered to patients. Research efforts are ongoing.)

2. Administer fluids to maintain hydration and urine output (p. 58). Monitor for onset of acute renal failure.

3. Tachycardia may be treated with metoprolol or propranolol. High doses of propranolol may be needed when one is treating tachycardia resulting from cocaine intoxication. One experiment reported that administration of 6 to 10 mg/kg given IV as a *pretreatment* prevented tachycardia and hyperthermia. Paradoxical hypertension has been reported with the use of propranolol in humans because of blockade of beta$_2$-receptor-mediated vasodilatation. This may require the use of a vasodilator such as phentolamine or sodium nitroprusside.

4. Lidocaine (in place of metoprolol or propranolol for ventricular tachycardias) at 1 to 2 mg/kg IV bolus followed by 25 to 75 µg/kg/min IV infusion (dogs) or 0.25 to 1.0 mg/kg IV bolus followed by 5 to 40 µg/kg/min IV infusion (cats).

5. Treat increased intracranial pressure if suspected (p. 29).

Enhancement of elimination

None is known to be effective.

CORAL SNAKES

Common species   Coral snakes

Mechanism of action   Elapid venom is primarily neurotoxic with curare-like symptoms.

Clinical signs   Signs can be seen within 1 to 7 hours after the bite but may not be seen until 18 hours after envenomation. Once present, signs progress rapidly. Bulbar paralysis with respiratory failure is seen resulting in death. Aspiration pneumonia is a common complication. Unlike colubrids (pit vipers), elapids must chew at the site of the bite for venom to be released; only mild to moderate tissue reactions and pain occur at the bite. Some bites may not result in envenomation (see Pit vipers, p. 223). In contrast to pit viper bites, severe and even fatal envenomation can result in the absence of significant local reactions.

Treatment   Antivenin, administered before the clinical signs appear, is recommended. Immobilization of the victim is important. Respiratory and ventilatory support is often needed. Antibiotics are given to control secondary infections. Morphine or other narcotics that depress respiration are contraindicated.

Signs

Bulbar paralysis (ptosis, ptyalism, palpebral hyporeflexia)
Possible lip wound
Tachypnea
Aspiration pneumonia
Lower motor neuron paresis or paralysis
Hemolysis or hemoglobinuria, or both
Electrocardiographic changes may be seen (ventricular tachycardia most commonly; other dysrhythmias less commonly)
Respiratory failure
Death

EMERGENCY TREATMENT

Procedures

1. Secure the airway and ventilate as necessary (pp. 5,9).
2. Administer supplemental oxygen (p. 7).
3. Secure venous access. Collect blood and urine for laboratory testing.
4. Administer antidotes

   Antivenin (*Micrurus fulvius,* equine origin, Wyeth-Ayerst, Radnor, Pa.). A minimum of 2 vials is given before appearance of signs. Antivenin is expensive (1995 cost—$220.23). Skin testing is necessary (as with Crotalidae antivenin). Antivenin will neutralize venom from the Texas (and Gulf Coast) coral snake (*M. f. tenere*) and possibly the south Florida coral snake (*M. f. barbouri*) but not that from the Sonoran or Arizona coral snake (*Micruroides euryxanthus euryxanthus*), from which no deaths have been reported. A recently developed Fab-based ovine antivenin for eastern coral snake (*M. fulvius fulvius*) envenomation is being investigated and may be available soon. This antivenin is reported to be more efficacious than previous products and with fewer side effects.

5. Broad-spectrum antibiotics are indicated if aspiration pneumonia occurs or if the bite wound appears to become infected. Sputum, bronchoalveolar lavage fluids, or wound cultures should be submitted for culture and sensitivity and minimal inhibitory concentration testing to guide antibiotic choice.

6. Corticosteroids are controversial. Routine administration of glucocorticoids is not recommended.

Suggested Reading

Antivenin Package Insert, Wyeth-Ayerst Laboratories, Inc., Radnor, Pa.

Harned H, Oehme F: Poisonous snake bites in dogs and cats, *Vet Med Small Anim Clin* 77:73-78, 1982.

Hudelson S, Hudelson P: Pathophysiology of snake envenomation and evaluation of treatments, Part 1, *Compend Cont Ed Pract Vet* 17(7):889-896, 1995.

Hudelson S, Hudelson P: Pathophysiology of snake envenomation and evaluation of treatments, Part 2, *Compend Cont Ed Pract Vet* 17(8):1035-1040, 1995.

Hudelson S, Hudelson P: Pathophysiology of snake envenomation and evaluation of treatments, Part 3, *Compend Cont Ed Pract Vet* 17 (11):1385-1396, 1995.

Kremer KA, Schaer M: Coral snake (*Micrurus fulvius fulvius*) envenomation in five dogs: present and earlier findings, *J Vet Emerg Crit Care* 5(1):9-15, 1995.

Peterson M, Meerdink G: Bites and stings of venomous animals. In Kirk RW, Bonagura JD, editors: *Current veterinary therapy,* ed 10, Philadelphia, 1989, Saunders.

CRAYONS

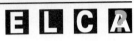

Sources

Children's toys, markers, shoe polish

Mechanism of action Children's crayons are wax and non-toxic. Some marking crayons may contain aniline dyes, which are toxic. Aniline dyes may also be found in shoe polish.

Clinical signs Apathy, dyspnea, vomiting, convulsions, and methemoglobinemia are seen if substances containing aniline dyes are ingested.

Treatment Emesis and gastric lavage, followed by catharsis are used. Breathing is monitored, and respiratory stimulation or ventilatory support may be needed. Oxygen is administered. Methylene blue or ascorbic acid is used to reduce the methemoglobin. Complete recovery is expected if the patient survives 24 hours after appropriate treatment is instituted.

Signs

Apathy
Dyspnea
Vomiting
Convulsions
Methemoglobinemia

EMERGENCY TREATMENT

Procedures

1. Secure the airway and ventilate as necessary (pp. 5, 9).
2. Administer supplemental oxygen (p. 7).
3. Secure venous access. Collect blood and urine for laboratory testing.

4. Control seizures (p. 24).
5. Treat methemoglobinemia if present (p. 181 and below).

Decontaminate

- Induce emesis *only* if the ingestion was within the last 60 minutes and the patient shows no clinical signs.
- Perform gastric lavage if the ingestion was within the last 2 to 4 hours.
- Give repeated doses of activated charcoal.
- Administer saline cathartic. Magnesium-containing solutions should be avoided.
- Consider whole bowel irrigation using CoLyte or GoLYTELY.

Administer antidotes or other indicated supportive care

1. Ascorbic acid 20 to 30 mg/kg PO or 20 mg/kg IV slowly
2. Methylene blue
   Dogs 3 to 4 mg/kg IV slowly if ascorbic acid has not been of benefit, or if no ascorbic acid has been given, see p. 373 for sodium nitrite and sodium thiosulfate.
   Cats 1.5 mg/kg has been reported to be beneficial to cats with nitrite-induced methemoglobinemia. Given in the absence of methemoglobinemia, methylene blue may cause Heinz-body formation.

Enhancement of elimination

Hyperbaric oxygen is useful if available
Exchange transfusions

Suggested Reading

Kirk RW, Bistner SI, Ford RB: *Handbook of veterinary procedures and emergency treatment,* ed 5, Philadelphia, 1990, Saunders.

CYANIDE

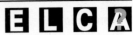

Sources Fires, cyanogenic plants (apricot pits, *Prunus* spp., *Sambucus* spp., cassava, etc.), photographic chemicals, plastic manufacture, laboratories, drugs (nitroprusside). It has been used as a rodent fumigant and in baits to kill wild animal pests such as the coyote. Hydrogen cyanide gas is a by-product of combustion of many substances found in homes; thus cyanide toxicity is common in animals trapped in burning buildings.

Mechanism of action Cyanide irreversibly combines with the ferric ion of cytochrome oxidase to form a stable complex. The blood can become oxygenated, but the cells are blocked from utilizing it. Increased respiratory rate and effort "super-oxygenate" the blood giving it a cherry red color.

Clinical findings Depends on the source and amount. Inhalation of large quantities of cyanide are rapidly fatal (minutes).
- Tachypnea, dyspnea, hyperpnea
- Signs of shock
- Bright red mucous membranes
- Shock and collapse
- Hypoxemia-induced mentation changes including confusion, dizziness (staggering), seizures, and coma.
- Agonal respirations followed by respiratory paralysis. Cyanosis may be noticed soon after onset of hypoventilation.
- Classic finding is the cherry red blood.
- Stomach contents may have a bitter almond smell.

EMERGENCY TREATMENT

Procedures

1. Remove the patient from the source of cyanide if possible. *Rescuers should wear self-contained breathing apparatus.*

2. Secure the airway and ventilate as necessary (pp. 5, 9).
3. Administer supplemental oxygen (p. 7).
4. Secure venous access. Collect blood and urine for laboratory testing.
5. Administer isotonic crystalloids as needed to support blood pressure and perfusion.
6. Control seizures (p. 24).

Decontaminate

1. If inhaled, remove the patient from the source. *Rescuers should wear self-contained breathing apparatus.*
2. If a known cyanide-containing substance was ingested within the last 15 minutes and no signs are present, induce vomiting.
3. If a known cyanide-containing substance was ingested within the last 15 to 60 minutes and no signs are present, perform gastric lavage.
4. Although cyanide is generally not adsorbed by activated charcoal, administration of activated charcoal may be of value if the toxin was ingested.
5. If there is dermal exposure (such as that from a fire or exposure to a chemical form of cyanide), bathe the animal thoroughly with soap and water. Avoid induction of hypothermia.

Administer antidotes or other indicated supportive care

1. 1.65 mL/kg 25% sodium thiosulfate IV.
2. *Only if the diagnosis of cyanide is certain* should sodium nitrite be administered (16 mg/kg IV). This drug may cause nitrite-induced methemoglobinemia, which could be fatal if cyanide poisoning is not present.
3. Hydroxocobalamin is an investigational drug that shows much promise in the treatment of cyanide toxicosis. It is currently not available in the United States.
4. Dicobalt edetate is used in the United Kingdom but is not available in the United States. Dicobalt edetate forms a nontoxic stable ion complex with cyanide.
5. Amyl nitrate is used as an antidote in humans, but literature regarding its use in dogs and cats was not found.

Enhancement of elimination

Hemodialysis may be of value in patients who have developed high thiocyanate (a less toxic compound from cyanide metabolism) levels.

DECONGESTANTS

Sources   Many over-the-counter cold and allergy preparations contain decongestants. The common decongestants include ephedrine, oxymetazoline, phenylephrine, pseudoephedrine, and phenylpropanolamine.

Mechanism of action   Most decongestants are sympathomimetic amines. The action produced by each compound depends on the adrenergic receptor or receptors that are activated. Phenylpropanolamine and phenylephrine are primarily alpha-adrenergic agonists though phenylpropanolamine also produces mild beta$_1$-adrenergic receptor stimulation and acts indirectly by enhancing norepinephrine release. Ephedrine and pseudoephedrine stimulate both alpha- and beta-receptors. The clinical signs are more closely related to beta-stimulation than alpha-stimulation with these two drugs.

Signs   Dogs are more frequently intoxicated than cats. Signs include restlessness, hyperactivity, pacing, and apparent hallucinations (flybiting, wincing, dodging invisible menaces). Most dramatic is the intensity with which these patients seem to "need" to keep in motion. Tachycardia is often noted but cannot be assumed because bradycardia may manifest as a response to hypertension. If blood pressure measurement is possible, moderate to severe hypertension will most likely be noted. Hyperactivity may progress to seizures. Mydriasis is common. Tachypnea with hyperventilation and hyperthermia are noted.

EMERGENCY TREATMENT ∎

Procedures

1. Secure the airway and ventilate as necessary (pp. 5, 9).
2. Administer supplemental oxygen (p. 7).
3. Secure venous access if possible (see note below). Collect blood for laboratory testing.
4. Control seizures (p. 24). NOTE: *in the experience of one of us (RWG), intravenous administration of diazepam has appeared to initiate hysteria and aggression resulting in worsening of signs. Although administration of acepromazine will stimulate extra-pyramidal motor pathways, thus lowering the seizure threshold, it has been more effective than diazepam (in my hands) in the treatment of hyperactivity associated with ingestion of deconges-tant sympathomimetic amines. It is administered intramuscularly at 0.05 to 0.1 mg/kg and repeated as needed every 20 to 30 min-utes until the patient calms enough to allow implantation of an intravenous catheter. Acepromazine has alpha-adrenergic re-ceptor blocking tendencies, which is useful in treatment.*
5. Treat hypertension (p. 22).
6. Treat hyperthermia if present (p. 25).

Decontaminate

1. Do not induce emesis unless the patient ingested the medication within the last 5 minutes. Perform gastric lavage (p. 52) if exposure was within the last 60 min-utes. Sustained-release types of these compounds are common; thus gastric lavage may be beneficial past the recommended 60 minutes.
2. Administer activated charcoal. Repeat dose every 3 to 4 hours.
3. Administer saline or osmotic cathartics (p. 56). Enemas may also be indicated.

Administer antidotes or other indicated supportive care

1. There are no known effective antidotes.
2. Administer fluids to maintain hydration and urine output (pp. 17, 58).

3. Monitor electrocardiogram for cardiac dysrhythmias and treat as indicated.
4. Treat increased intracranial pressure if suspected by neurologic examination (p. 29).

Enhancement of elimination

Urinary acidification (p. 59) may enhance elimination but may worsen renal damage if rhabdomyolysis accompanies intoxication.

Avoid

1. Avoid using propranolol for dysrhythmias or hypertension without first administering a vasodilator; paradoxic worsening of hypertension may result.
2. Do not use atropine to treat bradycardia or AV block associated with hypertension. The bradycardia is a protective reflex and, if removed, may worsen the hypertension.

DEET (*N,N*-diethyl-*m*-toluamide)

Sources Insect repellants such as Off, Deep Woods Off, and Cutters are examples of pure DEET (or deet) products. Hartz Blockade is a repellent and insecticide product containing DEET and fenvalerate (a pyrethroid, p. 229).

Mechanism of action Has not been fully elucidated.

Clinical signs Vomiting, tremors, excitation, ataxia and seizures have been reported in dogs and cats where deet was suspected as the toxic product. Irritation of the skin is also a possibility.

EMERGENCY TREATMENT

Procedures

1. Secure the airway and ventilate as necessary (pp. 5, 9).
2. Administer supplemental oxygen (p. 7).
3. Secure venous access. Collect blood and urine for laboratory testing.
4. Administer isotonic crystalloids as needed to support blood pressure and perfusion.
5. Control seizures (p. 24).
6. Treat hyperthermia if present (p. 25).

Decontaminate

*   Induction of emesis is relatively contraindicated.
*   Perform gastric lavage if the ingestion was within the last 2 hours.
*   Give repeated doses of activated charcoal.
*   Administer saline cathartic. Cathartics containing magnesium should be avoided.
*   Consider whole bowel irrigation using CoLyte or GoLYTELY.
*   Bathe the patient in liquid dishwashing detergent or mild shampoo. Continue for at least 15 minutes or until the odor is gone.

Administer antidotes or other indicated supportive care

There are no known antidotes.

Enhancement of elimination

There are no reported techniques that have been effective.

Suggested Reading

Dorman DC: Diethyltoluamide (DEET) insect repellent toxicosis, *Vet Clin North Am Small Anim Pract* 20(2):387-391, 1990.

Murphy MJ: Toxin exposures in dogs and cats: pesticides and biotoxins, *J Am Vet Med Assoc* 205(3):414-421, 1994.

Talcott PA, Dorman DC: Pesticide exposures in companion animals, *Vet Med* 92(2):167-181, 1997.

DETERGENTS

See also *Builders*

Sources Detergents contain surfactants and may be classified as anionic, cationics, nonionics, or zwitterionics (amphoterics).

Anionics Most common class; occur in laundry detergents, dish soaps, electric dishwasher detergents, and shampoos.

Cationics, including quaternary ammoniums Seen in fabric softeners, disinfectants, sanitizers, rust inhibitors in petroleum products.

Nonionics and zwitterionics Seen in dish soaps, shampoos, laundry detergents, and whiteners. They have a low order of toxicity.

Automatic dishwater detergents These are similar to builders and cationic detergents; toxicity ranges from moderate to high. The primary effect is from burns caused by the builders. The fatal oral dose in dogs is 0.5 to 2.5 g/kg of body weight.

Mechanism of action

Anionics High morbidity, very low mortality. These are considered to be of low to moderate toxicity except when they contain builders (see above and p. 106), which enhance toxicity. Electric dishwasher detergents have been reported to be of higher toxicity because of their reported higher pH. This has now been challenged in a study that found that the pH of these detergents was less than 12.5 (the pH traditionally considered to be associated with corrosive injury), and they were associated with very low morbidity and no mortality. When injuries do occur from exposure to anionic detergents, they are likely to be from the corrosive properties related to alkaline pH. Exposure of the eye to anionic detergents results in corneal erosion, ulceration, and opacity. Intravascular hemolysis has been reported in patients with hepatic insufficiency.

Cationics   High morbidity, low mortality. Lower concentrations of cationic detergents cause irritation to mucous membranes. Higher conentrations cause corrosive injury to mucous membranes and eyes. Cationics are readily absorbed from the GI tract. Quaternary ammonium compounds are reported to have a curare-like effect causing paralysis of striated muscle. Quaternary ammoniums are said to mimic organophosphate toxicity by inhibition of cholinesterase though conflicting literature can be found. Ocular exposure results in injuries ranging from mild irritation of ocular tissues to severe corneal ulceration.

Nonionics and zwitterionics   Low morbidity and very low mortality. Very low order of toxicity. Usually local irritation, which may result in vomiting and diarrhea in cases of ingestion.

Clinical signs (anionics)

GASTROINTESTINAL
Vomiting
Diarrhea
Abdominal pain

OCULAR
Mild irritation
Chemosis
Hyperemia of conjunctiva
Corneal erosion or ulceration

CORROSIVE INJURY
Oral ulcers
Hyperemia, irritation of mucous membranes
Esophageal irritation, erosion
Ptyalism
Dysphagia
Larnygeal edema with upper airway obstruction

INTRAVASCULAR HEMOLYSIS (RARE)
Anemia
Icterus

Hemoglobinemia, hemoglobinuria
Acute renal tubular damage resulting in acute renal failure

EMERGENCY TREATMENT

Procedures

1. Secure the airway and ventilate as necessary (pp. 5, 9).
2. Administer supplemental oxygen (p. 7).
3. Treat hypovolemia if present from vomiting and diarrhea.

Decontaminate

INGESTION
1. Administer milk or water.
2. Administer activated charcoal unless perforation is suspected.

OCULAR EXPOSURE
Flush eye with sterile saline (preferred) or water for 20 to 30 minutes.

DERMAL EXPOSURE
Flush the exposed area with water for 20 minutes.

Administer antidotes or other indicated supportive care

1. There are no known effective antidotes.
2. Administer fluids to maintain hydration and urine output (pp. 17, 58).
3. Monitor electrolytes and acid-base status (especially in cases of protracted vomiting and diarrhea) and correct abnormalities.
4. Monitor for development of intravascular hemolysis. If this should occur, administer fluids aggressively to induce brisk diuresis to prevent renal tubular damage. Monitor hematocrit and transfuse if it drops below 20%.

Enhancement of elimination

There are no known effective techniques.

Clinical signs (cationics and quaternary ammonium compounds)

SYSTEMIC SIGNS
Salivation
Vomiting, possibly hematemesis
Muscle tremors and fasciculations
Central nervous system depression
Respiratory depression
Seizures
Collapse
Coma
Muscle weakness, paralysis

OCULAR EXPOSURE
Mild redness
Severe corneal erosion, ulceration

DERMAL EXPOSURE
Hair loss
Skin irritation

EMERGENCY TREATMENT

Procedures

1. Secure the airway and ventilate as necessary (pp. 5, 9).
2. Administer supplemental oxygen (p. 7).
3. Secure venous access. Collect blood for laboratory testing. Administer fluids as needed to support blood pressure and perfusion. See p. 17.
4. Control seizures (p. 24).

Decontaminate

ORAL EXPOSURE
1. Administer milk, water, or egg whites.
2. Administer activated charcoal (contraindicated if esophageal or gastric perforation is suspected).
3. Induce vomiting *only if the concentration of cationic detergent is known to be less than 7.5%. Do not induce emesis* if the

cationic detergent concentration is >7.5% because this will likely increase corrosive injury to the esophagus and oropharynx.

OCULAR EXPOSURE
1. Flush the eye with copious quantities of water or sterile saline (preferred).
2. Treat corneal ulcers if noted.

DERMAL EXPOSURE
Bathe using warm water and soap. Rinse thoroughly.

Administer antidotes or other indicated supportive care

1. There are no known effective antidotes.
2. Administer fluids to maintain hydration and urine output (p. 58).
3. Monitor electrolytes. Correct imbalances.
4. Use atropine at (0.02 to 0.04 mg/kg IV, SQ, IM) to control parasympathetic signs (hypersalivation); repeat as needed but avoid atropine intoxication.
   Remember that atropine is NOT an antidote for detergent intoxications and is used only as needed to control parasympathetic signs.

Enhancement of elimination

There are no known effective techniques.

Clinical signs (nonionics and zwitterionics)

Vomiting
Diarrhea

EMERGENCY TREATMENT

Usually none required.
Monitor for electrolyte and fluid imbalances.
Flush eyes with saline or water for 15 to 30 minutes.

DIATOMACEOUS EARTH

Uses   Flea products

Common products   Diatomaceous earth

Mechanism of action   Diatomaceous earth (composed of diatoms, the siliceous exoskeletons of minute sea algae) kills fleas by abrasion of the cuticle and absorption of the protective waxy coating of the flea. Ingestion by pets is unlikely and has not been reported to cause toxicosis. Inhalation of the product (which is crystal silica) may induce lung disorders in pets and people (silicosis).

Signs   None unless inhaled. If inhaled, the patient may have signs related to lung disease.

EMERGENCY TREATMENT ▄

None necessary unless lung damage, which is treated with oxygen and ventilation if necessary.

Suggested Reading

Smith C: Searching for safe methods of flea control, *J Am Vet Med Assoc* 206(8):1137-1143, 1995.

DINOSEB

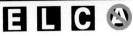

Source   Herbicide

Mechanism of action   Dinoseb (2-*sec*-butyl-4,6-dinitrophenol) prevents the electron transport–coupled oxidative phosphorylation of ADP to ATP (it uncouples oxidative phosphorylation).

Clinical signs   Signs of intoxication include tachypnea, weakness, disorientation, ataxia, and difficulty walking. Differential diagnosis includes organophosphate and organocarbamate toxicoses.

Treatment   Atropine or any agent that may contribute to hyperthermia is contraindicated. Treatment includes bathing to remove the toxicant; emesis, lavage, and catharsis; treatment of hyperthermia; avoidance of stress, which might increase body temperature; administration of fluids to prevent or treat shock, correct dehydration, and prevent electrolyte imbalances; administration of agents (such as dextrose or oral alimentation) to maintain a positive nitrogen balance; and administration of oxygen as needed.

EMERGENCY TREATMENT

Procedures

1.   Secure the airway and ventilate as necessary (pp. 5, 9).
2.   Administer supplemental oxygen (p. 7).
3.   Secure venous access. Collect blood and urine for laboratory testing.
4.   Control seizures (p. 24).
5.   Treat hyperthermia if present (p. 25). *Atropine is contraindicated.*
6.   Support hydration to maintain blood pressure or hydration and urine output with fluid therapy (pp. 17, 58).

Decontaminate

GI EXPOSURE (INGESTION)
- Induce emesis if recent ingestion if signs are not present (p. 50).
- Gastric lavage if signs are present after ingestion (p. 52).
- Administer activated charcoal and a saline cathartic; repeat PRN q4-6h (p. 54).

DERMAL EXPOSURE
Wash thoroughly with warm, soapy water. Wear rubber gloves when bathing the patient; avoid inducing hypothermia.

Administer antidotes or other supportive care

There are no known antidotes.

Suggested Reading

Ettinger SJ, Feldman EC: Toxicology. In *Textbook of veterinary internal medicine: diseases of the dog and cat,* ed 4, Philadelphia, 1995, Saunders, pp 312-326.

Fikes JD, Lovell RA, Metzler M: Dinoseb toxicosis in two dogs, *J Am Vet Med Assoc* 194(4):543-544, 1989.

Gerken D: Lawn care products. In Bonagura JD, Kirk RW, editors: *Current veterinary therapy,* ed 12, Philadelphia, 1995, Saunders.

Murphy M: Toxin exposures in dogs and cats: pesticides and biotoxins, *J Am Vet Med Assoc* 205(3):414-421, 1994.

Yeary R: Herbicides. In Kirk RW, editor: *Current veterinary therapy,* ed 9, Philadelphia, 1995, Saunders.

DIQUAT DIBROMIDE

Source Diquat dibromide is an active ingredient in herbicides.

Mechanism of action Diquat metabolism releases free radicals, which cause cellular membrane damage and cell death.

Clinical findings Animals poisoned with diquat have GI signs such as anorexia, vomiting, and diarrhea. Massive loss of body fluids occurs as they are "third spaced" in the gastrointestinal tract. Signs of acute renal failure including anuria, oliguria, or polyuria, isosthenuria, and renal tubular casts are noted with some frequency. CNS excitement occurs in severely poisoned animals.

EMERGENCY TREATMENT

Procedures

Treatment for diquat ingestion is much the same as for paraquat.

Decontaminate

1. Induce emesis (p. 50) if ingestion was within the last 30 to 60 minutes.
2. Perform gastric lavage if indicated (p. 52).
3. Administer adsorbent. Kaolin, clay, or bentonite is preferred over activated charcoal. Pulverized clay kitty litter is an appropriate adsorbent. If none of these products is immediately available, activated charcoal is preferable to waiting for acquisition of a clay.
4. Administer a saline or osmotic cathartic if ingestion was within the previous 12 hours.

Administer antidotes or other indicated supportive care

There are no known antidotes.
- Administer crystalloid fluids to maintain hydration and urine output.
- In diquat poisoning, the main problems are not associated with lung injury but with brain and kidney damage. Because acute renal failure is a common sequela, diuresis with mannitol, furosemide, and crystalloid fluids may be helpful. Monitor urine output.
- Other agents that have been used experimentally in diquat toxicosis include:
  Niacin

Riboflavin
Ascorbic acid
Superoxide dismutase
N-Acetylcysteine

Enhancement of elimination

- Diuresis may be helpful, but care must be taken to avoid adding to potential of development of pulmonary edema.
- Dialysis may be useful but may contribute to pulmonary edema.
- Hemoperfusion is effective in removing the toxin if begun early after exposure.

Avoid

Oxygen is *contraindicated* early in diquat poisoning. Oxygen administration may cause increased formation of oxyradicals.

ETHYLENE GLYCOL

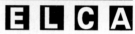

Sources   Antifreeze, color film processing solution

Mechanism of action   Ethylene glycol is metabolized by the liver using alcohol dehydrogenase in the first step of the pathway. Metabolites that are produced include glycoaldehyde (which causes CNS depression, including respiratory depression), glycolate (which causes metabolic acidosis), and oxalate (which combines with calcium to form calcium oxalate crystals, which precipitate in the renal tubules causing renal damage; oxalate also contributes to metabolic acidosis).

Many brands of antifreeze contain phosphorus rust inhibitors; monitor phosphorus and treat hyperphosphatemia if needed.

Clinical signs   The minimum lethal dose of undiluted ethylene glycol is 4.2 to 6.6 mL/kg for dogs (4.5 oz for a 20 lb dog) and 1.5 mL/kg for cats (1 tablespoon of ethylene glycol diluted

50:50 with water in radiator fluid in the average-sized cat). There are three stages of poisoning, the first two are often not noticed by owners (and may not be present if the animal is brought for treatment immediately after it has consumed the product).

Stage 1 occurs 30 minutes to 12 hours after ingestion and includes nausea, vomiting, depression, ataxia, seizures, and rarely coma and death. These signs are similar to acute alcohol intoxication and resemble drunkenness. Polyuria and polydipsia often occur within 1 hour after ingestion.

Stage 2 occurs 12 to 24 hours after ingestion and includes tachycardia and tachypnea.

Stage 3 occurs 24 to 72 hours after ingestion in dogs and 12 to 24 hours after ingestion in cats. This stage is characterized by oliguric renal failure; signs include severe depression, vomiting, diarrhea, azotemia, and oliguria.

Increased osmolality, increased osmol gap, and high anion gap metabolic acidosis (which is seen within 3 hours after ingestion) occur. Low urine specific gravity (<1.020) is also seen within 3 hours after ingestion. Calcium oxalate or hippuric acid crystals, or both, are occasionally but not always seen in the urine. The oxalate crystals can be the more common monohydrate form or the dihydrate form. Calcium oxalate crystals are occasionally seen in normal pets.

There is a test for ethylene glycol intoxication (PRN, Pharmacol Inc., Pensacola, Fla.) that can be used to support a diagnosis. This test will detect only ethylene glycol but not the toxic metabolites. Therefore the test must be run soon after ingestion to detect the ethylene glycol before metabolism. The test is not sensitive enough for cats. A positive test on cat blood means the cat has ingested a lethal dose and must be treated aggressively. A negative test on a cat is meaningless; cats are so sensitive to ethylene glycol that the color control used in the test has more than a feline lethal dose in it. A negative test on a dog indicates that the dog does not have lethal amounts of *ethylene glycol* in the circulation at the time of testing. It does not mean that the patient did not ingest antifreeze; it is possible that metabolism has reduced ethylene glycol levels lower than detectable by the test. The test cross-reacts with propylene glycol and other chemicals, and so it must be run on blood drawn *before* any medications are given (including activated charcoal). Antifreezes containing propylene glycol (Sierra, ARCO) are "safe" and are unpleasantly flavored to prevent ingestion. These "safer" compounds will not be metabolized to oxalate but could possibly cause problems related to the propylene glycol (Heinz body anemia).

Treatment   The toxin is removed from the GI tract if recently ingested. Intravenous fluids are used to correct dehydration and metabolic acidosis. Ethanol, which is preferentially metabolized by alcohol dehydrogenase, is the mainstay of treatment. 4-Methylpyrazole is antidotal in dogs. Sodium bicarbonate is used to correct metabolic acidosis.

Signs

STAGE 1
Polyuria, polydipsia
Nausea
Vomiting
Depression
Ataxia
Seizures
Increased osmolality, increased osmol gap, and high anion-gap metabolic acidosis
Hyperglycemia
Low urine specific gravity (<1.20)
Calcium oxalate crystals (occasionally)
Coma or death (rare in stage 1).

STAGE 2
Tachycardia, tachypnea

STAGE 3
Oliguric renal failure (azotemia, oliguria)
Severe depression
Vomiting
Diarrhea

EMERGENCY TREATMENT

Procedures

1. Secure the airway and ventilate as necessary (pp. 5, 9).
2. Administer supplemental oxygen (p. 7).

3. Secure venous access. Collect blood and urine for laboratory testing.
4. Administer isotonic crystalloids as needed to support blood pressure and perfusion. Monitor urine output, being especially vigilant for oliguria or anuria.
5. Control seizures (p. 24).
6. Treat hyperthermia if present (p. 25).

Decontaminate

- Induce emesis *only* if the ingestion was within the last 60 minutes and the patient shows no clinical signs.
- Perform gastric lavage if the ingestion was within the last 2 to 4 hours.
- Give repeated doses of activated charcoal.
- Consider appropriate use of saline cathartic.

Administer antidotes or other indicated supportive care

4-METHYLPYRAZOLE

Fomepizole (4-methylpyrazole) has recently been approved for use in dogs (Antizol-Vet, Orphan Medical, Minnetonka, MN 55305). This synthetic alcohol dehydrogenase inhibitor is considered to be as effective as ethanol (possibly more effective) but has fewer side effects; thus it is the recommended antidote for ethylene glycol ingestion in dogs. The 1.5 mL vial of fomepizole is diluted with 30 mL of 0.9% sodium chloride to be used as an injection (provided with the kit). A loading dose of 20 mg/kg is administered IV. At 12, 24, and 36 hours after the initial loading dose of Antizol-Vet, doses of 15, 15, and 5 mg/kg should be administered respectively. If ethylene glycol is still detected in the bloodstream of the dog after this, the clinician should continue to dose the dog with 5 mg/kg IV every 12 hours until ethylene glycol does not remain in the bloodstream or the animal has visibly recovered. *4-MP should not be used in cats.*

IV ETHANOL (ETHYL ALCOHOL)

- The preferred method of administration of ethanol is by constant IV infusion. For continuous IV infusion: Administer a loading dose of 600 mg/kg, followed by a continuous maintenance infusion of 100 mg/kg/hour. Administer this in fluids such as lactated Ringer's solution or half-strength saline at a rate suitable to provide one and one half times the maintenance needs (see Appendix B for

dog and cat daily fluid requirements, pp. 376 and 377).
Pure ethanol contains 754 mg/mL, and so 190 proof contains approximately 715 mg/mL.

- Using a 20% solution is recommended in some texts. It is given at 5.5 mL/kg IV q4h for 5 treatments and then q6h (dogs) for 4 treatments. Cats are treated with 5 mL/kg q6h for 5 treatments and then q8h for 4 treatments. IV ethanol is usually 100% effective *if* started within 1 hour after ingestion. By 4 hours after ingestion, therapy is less effective because of the rapid metabolism of ethylene glycol.

SODIUM BICARBONATE

Sodium bicarbonate is used to correct metabolic acidosis. The amount to give is based on the bicarbonate deficit.

$$\text{Bicarbonate deficit} = 0.3 \times \text{Body weight (kg)} \times \text{Base deficit}$$

Replace $\frac{1}{4}$ to $\frac{1}{2}$ of the calculated bicarbonate deficit slowly IV (over 1 hour); monitor the bicarbonate q4-6h and administer more as needed. If bicarbonate monitoring is not available, an alternative schedule of sodium bicarbonate administration has been recommended:

Dogs Sodium bicarbonate (5%) IP at 8 mL/kg q4h × 5 and then q6h for 4 additional treatments.

Cats Sodium bicarbonate (5%) IP at 6 mL/kg q6h × 5 and then q8h for 4 additional treatments.

Enhancement of elimination

Peritoneal dialysis (p. 61) is known to be highly effective in removing ethylene glycol if used early. The dose of IV alcohol should be doubled during peritoneal dialysis.

Suggested Reading

Grauer G, Thrall M: Ethylene glycol (antifreeze) poisoning. In Kirk RW, editor: *Current veterinary therapy,* ed 9, Philadelphia, 1986, Saunders.

Bahri L: 4-Methylpyrazole: an antidote for ethylene glycol intoxication in dogs, *Compend Cont Ed Pract Vet* 13(7):1123-1126, 1991.

Thrall MA, Grauer GF, Dial SM: Antifreeze poisoning. In Bonagura JD, Kirk RW, editors: *Current veterinary therapy*, ed 12, Philadelphia, 1995, Saunders.

FERTILIZERS

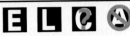

Sources   Numerous commercial products that are classified as fertilizers are available. Most are made up of a combination of nitrogen, phosphorus, and potassium compounds. Other ingredients, including trace elements, ammonia, insecticides, and herbicides, may be included in these products.

Mechanism of action   The effect of the fertilizer depends on the type of constituents found in the product.

Clinical findings

Gastrointestinal signs
   Vomiting
   Diarrhea
   Abdominal pain
Methemoglobin formation with nitrates or nitrites (p. 181).
Mucous membrane irritation
   Hyperemia
   Ulceration
Possible fever
Possible weakness, tremors
Possible seizures

Laboratory findings   Depend on the formulation of the product
   Chocolate brown blood (methemoglobinemia)
   Hyperkalemia
   Hyperphosphatemia
   Hyperosmolality
   Hyperammonemia
   Evidence of dehydration

EMERGENCY TREATMENT

Procedures

Stabilize the patient:
1. Secure the airway, administer supplemental oxygen, and ventilate the patient if necessary.
2. Treat hypotension or dehydration as necessary (p. 17). Monitor urine production because some fertilizers exert a diuretic effect necessitating higher administration rates of fluids to maintain hydration.
3. Control seizures (p. 24). Treat coma if necessary (p. 29).
4. Treat methemoglobinemia if necessary (p. 181).

Decontaminate

1. Administer milk or other demulcent for recent ingestion.
2. Induce emesis if ingestion was within the last 30 minutes. (Small animals will almost always vomit fertilizers anyway.)
3. Perform gastric lavage if necessary (p. 52). Consider scout radiographs of the stomach to ascertain if ingesta are present in the stomach.

Administer antidotes or other indicated supportive care

1. Treat other toxicoses present. Check the label of the product and see appropriate section in this book or call a regional poison control center.
2. Monitor electrolytes.
    Treat hyperkalemia if present (p. 41).
    Treat hyperphosphatemia.
    Treat hyperosmolality.
3. Control vomiting if necessary.
    Chlorpromazine
    Metoclopramide
    Trimethobenzamide
4. Consider H_2-blockers for gastritis.
    Cimetidine, ranitidine, famotidine
5. Consider sucralfate.
6. Administer analgesic for abdominal pain if necessary.

Enhancement of elimination

No technique is known to be helpful.

GARBAGE AND FOOD INTOXICATIONS

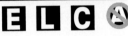

Sources   Food-related poisonings are more prevalent in the warmer months and during the holidays than at other times. Poisoning occurs as a result of ingestion of food contaminated by microorganisms or their toxins. Common organisms and toxins implicated in food poisoning include *Escherichia coli; Staphylococcus, Streptococcus,* and *Salmonella* spp.*; Clostridium perfringens* and *Clostridium botulinum* (see Botulism); and *Bacillus* spp.

Mechanism of action   Enterotoxemia causes altered gastrointestinal biochemical pathways and activation of autocoids (prostaglandins, kinins, etc.) that leads to altered motility, permeability, and CNS interactions.

Endotoxemia, which results from absorption of endotoxin released in the GI tract, may be seen as life-threatening endotoxic shock. Endotoxin is a lipopolysaccharide released from the cell wall of dead bacteria (mostly gram negative). Upon absorption from the gastrointestinal tract, the endotoxin acts through numerous mechanisms to initiate cascades or events that cause deleterious effects throughout the body. There are many texts that cover the syndrome quite well; the full syndrome is not covered in this text. Suffice to say that, untreated, endotoxemia is a severe, life-threatening disease that leads to shock, disseminated intravascular coagulopathy, pulmonary thromboembolism, acute respiratory distress syndrome, systemic inflammatory response syndrome (SIRS), multiple organ dysfunction syndrome (MODS), and death.

Clinical signs   Pets suffering enterotoxemia often vomit, usually within 3 hours after eating the contaminated or spoiled substance. Vomiting may remove the offending substance or substances, effecting a cure. Diarrhea, often bloody, may be seen if signs progress, and it develops 2 to 48 hours after food ingestion. Recovery normally occurs within 48 hours.

Protracted vomiting and diarrhea, along with permeability changes in the gastrointestinal tract caused by the toxin, may result in significant fluid losses and electrolyte imbalances. Early in the course of enterotoxicosis, hypermotility of the gastrointestinal tract may be noted. This may be followed in 12 to 72 hours by ileus and gas accumulation in the gut lumen. Gut stasis favors the growth of gram-negative bacteria, which may lead to endotoxemia.

Signs of endotoxemia are seen 5 to 48 hours after ingestion and include fever, vomiting, and possibly diarrhea. In severe intoxications, signs of endotoxic shock including depression, collapse, rapid-to-slow capillary refill time, hypotension, hypothermia or hyperthermia, early leukopenia and neutropenia followed by leukocytosis and neutrophilia with toxic neutrophils, hyperglycemia (early), or hypoglycemia (late), and oliguria may be seen.

Treatment   *Food intoxications can mimic serious problems such as gastric or intestinal torsions and foreign bodies. A thorough work-up including radiographs is warranted to ensure proper diagnosis and treatment!*

In cases where vomiting has occurred, the patient may have purged himself, thus requiring only supportive care (fluids, activated charcoal with a cathartic). If vomiting has failed to purge the stomach, treatment is by gastric lavage, repeated doses of activated charcoal, and perhaps use of a cathartic. Antiemetics may be necessary if vomiting continues after decontamination of the GI tract. Kaopectate can be used as an adsorbent or gastrointestinal protectant. Fluids are given as needed to treat hypovolemia, shock, or dehydration. Broad-spectrum antibiotics are given at the doctor's discretion. Enterotoxemia cases may appear to go well only to relapse. If relapse occurs, it usually does so within 48 hours. This may be related to onset of gut stasis and endotoxemia.

In treating endotoxemia, emesis, or lavage, and cathartics with or without enemas may be used to purge the GI tract if necessary. Treatment of endotoxic shock may be necessary (crystalloids and colloid fluids, corticosteroids [early], mannitol for oliguria, etc.). Broad-spectrum antibiotics are given.

Signs

Vomiting
Diarrhea (bloody)

Weakness

Possible abdominal pain

Hypermotility of gut followed by stasis, ileus, with or without gas distension

Collapse

Shock

Disseminated introvascular coagulation

EMERGENCY TREATMENT

Procedures

1. Secure the airway and ventilate as necessary (pp. 5, 9).
2. Administer supplemental oxygen (p. 7).
3. Secure venous access. Collect blood and urine for laboratory testing.
4. Control seizures (p. 24). Check for hypoglycemia and treat if necessary.
5. Administer isotonic crystalloids, colloids, or blood products as needed to support blood pressure, colloid oncotic pressure, and perfusion.
6. Treat hyperthermia if present (p. 25).

Decontaminate

1. Emesis has most often occurred. If the patient is symptomatic, induction of emesis will not likely be beneficial. If a pet has ingested food (within the last 30 to 60 minutes) that may have been contaminated or spoiled, induction of emesis may be indicated.
2. Gastric lavage may be beneficial in cases where quantities of ingesta remain in the stomach. A scout radiograph may be indicated to evaluate the appropriateness of gastric lavage.
3. Administration of activated charcoal is indicated. This should be repeated every 2 to 4 hours as needed.
4. Diarrhea (often bloody) often accompanies garbage-borne toxicities; thus cathartics would not be indicated. Frequently, however, ileus will be present, and administration of a cathartic such as magnesium sulfate or sorbitol may be beneficial (p. 56).

Administer antidotes or other indicated supportive care

1. There are no specific antidotes.
2. Antiemetics such as metoclopramide at 0.2 to 0.5 mg/kg PO, SC, IV q8h or as a continuous IV infusion at 0.01 to 0.02 mg/kg/hour or chlorpromazine at 0.05 mg/kg IV q4h if vomiting continues.
3. Broad-spectrum antibiotics.
4. Corticosteroids may be considered for endotoxic shock. Some references recommend prednisolone sodium succinate at 11 to 30 mg/kg IV or dexamethasone sodium phosphate at 2 to 8 mg/kg IV given *early* in the course of disease.
5. Nonsteroidal antiinflammatory drugs such as ketoprofen or flunixin meglumine have been recommended in treatment of endotoxemia. Again, early administration may prove beneficial but must be weighed against the potential side effects (gastrointestinal irritation, ulceration, and nephrotoxic effects). These drugs should not be given to a dehydrated animal.
6. If signs of disseminated intravascular coagulation or thromboembolic disease are noted, heparin therapy may be indicated.

Avoid

1. *Avoid* metoclopramide if obstruction is suspected.
2. *Avoid* chlorpromazine if pet is epileptic or seizuring.

GINSENG

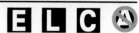

Sources   Dried roots of plants of the genus *Panax* are touted as a tonic for increasing strength and alleviating fatigue.

Mechanism of action   Saponins called ginsengosides are believed to be the active ingredients. The saponins decrease blood glucose and liver cholesterol, increase erythropoiesis, hemoglobin production, and iron absorption from the GI tract, stimulate the CNS, and increase blood pressure, heart rate, and GI motility. Toxicity is unlikely and has occurred only at extremely high levels. Supportive treatment (fluid therapy, seizure control) may be needed but is unlikely.

EMERGENCY TREATMENT

Procedures

1. Secure the airway and ventilate as necessary (pp. 5, 9).
2. Administer supplemental oxygen (p. 7).
3. Secure venous access. Collect blood and urine for laboratory testing.
4. Control seizures (p. 24). Check for hypoglycemia and treat if necessary.
5. Treat hypertension if necessary (p. 22).

Suggested Reading

Poppenga R: Risks associated with herbal remedies. In Bonagura JD, Kirk RW, editors: *Current veterinary therapy*, ed 12, Philadelphia, 1995, Saunders.

HASHISH

See *Marijuana*

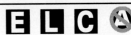

Source   Hashish is a resin from the marijuana plant, *Cannabis sativa*, which is dried and compressed into blocks. Hashish blocks can be refined further to hashish oil, which is 5 to 10 times more potent than the dried form. The active component is tetrahydrocannabinol (THC). Hashish may also contain opium.

Mechanism of action   Small animals may be poisoned by inhalation but are most commonly affected after ingestion.

THC is a CNS depressant that is quickly absorbed after ingestion. It causes euphoria initially followed by depression. It has potent antiemetic activity.

Clinical findings

Ataxia
Mydriasis, "glazed" eyes, with or without nystagmus
Hypothermia (rarely hyperthermia)
Tachycardia or bradycardia
Somnolence, depression, or coma are common; depression
  may be prolonged, with 18 to 36 hours not being unusual
Excitation is seen occasionally
Possible salivation
Possible tremors
Respiratory depression
Interestingly vomiting is sometimes seen.
Exposure to THC can be determined in the laboratory through
  analysis of urine. Consult the laboratory for sample submission.

EMERGENCY TREATMENT ∎

Procedures

1. Secure airway and support ventilation if respiratory depression warrants.
2. Secure venous access and administer crystalloids if necessary to prevent hypotension or dehydration.

Decontaminate

- Induce emesis if known ingestion occurred within the last 30 to 60 minutes. Because of the antiemetic activity of THC, this may not be successful.
- Perform gastric lavage if necessary (p. 52).
- Administer activated charcoal. Dose should be repeated every 4 to 6 hours as THC and its metabolites enter the enterohepatic circulation.
- Administer saline cathartic.

Enhancement of elimination

There are no techniques known to be effective.

HERBICIDES

See also *Dinoseb, Diquat,* and *Paraquat*

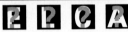

Sources Preemergent and postemergent products for weed control including Betasan (bensulide), Round-up (glyphosate), Aatrex (atrazine), Banvel (dicamba), Ortho-Paraquat/Gramoxone/Surefire/Cyclone/Prelude (paraquat). Herbicides are rarely responsible for severe toxicosis in pets, although GI signs may be seen. Most pets could not consume enough toxin from eating treated lawns. Rather, toxicity is more likely caused by ingestion of the product directly. The risk of canine lymphoma was reportedly increased (doubled) when owners applied 2,4-D ([2,4-dichlorophenoxy]acetic acid) several times per year, though the conclusions reached in this epidemiologic survey have been questioned. Oral and dermal exposure to lawn where diluted liquids or granules are properly applied are generally of neglible risk.

Mechanism of action 2,4-D causes anorexia, lethargy, myotonia, and metabolic acidosis when an acute lethal dose is ingested. Concentrated formulations are irritating and may produce gastroenteritis. The LD_{50} (medium lethal dose) for dogs is approximately 100 mg/kg; a 20 kg dog could consume this dose by ingesting only 10 mL of a liquid formulation containing 23% of the acid equivalent of 2,4-D; however, it is unlikely that an animal could consume a lethal dose after application of a properly diluted formulation. Mecoprop (MMCP) is toxicologically similar to 2,4-D. Atrazine and dicamba are not likely to be toxic unless chronic exposure occurs. Monosodium methane arsenate (MSMA), disodium methane arsenate (DSMA), and octyldodecyl ammonium salts of methyl arsenic acid are used as postemergents and do not have a high acute toxicity. Signs and treatment of acute arsenic poisoning are discussed elsewhere (p. 85).

Paraquat intoxication (p. 208) causes seizures, hyperexcitability, and incoordination. Surviving pets may die 3 to 5 days later from severe pulmonary congestion (pulmonary edema may develop within 1 to 3 days) or may develop pulmonary fibrosis in 7 to 10 days. Concentrated solutions are corrosive to the eyes and skin. Oxygen increases the toxicity and should be used sparingly as necessary. Forced diuresis is important because paraquat is a renal tubular toxin.

Glyphosate, simazine (similar to atrazine), and amitrole are believed to have low to neglible acute toxicity. Glyphosate has caused transient signs of ocular and dermal irritation after exposure to recently treated grass; signs resolve quickly when the product is rinsed from the pet.

Treatment   Treatment of 2,4-D poisoning includes activated charcoal and alkaline diuresis. Paraquat treatment is discussed on p. 209. Treatment of glyphosate poisoning would be necessary only in the event the pet drank directly from a concentrated formulation. Treatment would necessitate gastrointestinal decontamination and activated charcoal administration. Further treatment would be symptomatic and supportive.

EMERGENCY TREATMENT ■

Procedures for 2,4-D

1. Secure the airway and ventilate as necessary (pp. 5, 9).
2. Administer supplemental oxygen (p. 7).
3. Secure venous access. Collect blood and urine for laboratory testing.
4. Control seizures (p. 24).
5. Treat hyperthermia if present (p. 25).

Decontaminate

GI EXPOSURE (INGESTION)

Induce emesis if recent ingestion and if signs are not present (p. 50).

Gastric lavage if signs are present after ingestion (p. 52).

Administer activated charcoal and a saline cathartic; repeat PRN q4-6h (pp. 54, 56).

DERMAL EXPOSURE

Wash thoroughly with warm, soapy water. Wear rubber gloves when bathing the patient; avoid chilling the patient.

Administer antidotes and other supportive care

1. There are no known antidotes
2. Administer crystalloid fluids to maintain blood pressure, hydration, and urine output.

Enhancement of elimination

Ion trapping of the acid may be accomplished by alkalinization of the urine (p. 60).

HOPS

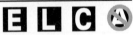

Sources   Hops are used in brewing beers and ales.

Mechanism of action   The exact mechanism of action has not been defined. Malignant hyperthermia has been reported, and it is hypothesized that the mechanism is related to uncoupling of oxidative phosphorylation.

Clinical signs   This syndrome has been reported in only a few dogs, most of which were greyhounds. After ingestion of hops, the patients developed signs of increasing temperature. Tachycardia, tachypnea, temperatures exceeding 106° F, seizures, and death were reported.

Panting

Tachycardia

Rapidly rising temperature (reported to be >2° F per 5 minutes)

Seizures

Death

EMERGENCY TREATMENT

Procedures

1. Secure the airway and ventilate as necessary (pp. 5, 9).
2. Administer supplemental oxygen (p. 7).
3. Secure venous access. Collect blood for laboratory testing. Administer fluids as needed to support blood pressure and perfusion. See p. 17.
4. Control seizures (p. 24).
5. Treat hyperthermia (p. 25).

Decontaminate

1. Induce emesis (p. 50) or perform gastric lavage (p. 52) if recently ingested.
2. Administer activated charcoal. It is unknown whether repeated doses are more effective than a single dose.
3. Administer saline or osmotic cathartics (p. 56). Enemas may also be indicated.

Administer antidotes or other indicated supportive care

1. There are no known effective antidotes.
2. Administer fluids to maintain hydration and urine output (p. 58).

Enhancement of elimination

There are no known effective techniques.

Suggested Reading

Duncan KL, Hare WR, Buck WB: Malignant hyperthermia-like reaction secondary to ingestion of hops in five dogs, *J Am Vet Med Assoc* 210(1):51-54, 1997.

HOUSEHOLD CLEANING PRODUCTS

See also *Acids and alkalis, Bleaches, Builders, Phenolics, Soaps*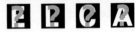

General information

Many brands of cleaners are available, and many of these cleaners contain multiple poisons. Therefore the decision regarding treatment may become complex. In general, treat the poison that is most toxic.

Surfactants and alkalis may dissolve mucous membranes and cause liquefaction necrosis; intravascular hemolysis can be seen as well. Alkalis continue to penetrate tissue until removed or inactivated by deeper tissues. Acids, formaldehyde, phenols, and other corrosives produce a coagulation necrosis; the coagulum acts as a barrier to further penetration, making acid injuries less serious than alkali injuries. Phenols may also produce a penetrating lesion and are hepato-, neuro-, and nephrotoxic. Oxalates bind calcium. A toxic mechanism has not been discovered for some products, including borates.

Antidote information is commonly found on many household cleaning products. The *Poisindex* (Micromedex, Inc., Denver, CO 80204-4506) and *Clinical Toxicology of Commercial Products* are handy references.

No attempt should be made to neutralize acids or alkalis by any of the commonly mentioned "antidotes," such as lemon juice, vinegar, antacids, or bicarbonate; these are ineffective and may cause further injury by the heat generated by the exothermic reactions. Water is generally sufficient in attempting to remove or dilute the poison.

Suggested Reading

Coppock R, Mostrom MS, Lillie LE: Toxicology of detergents, bleaches, antiseptics, and disinfectants, *Curr Vet Ther* X:162-170, 1989.

Gosselin RE, Smith RP, Hodge HC: *Clinical toxicology of commercial products*, ed 5, Baltimore, 1984, Williams & Wilkins.

Smith C: Searching for safe methods of flea control, *J Am Vet Med Assoc* 206(8):1137-1143, 1995.

Thompson JP, Senior DF, Pinson DM, Moriello KA: Neurotoxicosis associated with the use of hexachlorophene in a cat, *J Am Vet Med Assoc* 190(10):1311-1312, 1987.

HYDROGEN SULFIDE

Sources　Hydrogen sulfide is a highly toxic gas that is heavier than air. It is found in oil wells, refineries, tanneries, sulfur hot springs, hot asphalt fumes, mines, manure-holding pits, septic tanks, and sludge pools.

Mechanism of action　Hydrogen sulfide ions bind to cytochrome oxidase within mitochondria, thus blocking electron transport. This blockade results in cellular asphyxia similar to (but different from) the action of cyanide. It is also capable of causing direct irritation to mucous membranes.

Clinical findings

LOCAL EFFECTS
　Salivation
　Blepharospasm
　Cough
　Pneumonitis, noncardiogenic pulmonary edema

SYSTEMIC EFFECTS
　Tachypnea
　Nausea, vomiting
　Dizziness
　Confusion
　Seizures
　Coma

Shock
Collapse
Respiratory arrest
Death

EMERGENCY TREATMENT

Remove the patient from the source ONLY after proper precautions are taken to prevent poisoning of rescuers. High levels of gas may not have the distinctive "rotten egg" odor or may cause rapid onset of anosmia, thus the level of odor detected by the human nose is not indicative of actual levels. High levels of hydrogen sulfide gas cause rapid loss of consciousness and death.

Stabilize the patient.

Procedures

1. Secure the airway, administer oxygen, and ventilate the patient if necessary. See pp. 5, 9.
2. Perform cardiopulmonary cerebral resuscitation (CPCR) if necessary.
3. Control seizures (p. 24).
4. Treat hypotension (p. 17).
5. Observe for development of pneumonia or pulmonary edema. Treat as necessary. See p. 11.

HYMENOPTERA

Common species Bees, wasps, hornets, ants.

Mechanism of action The type of venom varies by species of insect. Phospholipase and hyaluronidase are common components. Honey bee, harvester ant, and paper wasp venom contains hemolysins; fire ant venom is necrotizing and contains hemolytic alkaloids. Field ant venom contains formic acid, which causes short-lived, intense pain.

Clinical signs   Stings and bites produce local inflammation and pain (which usually subsides within the hour). Intense regional edema can be seen. Multiple stings and bites can cause shock; allergic reactions (which can be fatal) may be seen in sensitized pets after one or more stings. When seen, anaphylaxis usually occurs within 30 minutes of the envenomation. Rarely, hemolysis, rhabdomyolysis, and liver or kidney failure can occur; monitoring laboratory values may be needed in severely affected animals.

In some insects, such as honey bees, the entire venom-stinger apparatus (the ovipositor of the female insect) is torn from the insect's body after stinging and remains attached to the victim. This apparatus contains muscle tissue that can continue contracting the venom sacs, injecting more venom into the pet. Removal with tweezers squeezes the venom sacs and injects more venom into the pet. The venom-stinger apparatus should be grasped between the stinger and the venom sac to prevent further envenomation. Alternatively, the stinger apparatus may be gently scraped (as with a credit card) rather than grasped and pulled from the pet. Some wasps and hornets may sting repeatedly because the venom-stinger appartus remains attached to the ovipositor.

Signs

Local inflammation and pain
Regional edema
Shock
Allergic reactions (angioedema, urticaria, anaphylaxis)
Hemolysis, rhabdomyolysis
Hepatic or renal failure
Death

Treatment   Shock and allergic reactions are treated with fluids, epinephrine (anaphylactic shock), and corticosteroids. Antihistamine can also be used (but is of no benefit in fire ant stings and of little benefit unless histamine release continues). Oxygen is used for dyspneic animals. Hemolysis, rhabdomyolysis, disseminated intravascular coagulation, and liver or kidney failure are treated as needed.

EMERGENCY TREATMENT ∎

Procedures

1. Secure the airway and ventilate as necessary (pp. 5, 9).
2. Administer supplemental oxygen (p. 7).
3. Secure venous access. Collect blood and urine for laboratory testing.
4. Administer isotonic crystalloids as needed to support blood pressure and perfusion.

Decontaminate

If the venom-stinger apparatus is still present, it should be gently scraped (with a credit card) rather than grasped and pulled from the pet.

Administer antidotes or other indicated supportive care

- Corticosteroids (dexamethasone sodium phosphate at 2 to 8 mg/kg IV slowly, or prednisolone sodium succinate at 11 to 30 mg/kg IV).
- Diphenhydramine at 0.5 to 2.2 mg/kg IM (or IV very slowly).
- Epinephrine 0.01 mg/kg IV, IM, for anaphylactic reactions.
- Broad-spectrum antibiotics in severe reactions and if evidence of infection or shock.
- Cool baths or compresses locally can be of temporary benefit, as may local application of a baking soda–water paste.

Suggested Reading

Cowell A, Cowell R: Management of bee and other Hymenoptera stings, *Curr Vet Ther* XII:226-228, 1995.

In Scott DW, Miller WH, Jr, Griffin CE, editors: Parasitic skin diseases. *Muller and Kirk's small animal dermatology,* ed 5, Philadelphia, 1995, Saunders, pp 461-462.

Peterson M, Meerdink G: Bites and stings of venomous animals, *Curr Vet Ther* X:177-185, 1989.

ILLEGAL DRUGS

See also *Amphetamines, Cocaine, Hashish, Marijuana, Narcotics,* and *PCP*

Domestic pets are rarely poisoned by illegal substances, except for dogs used for drug detection. Occasionally a pet is brought in for acute poisoning by an illicit substance. In addition to treating the pet, there may be legal ramifications that must be addressed, and the appropriate authorities may need to be notified. It is best to check with your local state board or local human hospitals to determine the specific medicolegal procedures that should be followed. We note that any perceived threat to the owner may make getting an accurate history difficult, making the task of identifying and treating the toxin more difficult.

Some pets may consume large quantities of the drug by ingesting plastic baggies often used for storing and reselling of illicit substances. These baggies, condoms, and balloons probably contain lethal doses, and they should be surgically removed as soon as the diagnosis is made. If surgical removal is not an option, whole bowel irrigation using polyethylene glycol (PEG) electrolyte solutions is advised (p. 55).

EMERGENCY TREATMENT ■

Amphetamines (p. 79), cocaine (p. 113), hashish (p. 146), marijuana (p. 176), narcotics (p. 189), PCP (p. 216)

Suggested Reading

Coppock R, Mostrom MS, Lillie LE: Ethanol and illicit drugs of abuse, *Curr Vet Ther* X:171-177, 1989.

Dumonceaux G, Beasley V: Emergency treatment for police dogs used for illicit drug detection, *J Am Vet Med Assoc* 197(2):185-187, 1990.

Kisseberth W, Trammel H: Illicit and abused drugs, *Vet Clin North Am Small Anim Pract* 20(2):405-418, 1990.

INSECT AND ANIMAL POISONING

See *Hymenoptera, Scorpions, Snakebites, Spider bites, Toad poisoning*

IRON

Sources   Most common exposure is from nutritional supplements (multiple-vitamin preparations with iron) that are ingested. There are also injectable forms of iron that are known to cause toxicity, but this is rare in dogs and cats. Iron may also be present in plant food preparations that have caused toxicity in dogs.

Mechanism of action   Ingestion of excess iron causes two main problems. First, iron has a direct corrosive effect on the mucosa of the stomach and small intestine. This may be so severe that necrosis results in perforation and peritonitis. In milder forms, it results in hemorrhagic gastroenteritis. Second, iron absorbed in excess of the total iron-binding capacity is distributed to the tissues where it enters cells to disrupt mitochondrial function, interfere with cellular respiration, and cause lactic acidosis. Free-radical formation is enhanced by increased availability of free iron, which results in additional cellular damage.

Clinical findings   The anaphylactic type of reaction seen with injectable iron is manifested by cardiovascular collapse and acute death. More commonly, the patient has signs associated with the ingestion of iron.

Signs associated with ingestion

Vomiting (may be bloody)
Diarrhea (may be bloody)
Drowsiness

These signs are noted up to 6 hours after ingestion. They are
   followed by a period of apparent recovery that is in turn fol-
   lowed by relapse.
Acute onset of shock
CNS depression
GI hemorrhage
Metabolic acidosis
Fulminant liver failure
Oliguria or anuria secondary to acute renal failure (from shock)

Laboratory findings

Serum iron concentrations will be elevated. Levels >350 µg/dL
   are considered to represent dangerous levels and require ini-
   tiation of chelation therapy.
Urine may appear very dark.

Radiographic findings

Radiographs may reveal radiodense objects or "sludge" from
   partially digested tablets.
Free abdominal fluid or gas may be seen if GI perforation has
   occurred.

Other tests of value

Diagnostic peritoneal lavage may help to establish the presence
   of GI perforation and peritonitis.
Blood gas and electrolyte determinations may reveal a wide
   anion-gap metabolic acidemia.

EMERGENCY TREATMENT

Procedures

Support the patient:
1.   Secure the airway and ventilate the patient if necessary.
2.   Administer supplemental oxygen if necessary
3.   Secure venous access.
4.   Administer epinephrine if anaphylaxis is suspected.
5.   Administer antihistamines if anaphylaxis is suspected.

6. Administer crystalloid fluids at shock doses if shock is present (p. 58).
7. Consider volume expansion with hypertonic saline (4 mL/kg 7% to 7.5% saline IV) or colloids (dextran 40 at 10 to 20 mL/kg IV, dextran 70 at 10 to 20 mL/kg IV, heta-starch at 20 mL/kg IV) if necessary.
8. Administer whole blood transfusion if necessary.
9. Administer sodium bicarbonate (p. 139) if pH <7.0.

Decontamination

- Early exposure: administer egg, water, or milk, and induce emesis.
- Administer magnesium hydroxide (milk of magnesia) to form precipitate, which is not absorbed.
- Perform gastric lavage. Move the lavage tube *gently* to and fro in the stomach while performing lavage to attempt to dislodge the concretions or tablets in the stomach.

Administer antidotes and other supportive care

If serum iron levels are greater than 350 µg/dL or if iron levels cannot be determined on a stat. basis, begin deferoxamine (Desferal) at 15 mg/kg/hour. Chelation will cause a reddish brown discoloration of the urine. Chelation therapy should continue until the urine color returns to normal. If serum iron levels are available, recheck in 4 hours. CAUTION: IV administration of deferoxamine is known to cause hypotension. Be observant for signs of hypotension and treat if necessary.

ISOPROPANOL (ISOPROPYL ALCOHOL)

Sources   Isopropanol (2-propanol, secondary propyl alcohol, dimethylcarbinol and petrohol) is used as an antiseptic and disinfectant and in skin lotions, hair tonics, after-shave lotions, perfumes and colognes, cleaning solvents, and sanitizers.

Mechanism of action   Isopropanol is a potent CNS depressant. It is twice as toxic as ethanol; intoxication can be seen after ingestion of less than 3.0 mL/kg. It is a gastrointestinal irritant when ingested. Isopropanol is readily absorbed from the GI tract; the rate of biotransformation is generally slower than that for ethanol. Inhalation can produce chemical pneumonia, pulmonary edema, and coma.

Clinical signs   The pet will appear drunk and often has an alcohol odor. Emesis, including hematemesis, retching, and cranial abdominal tenderness may be seen. Rapid CNS depression characterized by respiratory depression and coma occur. CNS stimulation may be observed preceding the depression if the product contains camphor, methyl salicylates, or naphthalenes. Shock can occur, as can ketonemia with uria (usually without glucosuria) and high anion-gap acidosis. Signs are similar to methanol, ethanol, and ethylene glycol intoxication.

Treatment   Although gastric lavage will probably not remove much isopropanol from the gut (because of alcohol's rapid absorption from the stomach), lavage is advised if large amounts were ingested within the past 2 hours. Emesis is not recommended because of the potential for rapid onset of CNS depression, which increases risk of aspiration. Dialysis is used in people.

Signs

Drunkenness
Alcohol odor
Emesis, hematemesis
Retching
Cranial abdominal tenderness
CNS depression (may follow CNS stimulation)
Respiratory depression
Coma
Shock
Ketonemia, ketonuria
High anion-gap acidosis
Increased osmolar gap

EMERGENCY TREATMENT

Procedures

1. Secure the airway and ventilate as necessary (pp. 5, 9).
2. Administer supplemental oxygen (p. 7).
3. Secure venous access. Collect blood and urine for laboratory testing.

Decontaminate

INGESTION
1. Perform gastric lavage if large ingestions within the past 2 hours.
2. Although isopropanol is not adsorbed well by activated charcoal, current literature recommends activated charcoal be administered.
3. Administer saline or osmotic cathartic. Cathartics containing magnesium should be avoided because of the potential for additional CNS depression from magnesium.

Administer antidotes and other supportive care

1. There are no known antidotes.
2. Blood gas determinations are important. CNS depression may induce respiratory acidosis. Isopropanol induces a wide anion-gap metabolic acidosis as well. The combination may cause profound acidemia.
3. Administer crystalloid or colloid fluids to support blood pressure, hydration, and urine output as needed.

Enhancement of elimination

1. Hemodialysis is helpful in removing the alcohol from the body, though this is rarely necessary because most patients can be treated successfully with supportive care alone.
2. Peritoneal dialysis is effective, but, because most patients can be treated successfully with supportive care alone, it is not likely to be worth the risks associated with it.

3. Hemoperfusion, multiple-dose activated charcoal, and forced diuresis are not helpful.

IVERMECTIN (AVERMECTINS)

E L C A

Sources Ivermectin (an avermectin) is mainly used in anthelminthics and heartworm preventives. Commercial products include Heartgard, Ivomec, Zimectrin, Equalen, Milbemycin (an avermectin).

Mechanism of action Ivermectin is a mixture of avermectin B_1a (>80%) and avermectin B_1b. Avermectins increase the activity of gamma-aminobutyric acid (GABA) receptors in the CNS of mammals (and in the peripheral nervous system in nematodes and arthropods) by increasing presynaptic release and enhancing postsynaptic binding of GABA in the inhibitory interneuron as well as by direct GABA agonist effects. GABA opens postsynaptic chloride channels allowing intracellular levels of negatively charged chloride ions to increase, which will hyperpolarize the cell membrane. Membrane hyperpolarization prevents depolarization of the cell in response to normal signals.

Clinical signs The most common signs of intoxication in the dog are ataxia, abnormal behavior, depression, vomiting, mydriasis, and ptyalism with hypersalivation. Other signs include disorientation, hyperesthesia, unresponsive or blank stare, paddling, hyperactivity, restlessness, stiffness, sleepiness, whining or groaning, head pressing or bobbing, aggression, chewing fits, apprehension, bradycardia, seizures, hyperthermia, weakness, breathing difficulties, and cyanosis. Severe intoxication is manifested by signs of shock (cyanosis, collapse, pallor, cold extremities, prolonged capillary refill time, and thready pulses), pulmonary edema, dyspnea, tachycardia, muscle tremors, coma, and death. In dogs where ivermectin has caused death of microfilarias, anaphylactic reactions may be the cause of the signs noted.

Signs in cats include ataxia, vocalization, disorientation, dementia, whole body tremors, mydriasis, apparent blindness (loss of menace reflex with slow and incomplete pupillary light reflexes), circling, head pressing, bradycardia, hypothermia, coma, and death.

Avermectins are active after oral or parenteral exposure. Clinical signs usually appear within hours of ingestion but may have delayed onset of up to 24 hours. Peak plasma levels are seen at 3 hours after ingestion. The reported half-life in dogs is reported to be 2 to 3 days. Several breeds are notably more susceptible to the effects of avermectins. The collie and collie crosses are most susceptible; the sheepdog has also been mentioned as a susceptible breed. Toxic dose is <200 µg/kg in susceptible animals, whereas more resistant animals reportedly showed no signs after administration of 2000 µg/kg. Cumulative toxicity is possible. Younger animals appear more susceptible.

Clinical findings

DOGS
Ataxia
Abnormal behavior
Depression
Vomiting
Mydriasis
Ptyalism, hypersalivation
Disorientation
Hyperesthesia
Unresponsive or blank stare
Paddling
Hyperactivity
Restlessness
Stiffness
Sleepiness
Whining or groaning
Head pressing or bobbing
Aggression
Chewing fits
Apprehension
Bradycardia
Seizures

Hyperthermia

Weakness

Breathing difficulties and cyanosis

Severe intoxication manifested by signs of shock (cyanosis, collapse, pallor, cold extremities, prolonged capillary refill time, and thready pulses)

Pulmonary edema

Dyspnea

Tachycardia

Muscle tremors

Coma and death

Anaphylaxis

CATS

Ataxia

Vocalization

Disorientation

Dementia

Whole-body tremors

Mydriasis

Apparent blindness (loss of menace reflex with slow and incomplete pupillary light reflexes)

Circling

Head pressing

Bradycardia

Hypothermia

Coma

Death

Diagnosis Diagnosis is based on clinical signs, history of exposure, onset interval, and dose. Plasma, liver, fat, and brain can be analyzed for avermectin levels. Brain tissue will provide the most meaningful data as detection of avermectins in brain tissues reveals passage of the toxin through the blood-brain barrier.

Treatment Probably the most important aspect of treatment is to recognize that recovery may be prolonged (weeks to months). In fact there is a report that a dog fully recovered after remaining comatose for 7 weeks. Treatment is symptomatic and supportive. Enteral or parenteral fluid and nutrition needs must be met on a daily basis. Aggressive nursing care is essential to prevent decubital ulcer formation.

EMERGENCY TREATMENT

Procedures

1. Secure the airway and ventilate as necessary (pp. 5, 9).
2. Administer supplemental oxygen (p. 7).
3. Secure venous access. Collect blood and urine for laboratory testing. Administer fluids as needed to treat hypotension and dehydraton.
4. Control seizures with phenobarital or pentobarbital. Avoid benzodiazepine tranquilizers (diazepam) because they also stimulate GABA receptors.
5. Treat increased intracranial pressure if suspected (p. 29).
6. Treat hyperthermia if present (p. 25).

Decontaminate

1. Remove toxins by induction of emesis (apomorphine) or gastric lavage if exposure was by ingestion.
2. Administer activated charcoal. Repeat dose every 3 to 4 hours. Although no studies have shown that multiple-dose activated charcoal will improve removal of ivermectin from enterohepatic circulation, the practice is known to cause no additional harm and is recommended until proved ineffective.
3. Administer enema, or saline or osmotic cathartics (p. 56).
4. At least one source suggests that one should consider surgical excision if the exposure to excess ivermectin was through recent (within past 30 to 60 minutes) subcutaneous injection and toxicosis is expected. There are no data to back up this suggestion.

Administer antidotes or other indicated supportive care

1. Physostigmine (a reversible cholinesterase inhibitor) has been used in severely poisoned (unresponsive) dogs with some success. It was administered very slowly IV at 0.06 mg/kg. The duration of action was short (30 to 90 minutes) but resulted in improved responsiveness and attempts by the patient to eat and drink.

2. Picrotoxin (a GABA antagonist) has also been used. When given IV, it may result in violent seizures that require treatment. Reports touting more rapid recovery after treatment with picrotoxin are anecdotal. Administration cannot be recommended as standard treatment.
3. Epinephrine is indicated for acute anaphylactic reactions.
4. Antihistamines are indicated if the source of ivermectin is Eqvalen (removed from market in 1984) because it contains polysorbate 80, a known histamine releaser in canines.
5. Atropine is indicated for bradycardia.

LEAD

Sources   Lead is found in old paints, some artist's paints, lead toys, drapery weights, sinkers, solder, wine bottle cork foils, battery plates, golf balls, improperly glazed ceramic dishes, used motor oil from engines that burn leaded gasoline, plumbing materials, lineoleum, tile, and lead smelters. The most common route of exposure is by ingestion, but lead is highly absorbable when heated to release fumes. Lead is absorbed from inhaled and topical exposure to leaded gasoline. Particulate lead may be inhaled from the exhaust of engines burning leaded gasoline.

Mechanism of action   Lead interferes with metabolic pathways of hemoglobin synthesis and normal erythrocyte maturation. Erythrocytes become more fragile and have reduced oxygen-carrying capacity. Ischemia may cause CNS signs. In addition, high concentrations of lead are known to cause cerebral edema and neuronal damage in the central nervous system. Peripherally, lead causes nerve demyelination and slower nerve-conduction velocities.

Clinical signs

Young dogs are most susceptible

NEUROLOGIC SIGNS
Central nervous system
  Seizures
  Dementia, hysteria
    Head pressing
    Champing of jaws
    Vocalizing
    Running aimlessly
    Biting at everything
    Circling
    Compulsive pacing

Peripheral nervous system
  Muscle spasms, opisthotonus
  Polyneuropathy (chronic lead poisoning)
    Quadriparesis
    Quadriparalysis
    Depressed spinal reflexes

OCULAR SIGNS
  Blindness
  Mydriasis
  Iridocyclitis
  Swelling of optic disk

GASTROINTESTINAL SIGNS
  Anorexia
  Vomiting
  Constipation often followed by diarrhea
  Apparent abdominal pain
  Tucked abdomen

Diagnosis

Complete blood cell count may be normal. Sometimes nucleated RBCs are found in the peripheral blood without corresponding polychromasia. Occasionally basophilic stippling is seen in the RBCs. Anemia is found occasionally.

URINE

Urine analysis may be normal or may show renal casts (hyaline or granular). Occasionally, small amounts of protein and glucose are found because of lead-induced renal damage.

URINE LEAD

Urine lead levels >0.75 ppm are suggestive of lead poisoning. Urine lead levels may be more accurate if the patient is treated with the chelator calcium disodium ethylenediaminetetraacetic acid (CaEDTA). A urine lead level is determined before chelation therapy is begun. CaEDTA is administered (see treatment below) and a 24-hour urine lead sample is collected. Urine lead levels >0.82 ppm 24 hours after chelation therapy is begun is diagnostic for lead poisoning.

BLOOD LEAD

Determination of blood lead levels is the most valuable laboratory test. Approximately 90% of absorbed lead is carried bound to erythrocytes. Therefore *analysis must be performed on whole blood,* not serum or plasma. Heparinized or EDTA tubes are submitted. Blood lead levels ≥0.6 ppm are diagnostic; levels ≥0.35-0.6 are considered diagnostic if accompanied by signs or other ancillary tests (see below). Blood lead levels do not correspond well with severity of signs. In cases of chronic plumbism, there is reported to be a high level (30%) of false negatives.

TISSUE LEAD

Liver and kidney lead levels >10 ppm are diagnostic for lead toxicosis. Some toxicologists consider lower levels and supportive signs to be conclusive for plumbism.

FECAL LEAD

Levels >35 ppm are suggestive.

RADIOGRAPHS

Metallic foreign bodies help support the possibility of lead poisoning; however, negative radiographic findings do *not* rule out lead poisoning. Rarely, radiographs of the epiphyseal plates (in dogs) reveal a "lead line."

Serum aminolevulinic acid (ALA) dehydratase inhibition and zinc protoporphyrin levels are sensitive tests but are expensive and do not replace blood lead in value.

EMERGENCY TREATMENT

Procedures

1. Secure the airway and assist ventilation if necessary (pp. 5, 9).
2. Secure venous access (p. 16).
3. Control seizures (p. 24).
4. Treat cerebral edema as necessary based on signs or CSF analysis that reveals cerebral inflammation. (See p. 29 for increased intracranial pressure.)
   a. Furosemide (1 to 5 mg/kg IV) followed by
   b. Mannitol (0.1 to 1.0 g/kg IV over 15 to 30 minutes)
   c. Corticosteroids
      • Methylprednisolone sodium succinate (25 to 30 mg/kg IV at entry followed by 12.5 to 15 mg/kg IV at 2 and 6 hours after entry; then 2.5 mg/kg/hour IV continuous infusion for 8 to 42 hours)
      • Dexamethasone sodium phosphate (2 to 3 mg/kg IV followed by 1 mg/kg SC q6-8h in tapering doses)

Decontaminate

1. Locate source and prevent further exposure.
2. Remove lead foreign bodies if present in GI tract or synovial spaces. Lead bullets or shot lodged in tissue are not usually associated with lead poisoning. They should, however, be removed if no other source of lead can be found in a patient with elevated blood lead levels and supportive signs.
3. Endoscopy
4. Surgery
5. Gastric lavage (not highly successful)
6. Catharsis with sodium sulfate or magnesium sulfate (0.5 mg/kg in a 10% solution in water by stomach tube). Not only does this promote evacuation of gastrointestinal foreign bodies, it also results in formation of a poorly absorbed lead salt (lead sulfate).

Administer antidotes and other supportive care

BEGIN CHELATION THERAPY

- Succimer (*meso*-2,3-dimercaptosuccinic acid, or DMSA) and 2,3-dimercapto-1-propanesulfonic acid, sodium salt (or DMPS) are newer chelators that show promise. Succimer (Chemet, McNeil Consumer Products Co., Fort Washington, PA 19034) has recently been made available in the USA, but DMPS is not yet available in this country. Succimer administered orally at 10 mg/kg q8h for 10 days has been found to successfully eliminate clinical signs of plumbism. It is believed to be less toxic than dimercaprol, calcium EDTA, or penicillamine.
- Administer dimercaprol (BAL). CaEDTA will increase lead excretion 20- to 50-fold. Occasionally this will make the patient worse. Administration of dimercaprol first may lessen this effect. Administer 10% dimercaprol in oil (2.5 mg/kg IM q4h on days 1 and 2, q8h on day 3 and then q12h). The dose may be increased to 5 mg/kg on day 1 only in acute, severe cases.
- Administer CaEDTA (25 mg/kg diluted to a concentration of 10 mg/mL in 5% dextrose in water given SC q6h for 5 days). CaEDTA may be nephrotoxic. Do not exceed 5 days of continuous therapy. Do not exceed a 2 g total daily dose.
- Administer penicillamine. Penicillamine (8 mg/kg PO q6h or 10 to 55 mg/kg q12h) may be administered orally in place of CaEDTA. It should be given on an empty stomach but may cause vomiting. Antiemetics may help resolve this complication.

ADMINISTER THIAMINE

1 to 2 mg/kg IM or 2 mg/kg PO q24h

ADMINISTER BROAD-SPECTRUM ANTIBIOTICS

Lead may be immunosuppressive.

CONTINUE THERAPY UNTIL BLOOD LEAD LEVELS ARE NORMAL

If lead poisoning is diagnosed early, before signs are severe or chronic, the prognosis for recovery is good. Even patients suffering polyneuropathy may fully recover. If the signs are severe, or CSF analysis is abnormal, full recovery is not so likely, but the patient may still recover to an acceptable state.

Suggested Reading

Ramsey DT, Casteel SW, Fagella AM, et al: Use of orally administered succimer (*meso*-2,3-dimercaptosuccinic acid) for treatment of lead poisoning in dogs, *J Am Vet Med Assoc* 208(3):371-375, 1996.

(+)-LIMONENE, LINALOOL, CRUDE CITRUS OIL EXTRACTS

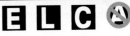

Sources   Insecticide, insect repellent, food additive, fragrance.

Mechanism of action   The mechanism of action of the citrus oil extracts has not been fully elucidated. It appears that both central and peripheral vasodilatation take place upon exposure. Linalool has a more prolonged action.

Clinical signs   Signs associated with toxicity of the crude citrus oil extracts include almost immediate hypersalivation, muscle tremors, ataxia, depression, and hypothermia. Although it appears that (+)-limonene has a wide margin of safety compared with linalool of other citrus oil extract, improper calculation of the dilution or careless use of the undiluted product has resulted in pronounced toxicosis. Most cats will recover in a matter of 6 to 12 hours, provided that the toxicosis was caused by (+)-limonene as the sole toxic agent. When other crude citrus oil extracts are the cause, the signs may be prolonged. Deaths have been reported.

EMERGENCY TREATMENT

Procedures

1.   Secure the airway and ventilate as necessary (pp. 5, 9).
2.   Administer supplemental oxygen (p. 7).

3.   Secure venous access. Collect blood and urine for laboratory testing.
4.   Administer isotonic crystalloids as needed to support blood pressure and perfusion.
5.   Control seizures (p. 24).
6.   Treat hypothermia if present (p. 30).

Decontaminate

- Bathe the cat in liquid dishwashing detergent. Continue for at least 15 minutes or until the odor is gone.
- Keep the patient in a warm, well-ventilated area.
- Induce emesis *only* if the ingestion was within the last 10 minutes and the patient shows no clinical signs.
- Perform gastric lavage if the ingestion was within the last 2 to 4 hours.
- Give repeated doses of activated charcoal.
- Administer saline cathartic. Magnesium-containing solutions should be avoided.
- Consider whole-bowel irrigation using CoLyte or GoLYTELY.

Avoid

Atropine is *not* indicated for ptyalism associated with this toxicity.

LOCAL ANESTHETICS

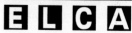

Sources   Creams for teething (Anbesol), cold sores, and hemorrhoids, sore throat sprays and lozenges (Vicks, Chloraseptic), benzocaine-containing suppositories, analgesic creams (Lanacane), and first-aid sprays, topical anesthetics (lidocaine, tetracaine, benzocaine).

Mechanism of action   A large amount of these products would need to be ingested to produce significant toxic effects for compounds containing lidocaine. However, methemoglobinemia, which can occur after oxidation of hemoglobin, is possible with topical application of even a small amount of benzocaine and tetracaine products; the cat is especially sensitive.

Clinical signs   Signs of methemoglobinemia include cyanosis, open-mouth breathing, convulsions, and dark brown blood.

EMERGENCY TREATMENT

Procedures

1. Secure the airway and ventilate as necessary (pp. 5, 9).
2. Administer supplemental oxygen (p. 7).
3. Secure venous access. Collect blood and urine for laboratory testing.
4. Administer isotonic crystalloids as needed to support blood pressure and perfusion.
5. Treat methemoglobinemia if present (p. 181).
6. Treat hyperthermia if present (p. 25).

Decontaminate

INGESTION
- Induce emesis *only* if the ingestion was within the last 60 minutes and the patient shows no clinical signs.
- Perform gastric lavage if the ingestion was within the last 2 to 4 hours.
- Give repeated doses of activated charcoal.
- Administer cathartic.

DERMAL EXPOSURE
- Wash thoroughly with warm, soapy water. Avoid chilling the patient.

Administer antidotes or other indicated supportive care

Antidotes for methemoglobinemia include ascorbic acid and methylene blue (p. 183).

Enhancement of elimination

Hyperbaric oxygen is useful if available.
Exchange transfusions.

Avoid

Handling. Keep manipulation and stress to a minimum. These patients may be extremely hypoxemic and therefore quite fragile.

Suggested Reading

Harvey J: Methemoglobinemia and Heinz-Body hemolytic anemia, *Curr Vet Ther* XII:443-446, 1995.

Krake A, Arendt T, Teachout D, et al: Cetacaine-induced methemoglobinemia in domestic cats, *J Am Anim Hosp Assoc* 21:527-534, 1985.

Wilkie DA, Kirby R: Methemoglobinemia associated with dermal application of benzocaine cream in a cat, *J Am Vet Med Assoc* 192(1):85-86,1988.

MACADAMIA NUTS

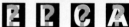

Signs of toxicity after ingestion of large quantity of macadamia nuts have been anecdotally reported in dogs in Hawaii, where the shelled nuts are readily available. Owners are usually quite disturbed because the symptoms are acute (onset can be quite rapid after ingestion) and can be dramatic. These dogs are said to present in various degrees of ataxia or hind-limb paresis. The signs usually resolve in 12 to 24 hours without treatment. The toxic element has not been researched.

No literature was found to confirm or refute this reported toxicity, but the above discussion regarding this topic was held in 1995 on Veterinary Information Network (Davis, California).

MARIJUANA

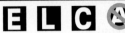

Source   Marijuana (*Cannabis sativa*) is a plant, the leaves, flowers, and seeds of which contain several cannabinoids, which are favored by some people for their psychoactive properties. A capsular form of the most potent cannabinoid (tetrahydrocannabinol, or THC) is now available for patients undergoing chemotherapy or who have glaucoma.

Mechanism of action   Whereas exposure in people is usually by the inhalant route, pets more commonly ingest the toxin. The toxic substance is the alkaloid tetrahydrocannabinol. It has antiemetic effects, making it useful for treating side effects associated with chemotherapy in people. These antiemetic effects unfortunately prevent most pets from vomiting the substance and effecting a self-cure. THC is rapidly absorbed after oral or inhalation exposure and is detoxified by the liver; only 6% to 20% of an oral dose reaches the systemic circulation. Most pets recover, though recovery may take 1 to 3 days.

Clinical signs   Signs in pets resemble those seen in people and include behavioral changes such as early euphoria, tachycardia, hypotension, muscle weakness, conjunctival injection, depression, stupor, ataxia, hypothermia, and rarely vomiting.

Treatment   In cases of recent ingestion of marijuana, vomiting may be induced if indicated. Activated charcoal and a cathartic are given. Further treatment is supportive and based on signs.

Clinical findings

Behavioral changes (early euphoria)
Tachycardia or bradycardia
Hypotension
Muscle weakness

Conjunctival injection
Depression
Stupor
Ataxia
Hypothermia
Tremors (rare)
Hypersalivation (not frequent)
Vomiting (rare)

EMERGENCY TREATMENT

Procedures

1. Secure the airway and ventilate as necessary (pp. 5, 9).
2. Administer supplemental oxygen (p. 7).
3. Secure venous access. Collect blood for laboratory testing if desired. Administer fluids as needed to support blood pressure and perfusion. See p. 17.

Decontaminate

1. Induce emesis (antiemetic properties may make this ineffective). Perform gastric lavage if indicated.
2. Administer activated charcoal. Repeat dose every 3 to 4 hours.
3. Administer saline or osmotic cathartics (p. 56). Enemas may also be indicated.

Administer antidotes or other indicated supportive care

1. There are no known effective antidotes.
2. Administer fluids to maintain hydration and urine output (p. 58).
3. Atropine may be indicated for pronounced bradycardia.

ENHANCEMENT OF ELIMINATION

There are no known effective techniques.

METALDEHYDE

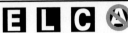

Sources   Common ingredient in molluscicides (snail or slug bait), which are available in kibbled, granular, powder, or liquid form. Be aware that baits may contain other toxins. Metaldehyde may also be present in fuels used in small heaters.

Mechanism of action   The precise mechanism of toxicity is unknown. What is known is that metaldehyde is metabolized to liberate acetaldehyde. Metabolism of acetaldehyde contributes to metabolic acidosis, which is worsened by muscle activity of tremors or seizures. It is unclear whether metaldehyde or acetaldehyde is responsible for the signs noted with metaldehyde toxicosis.

There is a detectable reduction in gamma-aminobutyric acid (GABA) in metaldehyde-poisoned patients. Levels of GABA were directly related to survivability. Levels of brain serotonin and norepinephrine are reduced. Seizural activity is more likely with more pronounced reductions.

Clinical findings   Usually begin showing signs within 15 minutes to 3 hours after ingestion.

EARLY SIGNS
Increased heart rate
Anxiety
Nystagmus (especially in cats)
Possible mydriasis
Hyperpnea, panting
Salivating, usually with the saliva being thick and frothy
Stiff-legged gait, ataxia
Possible vomiting

FOLLOWED BY
Muscular tremors that are only mildly and inconsistently induced by external stimuli, especially touch but rarely visual or auditory stimuli.
Possible diarrhea
Convulsions

EVENTUALLY

Continuous convulsions

Severe hyperthermia (temperatures >108°F)

Acidosis

Disseminated intravascular coagulopathy

Respiratory failure, cyanosis

Narcosis

Death—if the animal survives the acute episode, it may succumb to complications (including liver failure) in the next 3 to 5 days.

Diagnosis   Diagnosis of metaldehyde ingestion is usually made on the basis of clinical signs with or without known exposure. Stomach contents, urine, plasma, and tissue may be analyzed for the presence of metaldehyde.

EMERGENCY TREATMENT

Procedures

1. Secure the airway and provide ventilatory support if necessary.
2. Secure venous access.
3. Control seizures. If diazepam is ineffective, consider using barbiturates. Keep in mind that barbiturates compete with an enzyme that metabolizes acetaldehyde.
4. Treat hyperthermia (p. 25); monitor for signs of onset of disseminated intravascular coagulation, sepsis, etc.
5. Treat muscle tremors
   - *Diazepam* (0.5 to 1.0 mg/kg IV in increments of 5 to 20 mg to effect). It may also be administered rectally at a dose of 1 to 4 mg/kg in increments of 5 to 20 mg to effect for a rapid response.
   - *Methocarbamol* (up to 222.2 mg/kg IV PRN are reported in dogs; 44.4 mg/kg IV in cats).
   - *Acetylpromazine* (0.05 to 0.25 mg/kg IV) has been reported as effective in inducing sedation and does not appear to exacerbate the potential for seizures in metaldehyde toxicity.

6. Make certain that metaldehyde is the only ingredient. Some commercial products have been formulated so that an organocarbamate has been combined with the metaldehyde resulting in a combined toxicosis.

7. Administer crystalloid fluids for hemodynamic support or to maintain hydration.

8. Treat acidosis with buffering crystalloid solutions (lactated Ringer's solution, Normosol-R). If blood gas analysis is available, treat severe acidemia (pH <7.05) with sodium bicarbonate. The dose of bicarbonate required is calculated from the following equation:

$$HCO_3^- = 0.3 \times \text{Body weight (in kg)} \times \text{Base excess}$$

Administer one fourth to one half of the calculated dose intravenously over 15 to 30 minutes and reevaluate blood gas and blood pH values.

Decontaminate

- Administer milk and then induce emesis if the patient is known to have ingested the poison within the past 60 minutes and is showing no signs.

- If emesis is unwise, consider a rapid radiograph of the stomach to evaluate for the presence of ingesta. If no ingesta are present, administer activated charcoal and saline cathartics. If ingesta are present, perform gastric lavage (p. 52). Lavage using milk or sodium bicarbonate is reported to decrease absorption of metaldehyde.

- Administer activated charcoal and saline cathartics. Repeated doses of activated charcoal are not required because aldehydes do not commonly enter the enterohepatic circulation and are not resecreted into the GI tract.

METAL POISONING

See *Iron, Lead, Zinc*

METHANOL

See *Organic solvents and fuels*

METHYLENE CHLORIDE

See *Organic solvents and fuels*

METHEMOGLOBINEMIA

Sources Methemoglobin is an oxidized form of hemoglobin. Many drugs, chemicals, and some plants are capable of oxidizing hemoglobin to cause methemoglobinemia (Box 2-1).

Mechanism of action Agents that induce formation of methemoglobin oxidize ferrous to ferric hemoglobin. The abnormal hemoglobin cannot carry oxygen. Furthermore, the shape of the oxygen-hemoglobin dissociation curve is altered, aggravating cellular hypoxia. Many agents that induce formation of methemoglobin also cause Heinz body formation and hemolysis.

Clinical findings

Tachypnea
Cyanosis
Weakness
Tachycardia
Possible seizures
Shock
Acute death

AGENTS CAPABLE OF CAUSING METHEMOGLOBIN FORMATION

LOCAL ANESTHETICS
Benzocaine (Cetacaine, Lanacaine, Bicozine)
Lidocaine
Prilocaine

NITRATES AND NITRITES
Amyl nitrate
Sodium nitrite

MISCELLANEOUS
Hydrogen sulfide gas
Aniline dyes
Chlorates
Smoke inhalation (combustion by-products)
Sulfonamides
Organic solvents (toluene, benzene)
Nitrate-containing well water
Fertilizers
Mothballs

ANALGESICS
Acetaminophen
Phenazopyridine
Phenacitin

PLANTS (MORE COMMON IN RUMINANTS)
Astragalus
Oxytropis
Sorghum

DRUGS
Methylene blue
Methionine
Vitamin K_1

Laboratory findings

Dark (chocolate brown) blood; put a drop of blood on a filter
  paper and compare with known normal.
Normal hemogram unless accompanied by hemolysis or Heinz
  body formation.

Normal blood gas levels (blood gas instruments measure the amount of oxygen dissolved in plasma, which is usually normal in cases of methemoglobinemia).

Pulse oximetry will often reveal normal SpO_2.

EMERGENCY TREATMENT

Procedures

Stabilize the patient:
1. Secure the airway and administer 100% oxygen. Ventilate the patient if necessary. See p. 7.
2. Control seizures (p. 24).

Decontaminate

1. If inhaled, remove the patient from the source.
2. If ingested within the last 60 minutes and no signs are apparent, induce vomiting unless contraindicated (such as organic solvents, hydrocarbons). (See p. 50 for technique.)
3. If ingested within the last 2 hours and induction of vomiting is not performed, perform cautious gastric lavage. See p. 52.
4. Administer activated charcoal and cathartic.

Administer antidotes or other supportive care

1. Ascorbic acid 20 to 30 mg/kg PO or 20 mg/kg IV slowly
2. Methylene blue
   Dogs 3 to 4 mg/kg IV slowly if ascorbic acid has not been of benefit, or if no ascorbic acid has been given, see p. 373 for sodium nitrite and sodium thiosulfate.
   Cats 1.5 mg/kg has been reported to be beneficial with nitrite-induced methemoglogin.
   Given in the absence of methemoglobinemia, methylene blue may cause Heinz body formation.
3. Possible need for blood transfusions

Enhancement of elimination

Hyperbaric oxygen is useful if available
Exchange transfusions

MOTHBALLS

See *Naphthalene, Paradichlorobenzene*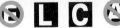

MUSHROOMS

 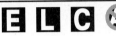

Sources Wild mushrooms are most common; "recreational" use of mushrooms may result in animal intoxication.

Mechanism of action Documented cases of mushroom toxicity are few in the veterinary literature. Many mushrooms have been identified as toxic, but the poisonous compound has never been identified. Identification of poisonous mushrooms is a difficult task, even for mycologists. For these reasons, we recommend that all mushroom ingestions be treated as potential lethal intoxications.

The mechanism of action of the various mushrooms depends on the toxin in that species of mushroom. The toxins that have been identified are best put into categories based on their specific effects. Mushrooms that contain complex polypeptides or cyclopeptides (amanitin, phalloidin) will cause cellular injury and death, resulting in kidney, liver, and heart damage and death (of the animal). Autonomic nervous signs (usually muscarinic) are caused by toxins isolated from some mushrooms. Toxins such as ibotenic acid, muscimol, or indoles similar to LSD will cause CNS effects including hallucinations. Gastrointestinal irritants are found in many species of mushroom.

Clinical signs The clinical signs noted depend on the type of toxin found in the ingested mushroom. Identification of an ingested mushroom is not likely; thus we offer the age-old adage: treat the patient, not the mushroom. There are a multiplicity of signs associated with (suspected) mushroom intoxications. The following signs have been reported with mushroom ingestion or suspected mushroom ingestion:

Seizures

Bizarre CNS signs—suspected hallucinations (hallucinations are reported in man)

Depression

Ataxia

Coma

Gastrointestinal upset

Abdominal pain

Colic

Nausea

Vomiting

Diarrhea

Intestinal cramps

Hyperthermia

Muscarinic signs

    Salivation

    Lacrimation

    Urination

    Defecation

Acute renal failure

Acute hepatic failure

Pronounced hypoglycemia

Circulatory collapse

Acute death

Hemolysis was reported in one case of mushroom ingestion in a dog.

EMERGENCY TREATMENT

Procedures

1. Secure the airway and ventilate as necessary (pp. 5, 9).
2. Administer supplemental oxygen (p. 7).
3. Secure venous access. Collect blood for laboratory testing. Administer fluids as needed to support blood pressure and perfusion. See p. 17.
4. Control seizures (p. 24).
5. Treat hyperthermia if present (p. 25).

Decontaminate

1. Induce emesis (p. 50) if exposure was by ingestion and vomiting has not occurred naturally. Perform gastric lavage (p. 52) if necessary.
2. Administer activated charcoal. Multiple-dose activated charcoal is recommended because positive identification of the toxin is almost never accomplished. Administration of multiple doses of activated charcoal may be helpful and is very unlikely to cause harm.
3. Administer saline or osmotic cathartics if indicated (p. 56).

Administer antidotes or other indicated supportive care

1. There are no known effective antidotes.
2. Administer fluids to maintain hydration and urine output (p. 58).
3. Monitor renal and hepatic function including blood glucose levels.

Enhancement of elimination

There are no known effective techniques.

NAPHTHA

See *Organic solvents and fuels*

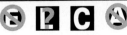

NAPHTHALENE (old-fashioned mothballs)

Sources Naphthalene is the active ingredient in old-fashioned mothballs, moth cakes, and moth crystals. It has also been used in toilet bowl deodorizers. The use of naphthalene has largely been replaced with paradichlorobenzene because naphthalene is at least 2 times more toxic than paradichlorobenzene. Naphthalene appears to be quite toxic to cats. Further, the National Animal Poison Control Center reported naphthalene as one of the top 25 causes of poisoning in dogs in 1992.

Mechanism of action Naphthalene induces gastrointestinal upset and vomiting. It also is known to stimulate the central nervous system. Hemolysis (from Heinz body anemia) is seen, especially in patients with glucose-6-phosphate dehydrogenase deficiencies.

Clinical findings

- The most common sign is vomiting.
- A typical odor of mothballs is usually noted emanating from the patient or its vomitus.
- Methemoglobinemia.
- Heinz body anemia with hemolysis and hemoglobinuria, resulting in pallor, tachycardia.
- CNS signs including seizures may been seen as a result of CNS stimulation.
- Rarely, signs of hepatitis, which occur 3 to 5 days after ingestion of naphthalene.

Laboratory findings

- Complete blood cell count most often reveals hemolytic anemia. Dehydration as a result of vomiting may offset the reduction of packed cell volume seen with mild anemia.
- Urine analysis may reveal hemoglobinuria.

Diagnosis

Usually based on history of ingestion or typical odor of moth-balls (patient breath, around mouth, in vomitus). There is no specific test for serum levels of naphthalene.

EMERGENCY TREATMENT

Procedures

1. Secure airway and support ventilation if required.
2. Secure venous access.
3. Control seizures (p. 24).
4. If anemia is causing signs of hypoxia, administer supplemental oxygen and give red blood cell transfusion.
5. Treat methemoglobinemia (p. 181) if suspected (mucous membranes are dark blue or brown).
6. Treat hemolysis or hemoglobinuria with intravenous crystalloids for hydration and consider alkalinization of the urine (pp. 58, 60) to prevent precipitation of hemoglobin in the kidneys.

Decontaminate

- Do not induce vomiting.
- Perform gastric lavage only if a known toxic amount was ingested within the last 30 to 60 minutes.
- Administer activated charcoal (p. 54).
- Administer saline cathartics (p. 56).

Enhancement of elimination

There is no role for hemodialysis or hemoperfusion in naphthalene ingestion.

NARCOTICS

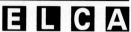

Sources   Narcotics (opiates) are derivatives of the poppy plant. Morphine is the base product that is chemically altered to produce codeine, hydromorphone, and oxymorphone. Other synthesized products include meperidine (Demerol), methadone (Dolophine), pentazocine (Talwin-V), butorphanol (Stadol, Torbutrol, and Torbugesic), and propoxyphene (Darvon). Diphenoxylate (Lomotil) and loperamide (Imodium) are other (antidiarrheal) products that may be involved in opiate poisoning.

Mechanism of action   Narcotics act by stimulating specific opioid receptors in the body.

Clinical signs   Early signs include drowsiness, ataxia, decreased pain, transient excitation (signs in cats are related more to excitation than to depression). Later signs include delirium, convulsions, miosis (mydriasis in cats), coma, respiratory depression, and pronounced hypotension. Death, which may occur within 12 hours, is from respiratory depression. Hypothermia is seen in dogs, whereas hyperthermia is often seen in cats.

Treatment   Emesis or lavage is indicated. Activated charcoal and a cathartic are indicated. *Because opiates can produce a slowing of the GI transit time, emesis, lavage, and use of activated charcoal should be accomplished regardless of the time of ingestion.* Naloxone (Narcan) is an effective antidote; it may need to be repeated because the half-life of most narcotics is greater than the half-life of naloxone. If a total dose of 10 mg of naloxone has been given with little response, it will be ineffective, and the diagnosis may need to be reevaluated.

Signs

EARLY
  Ileus
  Drowsiness

Ataxia
Decreased pain
Transient excitation (signs in cats are related more to excitation than to depression).

LATE

Delirium
Seizures (mainly with meperidine)
Miosis (mydriasis in late stages with hypoxemia)
Mydriasis in cats
Coma
Hypothermia, hyperthermia
Respiratory depression, cyanosis, pulmonary edema, pneumonia
Pronounced hypotension
Death, often from respiratory depression

EMERGENCY TREATMENT

Procedures

1. Secure the airway and ventilate as necessary (pp. 5, 9).
2. Administer supplemental oxygen (p. 7).
3. Secure venous access. Collect blood for laboratory testing. Administer fluids as needed to support blood pressure and perfusion. See p. 17.
4. Control seizures (p. 24).
5. Treat hyperthermia if present (p. 25) or prevent heat loss if hypothermia is present.

Decontaminate

1. Induce emesis only if patient is asymptomatic (p. 50) or perform gastric lavage if indicated (p. 52). Gastric lavage and activated charcoal may be effective several hours after oral exposure because of opioid-induced pylorospasm and hypomotility of the gastrointestinal tract.
2. Administer activated charcoal. Repeat dose every 3 to 4 hours.
3. Administer saline or osmotic cathartics (p. 56). Enemas may also be indicated.

Administer antidotes or other indicated supportive care

1. Naloxone (Narcan) is the preferred antidote (*dog*: 0.02 to 0.04 mg/kg IV prn; *cat*: 0.05 to 0.1 mg/kg IV). Other antagonists include levallorphan and nalorphine. The antagonists have a shorter duration of action than that of most opiates; therefore repeat doses are often indicated.
2. Administer fluids to maintain hydration and urine output (p. 58).
3. Treat increased intracranial pressure if suspected (p. 29).
4. Meperidine-induced seizures may be refractory to opiate antagonists. Phenobarbital or pentobarbital may be required.

Enhancement of elimination

There are no known effective techniques.

NICOTINE

E L C A

Common products   Mostly found in cigarettes (especially butts) but also may be caused by ingestion of snuff, nicotine gum, certain plants (mescal bean), and certain insecticides.

Mechanism of action   Nicotine mimics the action of acetylcholine at ganglia of the autonomic nervous system, neuromuscular junctions of the skeletal system, and some synapses in the central nervous system.

Clinical signs   The onset of signs is rapid after ingestion. Patients will become excited or hyperactive. Often salivation, vomiting, and diarrhea are seen. Patients are often tachypneic. Urination and lacrimation may be seen. With higher doses or longer exposures, the patient will begin to have tremors or muscular twitches, will be unable to stand, and may experience rapid shallow respirations followed by slow respiration. Tachycardia, collapse, coma, and death will follow.

EMERGENCY TREATMENT

Procedures

1. Secure the airway and ventilate as necessary (pp. 5, 9).
2. Administer supplemental oxygen (p. 7).
3. Secure venous access. Collect blood and urine for laboratory testing.
4. Administer isotonic crystalloids as needed to support blood pressure and perfusion.
5. Control seizures (p. 24).
6. Treat hyperthermia if present (p. 25).

Decontaminate

- Induce emesis *only* if the ingestion was within the last 60 minutes and the patient shows no clinical signs.
- Perform gastric lavage if the ingestion was within the last 2 to 4 hours.
- Give repeated doses of activated charcoal.
- Administer saline cathartic. Magnesium-containing solutions should be avoided.
- Consider whole-bowel irrigation using CoLyte or GoLYTELY.

DERMAL EXPOSURE (INSECTICIDES)

Wash with warm water, dishwashing liquid, or unmedicated shampoo. Rinse thoroughly.

Administer antidotes or other indicated supportive care

Atropine is indicated for parasympathetic signs. The dose should be titrated to effect; often amounts equal to those used in organophosphate intoxication will be required.

Enhancement of elimination

Acidification of the urine (p. 59) may shorten the time of recovery in patients by promoting urinary excretion. This should not be attempted when the patient is acidemic (pH <7.3).

Avoid

Avoid antacids because nicotine is better absorbed from an alkaline stomach.

NONSTEROIDAL ANTIINFLAMMATORY DRUGS (NSAIDs)

See also *Acetaminophen, Aspirin*

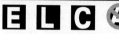

Sources Many analgesics, antipyretics, antiinflammatory drugs belong to this class of drug. Examples include indomethacin, piroxicam (Feldene), ibuprofen (Motrin, Advil, Nuprin, Vick's DayQuil), phenylbutazone (Bute, Butazolidin), naproxen (Naprosyn, Aleve).

Mechanism of action NSAIDS inactivate cyclooxygenase and therefore inhibit production of protective prostaglandins of the E-series. Reduced prostaglandin production results in reduced blood flow to the GI tract, reduced secretion of gastric mucus, and GI tract ischemia and ulceration (which may perforate). Prostaglandin inhibition also reduces blood flow to the kidneys resulting in renal papillary necrosis and acute renal failure. Newer NSAIDS such as carprofen are touted to have fewer toxic side effects because of decreased inhibition of prostaglandin synthesis and yet offer effective antiinflammatory action.

Clinical signs Abdominal pain, lethargy, anemia, melena, and hematemesis are most commonly seen with GI irritation and ulceration. If perforation has occurred, clinical signs may include abdominal pain, perhaps a fluid wave, shock, injected sclera, brick-red mucous membranes, and tachycardia. Temperature may be elevated or depressed. Pulses may be bounding or weak and thready.

Clinical signs associated with acute renal failure include hyposthenuria or isosthenuria, renal tubular cell casts in the urine sediment, or glucosuria without hyperglycemia. Urine gamma-glutamyltransferase (GGT) will be elevated. These early signs of acute renal failure will be followed by increasing BUN and creatinine, electrolyte disturbances, and possibly oliguria or more rarely polyuria. Occasionally, increased alanine amino-transferase (ALT) and alkaline phosphatase (ALP) may be seen.

Signs

Abdominal pain
Lethargy
Anemia
Melena, hematochezia
Hematemesis
Increased BUN and creatinine
Hyposthenuria or isosthenuria
Renal tubular casts
Glucosuria without hyperglycemia
Increased ALT and ALP
Hypoventilation or apnea in some cases
Acid-base disorders (sometimes initial alkalemia with later metabolic acidemia)
Signs of peritonitis if perforation
Coma, rarely seizures

Treatment   Treatment involves preventing or correcting GI ulceration, perforation, and acute renal failure. There is no specific antidote for NSAIDs.

EMERGENCY TREATMENT

Procedures

1. Secure the airway and ventilate as necessary (pp. 5, 9).
2. Administer supplemental oxygen (p. 7).
3. Secure venous access. Treat shock if needed. Collect blood and urine for laboratory testing. Obtain data base including biochemical profile, electrolytes, venous or arterial blood gases, and urinalysis.
4. Control seizures if necessary.
5. Insert a urethral catheter and administer crystalloids to maintain urine output of at least 2 to 3 mL/kg/hour in the dog and 1 to 2 mL/kg/hour in the cat. Rapid development of oliguria or anuria associated with NSAID

overdose dramatically increases the danger of overhydration. Patients must be monitored closely. Monitor central venous pressure if possible.

6. Perform serial monitoring of the urine to detect evidence of acute renal failure.

IF PERFORATION IS SUSPECTED

- Confirm with abdominocentesis. Consider diagnostic peritoneal lavage if abdominocentesis fails to confirm yet suspicion is high.
- Support the patient and perform exploratory surgery to repair perforation.
- Perform thorough abdominal lavage using large quantities of sterile saline
- Continue treatment with open abdominal techniques or intermittent abdominal lavage and active drainage.
- Provide IV broad-spectrum antibiotics.

IF RENAL DAMAGE IS SUSPECTED BASED ON URINE ANALYSIS

- Treat acid-base and electrolyte imbalances:
    a. Fluid therapy with crystalloids will usually correct the acid-base problems. If severe acidemia is present (pH <7.1), administer sodium bicarbonate.
    b. Treat hyperkalemia if present (p. 41).
- Continue crystalloids to maintain urine production of at least 2 to 3 mL/kg/hour in the dog and 1 mL/kg/hour in the cat.
- Administer furosemide (Lasix) dopamine, or mannitol, or all three, to maintain urine production as above.
- Monitor CVP, blood pressure, and urine output.

Decontaminate

- Induce emesis if recent ingestion (2 to 4 hours) or if signs are not present (p. 50).
- Gastric lavage if signs are present after ingestion (p. 52).
- Adminster activated charcoal and a saline cathartic; repeat PRN q4-6h (pp. 54, 56).

Administer antidotes or other indicated supportive care

- Protect the GI tract:
    a. Administer sucralfate.

b. Administer misoprostol (Cytotec) at 1 to 5 µg/kg q8-12h PO (dog only) for ulcer prophylaxis.
c. Administer omeprazole at 0.7 mg/kg q24h PO dog only.
d. H_2-receptor antagonists have *not* been shown to be of benefit as a prophylactic therapy against NSAID-induced GI ulcers.

Enhancement of elimination

Call the poison control center for advice concerning the specific NSAID in question.

Avoid

Gentamycin and other nephrotoxic drugs.

Suggested Reading

Engelhardt J, Brown S: Drug-related nephropathies, Part 2: Commonly used drugs, *Compend Cont Ed Pract Vet* 9(3):281-288, 1987.

Gfeller RW, Sandors AD: Naproxen-associated duodenal ulcer complicated by perforation and bacteria- and barium sulfate–induced peritonitis in a dog, *J Am Vet Med Assoc* 198(4):644-646, 1991.

Kore A: Ibuprofen.In Kirk RW, Bonagura JD, editors: *Current veterinary therapy*, ed 11, Philadelphia, 1992, Saunders.

Matz M: Gastrointestinal ulcer therapy. In Bonagura JD, Kirk RW, editors: *Current veterinary therapy*, ed 12, Philadelphia, 1992, Saunders.

Murphy M: Toxin exposures in dogs and cats: drugs and household products, *J Am Vet Med Assoc* 205(4):557-560, 1994.

Spyridakis LK, Bacia JJ, Barsanti JA, Brown SA: Ibuprofen toxicosis in a dog, *J Am Vet Med Assoc* 189(8): 918-919, 1986.

Thomas N: Piroxicam-associated gastric ulceration in a dog, *Compend Cont Ed Pract Vet* 9(10):1004-1030, 1987.

Vasseur PB, Johnson AL, Budsberg SC, et al: Randomized, controlled trial of the efficacy of carprofen, a nonsteroidal anti-inflammatory drug, in the treatment of osteoarthritis in dogs, *J Am Vet Med Assoc* 206(6):807-811, 1995.

ONION AND GARLIC TOXICITY

Sources   Food, flea products (garlic), health food products (garlic)

Mechanism of action   The active ingredient in oil of onion is allyl propyl disulfide; the active ingredient in oil of garlic is a similar compound called "allicin." Onions act as oxidizing agents that cause Heinz body anemia. Garlic appears to be safe, but anemia has been observed in chronic toxicity studies. Garlic may cause contact dermatitis or imitate an asthmatic attack.

Clinical signs   Signs are secondary to anemia and include pale mucous membranes, tachycardia, tachypnea, lethargy, and weakness. Vomiting, diarrhea, and hematuria or hemoglobinuria secondary to intravascular hemolysis can be seen. Microscopically, Heinz bodies, leptocytes, and poikilocytes may be observed.

Treatment   No specific antidote exists. Treatment is supportive and is an attempt to reduce the oxidative effects of the active ingredient and prevent renal damage caused by hemoglobinuria.

EMERGENCY TREATMENT

Procedures

1.   Secure the airway and ventilate as necessary (pp. 5, 9).
2.   Administer supplemental oxygen (p. 7).
3.   Secure venous access. Collect blood and urine for laboratory testing.
4.   Administer isotonic crystalloids as needed to support blood pressure and perfusion.
5.   Perform type and major and minor crossmatch and administer fresh, whole blood, stored blood, packed red

blood cells if packed cell volume is less than 15% to 20%. Nonstromal hemoglobin solutions are near marketing in veterinary medicine. These may be used without blood typing and crossmatching when available.

Decontaminate

- Induce emesis if the ingestion was within the last 60 minutes and the patient shows no clinical signs.
- Perform gastric lavage if the ingestion was within the last 2 to 4 hours.
- Administer saline cathartic.

Administer antidotes or other indicated supportive care

1. Administer crystalloid fluids to induce brisk diuresis to avoid renal damage caused by hemoglobinuria. Monitor urine output and central venous pressure.
2. Monitor blood gases and urine pH. It is imperative that acidic urine not be allowed because acidic urine will promote renal damage from hemoglobinuria. Correct with sodium bicarbonate as needed (p. 139).

Enhancement of elimination

There are no known effective measures.

Avoid

Many baby foods are reported to contain onion. Avoid feeding these baby foods to recovering patients.

Suggested Reading

Murphy M: Toxin exposures in dogs and cats: pesticides and biotoxins, *J Am Vet Med Assoc* 205(3):414-419, 1994.

Poppenga R: Risks associated with herbal remedies. In Bonagura JD, Kirk RW, editors: *Current veterinary therapy*, ed 12, Philadelphia, 1995, Saunders.

Solter P, Scott R: Onion ingestion and subsequent Heinz body anemia in a dog: a case report, *J Am Anim Hosp Assoc* 23:544-546, 1987.

ORGANIC SOLVENTS AND FUELS

   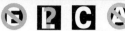

Sources This section includes many chemicals that are found in solvents, degreasing agents, dry cleaning agents, and fuels for camp stoves, warmers, etc. Acetone, benzene, benzol, methanol, methylene chloride, naphtha, trichloroethane, trichloroethylene, toluene, toluol, xylene, and xylol are examples included in this category.

Mechanism of action Nearly all these compounds cause pulmonary injury from direct effects with inhalation or systemic effects from ingestion and inhalation. Pulmonary aspiration is one of the greatest concerns in patients exposed to these compounds. Aspiration of very small amounts will likely induce chemical pneumonia. Most of these agents also have direct CNS-depressant effects. They are reported to be irritating to the skin, eyes, and mucous membranes. Further, they are known to sensitize the myocardium to catecholamines, thus increasing cardiac dysrhythmias. Hypoxemia may be seen if the patient was exposed to the compound in an enclosed space. Hepatic and renal injury may occur by undefined mechanisms.

Signs Inhalation or exposure to fumes causes conjunctivitis, nausea, vomiting, depression, wheezing, cyanosis, weak pulse, convulsions, and collapse. Signs noted after ingestion include nausea, vomiting, diarrhea (hemorrhagic at times), fixed pupils, ataxia, depression, and coma. Hemolysis and methemoglobinemia have been reorted with exposure to naphthalene and toluene.

Treatment Treating poisoning by inhalation requires removing the patient from the source, administering oxygen (when available), and washing the eyes copiously with water. Treating poisoning by ingestion involves oxygen therapy, treatment for aspiration or chemical pneumonia (see discussions of bronchospasm, p. 13, and pulmonary edema, p. 11), cautious gastric lavage, activated charcoal, and a cathartic. Epinephrine and other catecholamines should be avoided if possible because of the possible sensitization of the myocardium by these agents.

Signs

INHALATION	INGESTION
Conjunctivitis	Nausea
Nausea	Vomiting
Vomiting	Diarrhea (possibly bloody)
Depression	Fixed pupils
Cyanosis	Ataxia
Weak pulse	Depression
Convulsions	Methemoblobinemia
Collapse	Hemolysis
	Coma

EMERGENCY TREATMENT

Procedures

1. Secure the airway and ventilate as necessary (pp. 5, 9).
2. Administer supplemental oxygen (p. 7).
3. Secure venous access. Collect blood and urine for laboratory testing.
4. Administer isotonic crystalloids as needed to support blood pressure and perfusion.
5. Control seizures (p. 24).
6. Treat bronchospasm (p. 13), pulmonary edema (p. 11), methemoglobin (p. 11).

Decontaminate

- If exposure is by inhalation, remove the source or move the patient to a well-ventilated environment.
- *Do not induce emesis.*
- Perform cautious gastric lavage if the ingestion was within the last 1 to 2 hours. Take care not to allow aspiration of gastric contents during procedure.
- Give activated charcoal.
- Administer saline or sorbitol cathartic. Magnesium-containing solutions should be avoided.

- If exposure is dermal, bathe the patient in warm, soapy water or mild dishwashing detergent (Dawn) and rinse well with warm water. Perform this in a well-ventilated room. Avoid inducing hypothermia.

Administer antidotes or other indicated supportive care

1. There are no known antidotes.
2. Treat chemical pneumonia with oxygen, ventilation, nebulization, and coupage ('percussion of the thorax to aid in the removal of secretions'). Broad-spectrum antibiotics are not indicated prophylactically but may become necessary if the chemical pneumonia initiates bacterial infection. Monitor blood counts, sputum, and pulmonary washings as necessary to determine the need for antibiotics.
3. Monitor ECG and treat cardiac dysrhythmias. CAUTION: These agents cause increased myocardial sensitivity. Use of epinephrine or other sympathomimetic amines may induce or aggravate cardiac dysrhythmias.
4. Monitor urine output and renal parameters to observe for onset of acute renal failure.
5. Monitor for evidence of hepatic injury and treat accordingly.
6. Treat methemoglobinemia if present (p. 11).

Enhancement of elimination

There are no techniques that are effective.

Avoid

Catecholamines

Suggested Reading

Kirk RW, Bistner SI, Ford RB: *Handbook of veterinary procedures and emergency treatment*, ed 5, Philadelphia, 1990, Saunders.

Osweiler GD, Carson TL, Buck WB, Van Gelder GA: *Clinical and diagnostic veterinary toxicology*, ed 3, Dubuque, Iowa, 1985, Kendall/Hunt.

ORGANOCARBAMATE POISONING

See *Acute organophosphate and
organocarbamate poisoning*, p. 73

ORGANOCHLORINES
(CHLORINATED HYDROCARBONS)

Sources Insecticides. Organochlorine insecticides are not so commonly used as organophosphates. Possible products include DDD (Rhothane, TDE), DDT, Perthane, methoxychlor, toxaphene, chlordane, lindane, aldrin, dieldrin, heptachlor, and mirex.

Mechanism of action These compounds are highly lipid soluble and remain stored in the body for long periods of time. Skin and GI absorption occur; minimal biotransformation occurs. These insecticides allow an increase in intracellular sodium and potassium, which results in a decreased membrane potential. This hypopolarized membrane is more easily stimulated (lowered threshold), resulting in rapid and repeated neuronal discharge.

The cyclodene type of organochlorines (aldrin, dieldrin, chlordane, heptachlor, toxaphene) are more acutely toxic than the DDT type of organochlorines. They act by competitively inhibiting the binding of GABA at its receptors.

Some organochlorine compounds may increase myocardial sensitivity to the arrhythmogenic effects of catecholamines. Many of these compounds are metabolized to compounds that are injurious to the liver and kidneys.

Clinical signs Signs can be from acute or chronic intoxication. Acute signs resemble pyrethrin and organophosphate intoxication and include salivation, vomiting and nausea, restlessness, hyperexcitability, incoordination, muscle spasms, convulsions, seizures, respiratory failure, death. Seizures are often described as spinning on one foot or rolling and falling over backwards. Rarely the patient is presented in a depressed mental state. Excitation often results in an increased body temperature. Chronic exposure is seen as anorexia, weight loss, emaciation, tremors, convulsions, coma. Liver failure is possible. Cats are more sensitive than dogs.

Treatment   Treatment is supportive and includes removal of the toxin and symptomatic therapy. Seizures are controlled with anticonvulsants.

Signs

ACUTE
Salivation
Vomiting
Nausea
Restlessness
Hyperexcitability
Incoordination
Muscle spasms
Convulsions
Seizures
Hyperthermia
Respiratory failure
Death

CHRONIC
Anorexia
Weight loss
Emaciation
Tremors
Convulsions
Coma

EMERGENCY TREATMENT

Procedures

1.   Secure the airway and ventilate as necessary (pp. 5, 9).
2.   Administer supplemental oxygen (p. 7).

3. Secure venous access. Collect blood and urine for laboratory testing.
4. Control seizures (p. 24).
   Seizure control is often necessary for 24 hours or more. Phenobarbital may stimulate mixed function oxidase activity to shorten the half-life of organochlorine compounds.
5. Treat hyperthermia if present (p. 25).
6. Administer crystalloid fluids to maintain hydration, perfusion, and urine output.

Decontaminate

GI EXPOSURE (INGESTION)
- Induce emesis if recent ingestion (30 to 60 minutes) if signs are not present (p. 50).
- Perform gastric lavage if signs are present after ingestion (p. 52).
- Administer activated charcoal and a saline cathartic (p. 56).

Administer antidotes and other supportive care

There are no known effective antidotes.

DERMAL EXPOSURE
Wash thoroughly with warm, soapy water. Wear rubber gloves when bathing the patient; avoid inducing hypothermia.

Enhancement of elimination

There are no known effective methods. Organochlorine insecticides are eliminated in the urine after hepatic metabolism; diuresis is *not* effective. Repeat doses of activated charcoal are not likely to enhance elimination.

Suggested Reading

Morgan RV: *Handbook of small animal practice*, ed 2, New York, 1992, Churchill Livingstone, p 1097.

ORGANOPHOSPHATE-INDUCED DELAYED NEUROPATHY

(For acute toxicity, see p. 73)

Sources Insecticides and anthelminthics including malathion, parathion, Diazinon, carbaryl (Sevin), bendiocarb (Ficam), propoxur (Baygon, Sendran), chlorpyrifos (Dursban), methyl-carbamate, chlorfenvinphos (Dermaton Dip), cythioate (Proban), dichlorvos (Vapona), dioxathion, fenthion (ProSpot), ronnel, phosmet, DFP, fenitrothion, EPN, cyanofenphos (Amaze, Oftanol), trichlornate, mipafox, trichlorfon, tri-*ortho*-cresol phosphate (TOCP).

Mechanism of action Inhibits acetylcholinesterase acutely. After single or multiple doses with dermal or oral exposure, a delayed neurotoxicity may be seen. Signs vary with the dose and duration of exposure but can be seen within 7 to 14 days or as late as weeks to months after exposure. The brain and spinal cord contain neurotoxic esterases that can bind to organophosphates. The complex undergoes a time-dependent aging process. When aged, the complex becomes neurotoxic destroying axons and myelin sheaths (a "dying-back" phenomenon). Long peripheral nerves farthest from the spinal cord are most vulnerable. Motor and sensory nerves are affected.

Clinical signs Varying degrees of posterior paralysis are seen. Also, goose-stepping, high-stepping, weakness, ataxia, ascending paralysis (usually flaccid). Lower motor neuron signs and muscle atrophy are seen. Death is from respiratory paralysis.

Treatment None; some improvement may occur.

Suggested Reading

Miller M: Organophosphate toxicity in domestic animals, Part 2: Delayed effects, *Vet Med Small Anim Clin* 78:771-784, 1983.

OVER-THE-COUNTER MEDICATIONS: COLD AND ALLERGY REMEDIES

See also *Acetaminophen and phenacetin,*
Antihistamines, Aspirin, Decongestants,
Nonsteroidal antiinflammatory drugs,
Vitamins

There are numerous over-the-counter products that are used to treat colds and allergies in humans. These products contain one or more of the following general types of drugs:

- Analgesic and antipyretic (such as acetaminophen or phenacetin, aspirin (acetylsalicylic acid), nonsteroidal antiinflammatory drugs (NSAIDs) (Ibuprofen, Naproxasyn)
- Antitussive (such as dextromethorphan)
- Antihistamine (chlorpheniramine, brompheniramine, diphenhydramine, doxylamine)
- Decongestant (ephedrine, oxymetazoline, phenylephrine, pseudephedrine, phenylpropanolamine)
- Expectorant (guaifenesin)

Although fatal intoxication is (thankfully) not common, these products are responsible for a significant number of cases of small animal poisoning. They are administered by well-intentioned owners or ingested accidently and often produce undesirable effects. In one author's practice (RWG) the most common class of ingredient causing acute signs is the sympathomimetic amine decongestant (p. 122). The class responsible for the second most frequent presentation is the analgesic class. These drugs are frequently less acute but cause more serious complications. In general, treatment is supportive, and most animals recover from intoxication with these products.

Common products   Tylenol, Vick's NyQuil, Sine-Off, Sine-Aid, Actifed, Sudafed, Tylenol Sinus, Tylenol Allergy Sinus, Tylenol Cold, Vick's 44, Alka-Seltzer Plus, Excedrin, Anacin, Anacin 3, Comtrex, Triaminic, Drixoral, Chlor-Trimeton, and many others.

EMERGENCY TREATMENT

See specific type of drug (such as Acetaminophen, Antihistamine, Decongestant).

PARADICHLOROBENZENE (mothballs)

See also *Naphthalene*

Sources Paradichlorobenzene is the active ingredient in most moth cakes and moth crystals and is being substituted for naphthalene in mothballs. It has also been used in toilet bowl, diaper pail, and restroom deodorizers.

Mechanism of action Paradichlorobenzene is an organochlorine insecticide of relatively low toxicity. Ingestions may cause CNS excitement and seizures as a result of partial depolarization of nerve cell membranes. It is metabolized to a phenol that is hepatotoxic.

Clinical findings

- The most common sign is vomiting.
- A typical odor of mothballs is usually noted emanating from the patient or its vomitus.
- CNS signs including seizures may been seen as a result of CNS stimulation.
- Rarely, signs of hepatitis

Diagnosis

Usually based on history of ingestion or typical odor of mothballs (patient's breath, around mouth, in vomitus).

EMERGENCY TREATMENT

Procedures

1. Secure airway and support ventilation if required.
2. Secure venous access.
3. Control seizures or CNS signs (p. 24). If seizures are present, seizure control may be required for 24 hours or longer.
4. Monitor liver function.

Decontaminate

- Do not induce vomiting.
- Perform gastric lavage only if a known toxic amount was ingested within the last 30 to 60 minutes.
- Administer activated charcoal (p. 54).
- Administer saline cathartics (p. 56).

PARAQUAT

 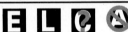

Source   Herbicide

Mechanism of action   Paraquat accumulates in the lungs where it readily accepts an electron to become a free radical. When this free radical is oxidized, it gives up an electron as a superoxide radical, which is extremely unstable and spontaneously breaks down to the highly reactive, singlet oxygen. Singlet oxygen reacts with and destroys phospholipid cellular membranes. Hydroxyl radicals and arachidonic acid are liberated, leading to further membrane damage and subsequent cellular death.

Clinical findings It appears that more dogs are poisoned than cats; most common exposure is through ingestion. Massive ingestions may cause acute signs including CNS excitation, convulsions, vomiting, diarrhea, and respiratory distress. More commonly, there is a delay in onset of signs of 1 to 3 days after exposure. Surfaces exposed to paraquat are often irritated and possibly ulcerated. Initial signs are usually vomiting and lethargy. Dehydration is common. Respiratory signs begin 2 to 7 days after exposure. Dogs become tachypneic and dyspneic with moist crackles. Cyanosis is often seen. The breathing pattern may be rapid and shallow or rapid and deep. The pulmonary damage is progressive but dose dependent. If the pet survives initially, the lungs may still fail because of pulmonary fibrosis. Death from acute effects usually occurs within 7 days. Death from chronic effects may occur after as many as 21 days.

Radiographs may reveal pulmonary edema or pneumomediastinum initially. If the animal survives the initial phase where pulmonary edema is common, the lungs may become fibrotic, taking on a more pronounced interstitial radiographic pattern.

Diagnosis History of exposure and signs of toxicity are usually all that is available to the veterinarian for antemortem diagnosis. Urine may be analyzed to confirm exposure but must be done in the first 2 days after exposure to be of most value. Postmortem examination of tissues may help establish the diagnosis. Analysis of the suspected source of exposure is possible in commercial laboratories. Paraquat on plants will degrade in sunlight in approximately 3 weeks.

EMERGENCY TREATMENT ∎

Procedures

1. The most important aspect of treatment is to remove ingested paraquat.
2. Induce emesis (p. 50) if ingestion was within the last 30 to 60 minutes.
3. Perform gastric lavage if indicated (p. 52).

4. Administer adsorbent. Kaolin, clay, or bentonite are preferred over activated charcoal. Pulverized-clay kitty litter is an appropriate adsorbent. If none of these products is immediately available, activated charcoal is preferable to waiting for acquisition of a clay.
5. Administer a saline or osmotic cathartic if ingestion was within previous 12 hours.

Administer antidotes or other indicated supportive care

There are no known antidotes.
Other agents that have been used experimentally in paraquat toxicosis include:

Niacin
Riboflavin
Ascorbic acid
Superoxide dismutase
N-Acetylcysteine

Enhancement of elimination

- Diuresis may be helpful, but care must be taken to avoid adding to problems of pulmonary edema.
- Dialysis may be useful but may contribute to pulmonary edema.
- Hemoperfusion is effective in removing the toxin if begun early after exposure.

Avoid

- Oxygen is *contraindicated* early in paraquat poisoning. Oxygen administration may cause increased formation of oxyradicals.
- Clients should be made aware that the prognosis in cases of paraquat poisoning is poor.

PCP

See *Phencyclidine*

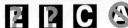

PENITREM A

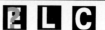

Sources   A neurotoxin often found in moldy food, garbage, grains, and nuts including walnuts, almonds, and peanuts.

Mechanism of action   Although there is little in the literature that gives specific actions, there is a suggestion that penitrem A acts to increase resting potential, increase transmission of impulses across motor end plates, and increase duration of depolarization of affected nerves. It is also suggested that penitrem A may inhibit glycine (a neurotransmitter) in the spinal cord, much like strychnine.

Clinical signs   Ingestion of moldy nuts or garbage that contains the tremorogenic substance penitrem A results in rapid onset of signs. Signs include hypersalivation, drooling, panting, restlessness, and mild incoordination. Urination may be seen. Higher doses cause muscle tremors that may progress to pronounced tonic spasms (resembling strychnine), hyperthermia, seizures, and death. The muscle tremors may be worsened by external stimuli such as loud noises and touch (much like strychnine), but this is not so consistent as in strychnine poisoning. That is to say, with penitrem A, a touch may cause tonic spasms once or twice out of several touches, whereas strychnine-poisoned dogs will have a spasm with every stimulus. Excessive muscle activity may result in hyperthermia, rhabdomyolysis, dehydration, and exhaustion. Hyperglycemia has been reported, possibly caused by catecholamine release. In lactating bitches, the signs of penitrem A ingestions have been confused with those for eclampsia.

Treatment   If the toxin was ingested within the last 15 to 30 minutes and the patient is showing no signs, emesis should be induced. Activated charcoal and cathartic are advised.

If the patient is showing signs, *emesis is contraindicated*. The patient should be anesthetized and a gastric lavage performed to remove the molded ingesta. Activated charcoal is indicated, as is sorbitol or osmotic cathartic.

We note that, on several occasions, client funds have precluded aggressive treatment listed above, but treatment with activated charcoal, acepromazine, and intravenous methocarbamol have resulted in satisfactory recovery. Whether this would work in all cases is not scientifically studied and therefore not recommended as first-line treatment.

Clinical findings

Hypersalivation, ptyalism
Restlessness
Muscle tremors
Hyperreactivity to external stimuli
Tonic spasms
Seizures
Death

EMERGENCY TREATMENT

Procedures

1. Secure the airway and ventilate the patient as needed (pp. 5, 9).
2. Control excessive muscle activity, tremors, spasms, seizures (p. 24).
3. Secure venous access. Administer crystalloids as necessary to support blood pressure and perfusion.

Decontaminate

1. Remove toxin by induction of emesis if ingestion was recent (within the last 5 to 15 minutes) and the patient is showing *no* signs.
2. Perform gastric lavage if ingestion was within the last 60 minutes. Consider radiograph of stomach.
3. Administer activated charcoal. It is unknown if repeating administration of activated charcoal has any advantage.
4. Administer saline or sorbitol cathartics (p. 56).

Administer antidotes or other indicated supportive care

1. Although acepromazine is known to lower seizure threshold in animals, it may be used with caution to control tremors associated with penitrem A.
2. Intravenous administration of methocarbamol has been used with success in control of penitrem A–induced tremors.
3. Administer crystalloids to maintain hydration and urine output.

PENNYROYAL OIL POISONING

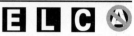

Uses   Flea control, fragrance, and flavoring agent.

Common products   Pennyroyal oil, found in many health food stores.

Mechanism of action   Pennyroyal oil is derived from the leaves and flowering tops of pennyroyal plants (a member of the Labiatae family, also called "squaw mint" or "mosquito plants"). Pulegone is the toxic ingredient in pennyroyal oil; pulegone is biotransformed in the liver to menthofuran, a toxin. Effects are dose related. Pulegone constitutes 85% of pennyroyal oil and causes hepatocellular necrosis.

Clinical signs   Signs may be seen after dermal or oral exposure and may include nausea, emesis, dyspnea, GI bleeding, seizures, coma, coagulation abnormalities, DIC, hepatic necrosis, and death.

Treatment   No antidote is available. Immediate induction of emesis and administration of activated charcoal and a cathartic are indicated. Animals should be bathed repeatedly until no residue of the oil remains. Additional fluid therapy for support and anticonvulsants for seizures are used.

Because of the possibility of hepatic failure and disseminated intravascular coagulation, these conditions should be detected early by repeated blood profiles and urinalyses; treatment is directed toward either of these conditions as they develop. Blood loss can be treated with blood or plasma as needed.

Signs

Nausea
Emesis
Dyspnea
GI bleeding
Seizures
Coma
Coagulation abnormalities (disseminated intravascular coagulation)
Hepatic necrosis
Death

EMERGENCY TREATMENT

Procedures

1. Secure the airway and ventilate as necessary (pp. 5, 9).
2. Administer supplemental oxygen (p. 7).
3. Secure venous access. Collect blood and urine for laboratory testing.
4. Control seizures (p. 24).
5. Treat hyperthermia if present (p. 25).
6. Administer fluids to maintain perfusion, hydration, and urine output.

Administer antidotes and other indicated supportive care

- There are no effective antidotes
- Blood, plasma, or fresh frozen plasma if disseminated intravascular coagulation or other coagulopathy develops.

Decontaminate

GI EXPOSURE (INGESTION)
- Induce emesis if recent ingestion and if signs are not present (p. 50).
- Gastric lavage if signs are present after ingestion (p. 52).
- Adminster activated charcoal and a saline cathartic; repeat PRN q4-6h (p. 56).

DERMAL EXPOSURE
Wash thoroughly with warm, soapy water. Wear rubber gloves when bathing the patient; avoid chilling the patient.

Suggested Reading

Poppenga R: Risks associated with herbal remedies. In Bonagura JD, Kirk RW, editors: *Current veterinary therapy*, ed 12, Philadelphia, 1995, Saunders.

Sudekum M, Poppenga RH, Raju N, Braselton WE Jr: Pennyroyal oil toxicosis in a dog, *J Am Vet Med Assoc* 200(6):817-818, 1992.

PERSIMMON TOXICITY

Common products   Persimmons

Uses   Fruits

Mechanism of action   Unsure, but several cases have been reported of intestinal obstruction by the seeds and bacterial enteritis.

Clinical signs   Intestinal necrosis with subsequent peritonitis was reported post mortem in lories. Larger birds (Amazon parrots) have ingested persimmons without signs.

Treatment   None; diagnosed post mortem.

PHENCYCLIDINE (PCP)

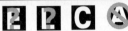

Sources Phencyclidine is a dissociative anesthetic agent that is easily synthesized and produced illegally. Known as "angel dust," "hog," or "PCP," it is commonly sold on the illegal market as a "recreational" drug. It is sold in powder, tablet, crystal, liquid, and leaf mixture forms with purity running from 5% to 90%.

Mechanism of action PCP causes stimulation or depression of the CNS, but the mechanism of action is obscure.

Clinical findings

CNS depression or excitation
Mydriasis, nystagmus
Sniffing activity
Tonic-clonic convulsions
Hypersalivation
"Fly biting" or "jaw snapping"
Opisthotonus
Tachycardia
Elevated blood pressure and increased cardiac output
Hyperthermia is common
Acidemia
Respiratory failure
Cardiac dysrhythmias
Hypotension
Myoglobinuria
Death

Laboratory findings

- Evidence of acute renal failure (such as renal tubular casts, isosthenuria, oliguria, anuria, glycosuria without hyperglycemia, proteinuria)
- Hypoglycemia may be seen.
- Increased serum aspartate aminotransferase (SAST) and creatine phosphokinase
- Myoglobinuria

EMERGENCY TREATMENT

Procedures

1. Secure the airway and assist ventilation if necessary.
2. Treat seizures (p. 24), coma (p. 29), rhabdomyolysis and myoglobinuria (p. 26), hypertension (p. 22), and hyperthermia (p. 25) as necessary.
3. Maintain hydration with crystalloid fluids.
4. Support renal function with fluids, furosemide, or dopamine drip (1 to 3 µg/kg/min).
5. Sedate the patient if CNS stimulation or hyperactivity is a problem. Diazepam may be used. Although acepromazine is known to lower the seizure threshold, it may be useful in sedating the patient as well as treating hypertension.

Decontaminate

- Emesis or gastric lavage is of little value because of the rapid absorption of PCP.
- Administer activated charcoal. Repeat the dose every 2 to 4 hours.
- Administer a cathartic (p. 56).

Administer antidotes or other supportive care

There are no known specific antidotes or drugs for the treatment of PCP intoxication.

Enhancement of elimination

- Forced diuresis may promote elimination of the drug through renal excretion.
- Although urinary concentrations of PCP are increased with urinary acidification, there is no evidence that this results in enhanced elimination. Furthermore, urinary acidification may increase the risk of renal damage and subsequent failure in patients with myoglobinuria. It is not recommended.

PHENOLICS

Sources Phenol and phenolic compounds are coal-tar derivatives found in disinfectants, drugs and foods (benzoic acid), caustics (phenol), keratolytics (phenol and resorcinol), soaps (3% hexachlorophene, pHisoHex), and antiseborrheic shampoos and other products (phenol and coal tar).

Mechanism of action Phenols denature and precipitate proteins of all cells. They are extremely corrosive and produce penetrating lesions. In lower doses, phenols and phenolic compounds cause direct stimulation of the respiratory center of the brain. The result is hyperventilation and respiratory alkalosis. Metabolic compensation for the respiratory alkalosis results in renal excretion of bicarbonate. The phenols are mildly acidic and disrupt carbohydrate metabolism. The respiratory alkalosis is followed by metabolic acidosis. Phenols are absorbed rapidly from the GI tract as well as percutaneously. Cats, certain reptiles, and birds are highly sensitive to phenols. Phenolics are caustic to mucous membranes, causing visible corrosion. Most pets will not ingest enough product to cause esophageal injuries. Cutaneous exposure with concentrated products results in corrosive injury that is initially white in color followed by the development of dry dermal eschar formation. Severe corneal injury including ulceration and penetration result from contact with phenolic compounds. Hexachlorophene causes demyelination and spongiosis of white matter.

Clinical signs Profuse ptyalism, anorexia, emesis, panting, and ataxia are seen. As time progresses, muscle fasciculations, shock, and unconsciousness may develop. Mucous membranes may be dark because of respiratory depression and methemoglobinemia. Hepatic and renal damage are seen within 12 to 24 hours.

Toxicity with hexachlorophene is most commonly seen in young puppies and kittens bathed with pHisoHex. This product is slightly water insoluble and remains on the skin after bathing, which allows skin penetration. Signs of hexachlorophene toxicity include weakness, trembling, lethargy, shock, muscle tremors, hypothermia, tachycardia, tachypnea.

Excretion of phenolic metabolites may discolor the urine green or black; addition of ferric chloride to the urine turns it purple or blue.

Treatment   *Phenolic intoxications are true emergencies.* Owners should be instructed to administer water, milk, or egg whites before transport to the veterinary hospital. Emesis should not be induced nor should gastric lavage be attempted if esophageal injury is suspected. Otherwise gastric lavage and activated charcoal are the treatment of choice. N-Acetylcysteine (Mucomyst) may prevent renal and hepatic injury. Ascorbic acid or methylene blue is used to correct methemoglobinemia. Respiratory alkalosis followed by metabolic acidosis is often seen and treated as needed; oxygen is given as necessary. Exposed skin should be washed with soap and water.

Neurologic signs seen in experimental hexachlorophene poisoning in cats were treated with 30% urea and resulted in a rapid decrease in CSF pressure; cats did not respond to treatment with prednisolone or acetazolamide. Experimentally, adult cats given 20 mg/kg/day developed neurologic signs within 2 weeks of daily administration; paralyzed cats that did not develop coma completely recovered within 4 to 6 weeks after treatment with urea and supportive care.

Signs

Profuse salivation
Anorexia
Emesis
Panting
Respiratory stimulation followed by depression
Ataxia
Muscle fasciculations
Shock
Unconsciousness
Dark mucous membranes
Green or black urine

EMERGENCY TREATMENT

Procedures

1. Carefully secure the airway and ventilate as necessary (pp. 5, 9).
2. Administer supplemental oxygen (p. 7).
3. Secure venous access. Collect blood and urine for laboratory testing.
4. Administer isotonic crystalloids as needed to support blood pressure and perfusion.
5. Treat methemoglobinemia if present (p. 181).
6. Treat hyperthermia if present (p. 25).

Decontaminate

INGESTION
- Do not induce vomiting.
- Perform gastric lavage if ingestion was within the last 2 hours and oral examination (and perhaps esophagoscopy) reveals no severe corrosive injury or perforation.
- Give repeated doses of activated charcoal (may be effective for hexachlorophene toxicity because it is excreted in the bile).
- Administer saline cathartic.

DERMAL EXPOSURE
- Wash the patient in polyethylene glycol or glycerol followed by thorough washing with dishwashing liquid and copious rinsing. *Caregivers should wear protective gloves, clothing, and face shields.*
- Injured areas should be covered with bandages soaked in 0.5% sodium bicarbonate.

OCULAR EXPOSURE
- Irrigate the eye in isothermic, sterile 0.9% saline for 30 minutes.
- Treat corneal ulcers with generally accepted treatment options.

Administer antidotes or other indicated supportive care

- Mucomyst may be indicated to help avoid renal and hepatic damage.

Enhancement of elimination

There are no known effective techniques.

PINE OILS

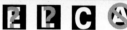

Sources   Sanitizers, disinfectants.

Mechanism of action   The lethal dose for small mammals is estimated at 1.0 to 2.5 mL/kg; a lower dose can result in severe intoxication. Pine oils are directly irritating to mucous membranes. They are readily absorbed from the GI tract resulting in severe gastrointestinal signs. Renal cortical damage and CNS depression also occur.

Clinical signs   The odor of pine oil is often present; pronounced oral and pharyngeal irritation are usually seen. Vomiting, retching, progressive CNS signs including hyperesthesia, weakness, ataxia, and coma occur. Tachycardia, hyperthermia, and nephritis occur as well. Vomiting usually occurs after ingestion. Pulmonary damage results from aspiration or chemical pneumonia from absorption of pine oil from the GI tract and subsequent deposition in the lung.

Treatment   Owners should be advised to promptly administer water, milk, or egg whites. The patient should be transported to the hospital where it should be hospitalized and observed closely for at least 24 hours. Since aspiration pneumonia is a real danger and the onset of CNS depression can be rapid, induction of emesis is contraindicated (though nearly all patients will vomit after ingestion because of the irritating nature of pine oils). Gastric lavage may be a feasible treatment option but must be weighed against the risk of causing aspiration pneumonia. Activated charcoal and cathartics are given. Maintaining fluid and electrolyte balances is essential.

Signs

Pine oil odor
Pronounced oral and pharyngeal irritation
Retching, vomiting, hematemesis
Hyperesthesia
Pulmonary edema, dyspnea, tachypnea
Pneumonia
Severe CNS depression
Weakness
Ataxia
Tachycardia
Hyperthermia
Unresponsive pupils
Coma
Death

EMERGENCY TREATMENT

Procedures

1. Secure the airway and ventilate as necessary (pp. 5, 9).
2. Administer supplemental oxygen (p. 7).
3. Secure venous access. Collect blood and urine for laboratory testing.
4. Administer isotonic crystalloids as needed to support blood pressure and perfusion.
5. Treat pulmonary edema if present (p. 11).
6. Control seizures (p. 24).
7. Treat hyperthermia if present (p. 25).

Decontaminate

INGESTION

- Nearly all animals will vomit after ingestion of pine oil containing disinfectants. Induce emesis *only* if the inges-

tion was within the last 5 to 10 minutes and the patient shows no clinical signs; otherwise induction of emesis is contraindicated.
- Give water or milk as a diluent.
- Give activated charcoal.
- Administer saline or osmotic cathartic. Magnesium-containing solutions should be avoided.
- Gastric lavage is a risk. Perform only when the benefits of gastric emptying are believed to be greater than the risk of aspiration. In general, gastric lavage should be limited to patients who are known to have ingested large quantities of pine oil disinfectants within the last hour.

DERMAL EXPOSURE
- Bathe thoroughly with soap and water. Rinse well.

OCULAR EXPOSURE
- The eye should be irrigated with copious quantities of sterile isothermic isotonic saline or water for 20 to 30 minutes.
- Ocular damage should be treated using generally accepted treatment options.

Administer antidotes or other indicated supportive care

There are no known antidotes.

Enhancement of elimination

Resin hemoperfusion is most effective followed by charcoal hemoperfusion. Hemodialysis is minimally effective.

PIT VIPERS

Common species   Copperheads, rattlesnakes, water moccasins (cottonmouths)

Mechanism of action   The mechanism of action of snake venom depends mainly on the type of venom. Refer to the list of suggested readings. In general, snake venom contains hyaluronidase (which allows the venom to spread and penetrate tissues) and phospholipase A (which disrupts cell membranes, uncouples phosphorylation, and releases vasoactive amines). Enzymatic and nonenzymatic polypeptides are cardiotoxic and neurotoxic and contribute to release or activation of tissue peptidases.

Many venoms have procoagulant properties, and many have anticoagulant properties. Some venoms cause defibrination of plasma. The overall effects of severe envenomation by pit vipers is usually an overall anticoagulative state.

Clinical signs   Most bites involve the head, face, or neck; clinical experience dictates a poorer prognosis for bites involving the trunk (abdomen, thorax). Severe hypotension occurs because of blood pooling in the hepatosplanchnic bed in dogs and the lungs and thoracic vessels in cats. Local edema is noticeable as a result of vascular destruction, allowing massive leakage of red blood cells and plasma. Ecchymosis often is seen at the site of the bite within 30 to 60 minutes; if envenomation did not occur, no ecchymosis and only minor edema (if any) is noticed. Pain is usually severe after envenomation. It must be noted that the bite of the Mojave rattlesnake may have minimal local signs but may result in life-threatening paresis, paralysis, and respiratory failure.

Echinocytes (red blood cells resembling World War II sea mines) appear in the majority of envenomated dogs. They are seen on peripheral blood smears within 24 hours after the bite if envenomation occurs. They disappear from the blood within 48 to 72 hours. Hypokalemia often occurs with envenomation (indicating the need for supplementation during treatment with IV fluids). Hyperkalemia may be seen with venoms that cause extensive necrosis and hemolysis.

Envenomation does not always occur (bites may lack venom up to 25% of the time). The severity of envenomation is related to the time of the year (the peptide fraction is higher in the spring, and the enzyme fraction is higher in the fall), the volume of venom present since the previous bite, the aggressiveness of the snake, the size of the victim, the location of the bite, the number of bites, and the amount of victim activity after the bite (venom is absorbed through the lymphatics; excessive muscular movement causes the venom to spread faster). The amount of venom is *not* related to the size of the snake. Patients must be monitored frequently for signs of envenomation. With minimal or no envenomation there are few or no local signs, no systemic signs, and normal laboratory findings; with moderate to severe envenomations there are usually pronounced local signs, including edema, pain, and ecchymosis, and systemic signs as well as laboratory abnormalities that might indicate disseminated intravascular coagulation, renal failure, hepatic failure, or coagulopathies.

Systemic signs may take 24 to 72 hours to develop in mild envenomations, and so the animal should be observed closely.

Treatment   Restricting patient movement is essential to slow the spread of the venom; antihistamines can be used to calm the victim and prevent allergic reactions to the antivenin. Antivenin is recommended to counteract the venom. The use of antivenin is controversial, and many veterinarians choose not to use it. However, it is recommended in moderate to severe envenomations and in patients showing systemic signs. Antibiotics are used to prevent secondary infections. Although the package insert (of commercial antivenins) suggests using corticosteroids, their use is controversial. Because there are reports of increased morbidity and mortality when corticosteroids are used in treating envenomations, we believe they should be avoided. Local first-aid measures, such as applying tourniquets and incising wounds to aspirate venom, should be avoided. Repeated laboratory assessments (complete blood cell count [platelet count, in particular], coagulation profile, urinalysis) to check for coagulopathies and renal failure and monitoring the bite for development or progression of edema are important. Nonsteroidal antiinflammatory drugs are contraindicated in the acute phase of treatment (first 24 hours) because of the variable components of the venom and the anticoagulant effects of NSAIDs.

Clinical signs   (extremely variable)
Hypovolemic shock
Nausea, vomiting
Mental confusion
Dyspnea, tachypnea, hypoventilation
Muscular weakness, paresis, paralysis
Bleeding disorders, (disseminated intravascular coagulation, defibrination), petechiae, ecchymosis
Tachycardia, ventricular dysrhythmias
Anemia (bleeding diathesis, hemolysis)
Pain, swelling, tissue edema, myonecrosis, sloughing

EMERGENCY TREATMENT

Procedures

1. Secure the airway and ventilate as necessary (pp. 5, 9), especially in the case of Mojave rattlesnake bite.
2. Administer supplemental oxygen (p. 7).
3. Secure venous access. Collect blood and urine for laboratory testing.
4. Administer isotonic crystalloids as needed to support blood pressure and perfusion.
5. Treat hemolysis, hemoglobinuria, acute renal failure as needed.
6. Immobilize the pet and affected area to slow venom spread.

Administer antidotes or other indicated treatments

- Antivenin (Antivenin [Crotalidae] Polyvalent [Equine origin], Fort Dodge Laboratories, Inc., Fort Dodge, Iowa (1-800-677-3728) or Wyeth-Ayerst (1-800-666-7248). At least 1 vial is given IV if needed; the smaller the patient, the more antivenin is usually needed. The need for administration of additional vials is indicated by progression rather than arrest or regression of clinical or laboratory findings.
- Administer blood products as needed based on detection of anemia or coagulopathies. Fresh whole blood, stored whole blood, or packed red blood cells are indicated for acute anemia. Fresh whole blood, fresh plasma, fresh frozen plasma, or cryoprecipitate may be indicated for coagulopathies.
- Although glucocorticosteroids are known to block phospholipase A_2 (a common component of pit viper venom), their use remains controversial. Literature can be found to support both sides of the controversy. No clear-cut benefit or detriment has been clearly shown. For the time being, we would recommend that administration of glucocorticoids be avoided or, at the very least, limited for use on patients who are in shock or have had hypersensitive reactions to the antivenin.

- Broad-spectrum antibiotics are indicated in most cases.
- Antihistamine use is also controversial, though recent literature seems to promote the use of diphenhydramine to calm the animal and may play a role in the rare instance of histamine-mediated swelling. Antihistamines are indicated in the case of allergic reaction to the antivenin and may be given before antivenin to lessen the incidence or severity of allergic reaction.
- Analgesia. The majority of pit viper envenomations (with the exception of the Mojave rattlesnake) result in intense pain to the patient. The use of pain-relieving drugs is indicated. NSAIDs with known anticoagulant effects (such as aspirin) should be avoided.
- Wound excision or fasciotomy are rarely indicated.

Monitor

- For coagulopathies: fibrin degradation products, activated clotting times, platelet counts.
- For cardiac dysrhythmias.
- For signs of acute renal failure: urine output, urine sediment for presence of renal tubular casts, glycosuria without concurrent hyperglycemia, proteinuria, increasing BUN and creatinine (late signs).
- For progression of swelling: measure the bite site above and below and record every 15 minutes. If the site is on the torso, shave the hair and mark the boundaries of swelling with a marker. Repeat every 15 minutes. If swelling is in the neck area, prepare for emergency tracheotomy.

Enhancement of elimination

There are no known effective techniques.

Avoid

- Electrical shock therapy does not work.
- Respiratory depressant analgesic drugs, especially in animals exhibiting weakness.
- Acidosis, especially when rhabdomyolysis or hemoglobinuria is present. More severe renal complications will result.

Notes on antivenin   To be most effective, antivenin should be given within 4 hours of the bite. It is less effective after 8 hours and may be ineffective after 12 hours; however, in severe envenomation, antivenin may be helpful even if 24 hours has elapsed since the bite. Maximum blood levels may not be reached for 8 hours after IM administration.

The pet is skin tested before administration following package directions. If the skin test is positive, antivenin may still be given with careful monitoring of the pet. Antivenin should be given slowly to prevent allergic reactions (monitor the pinnae for erythema, which is an early sign of an allergic reaction). Antivenin is always given slowly to avoid activating the complement cascade.

If a reaction occurs during administration, stop the antivenin, give diphenhydramine IV very slowly at 0.5 to 2.2 mg/kg, wait several minutes, and restart antivenin slowly observing for another reaction. If a second reaction occurs, stop administration and consult a specialist. Antivenin is expensive (1997 cost, $178).

One of us (RWG) administers 1 vial of antivenin initially when indicated. If systemic signs remain (ongoing shock, tachycardia, decreasing platelet counts performed q2-6h, cardiac dysrhythmias, continued swelling of the wound) on serial examinations, additional vials are administered.

Suggested Reading

Antivenin (Crotalidae) Polyvalent package insert, Fort Dodge Laboratories, Inc., Fort Dodge, Iowa 50501; 1-800-677-3728.

Antivenin package insert, Wyeth-Ayerst Laboratories, Inc., Radnor, PA 19355, 1-800-666-7248.

Brown DE, Meyer DJ, Wingfield WE, Walton RM: Echinocytosis associated with rattlesnake envenomation in dogs, *Vet Pathol* 31:654-657, 1994.

Driggers T: Venomous snakebites in horses, *Compend Cont Ed Pract Vet* 17(2):235-241, 1995.

Hudelson S, Hudelson P: Pathophysiology of snake envenomation and evaluation of treatments, Part 1, *Compend Cont Ed Pract Vet* 17(7):889-896, 1995.

Hudelson S, Hudelson P: Pathophysiology of snake envenomation and evaluation of treatments, Part 2, *Compend Cont Ed Pract Vet* 17(8):1035-1040, 1995.

Hudelson S, Hudelson P: Pathophysiology of snake envenomation and evaluation of treatments, Part 3, *Compend Cont Ed Pract Vet* 17(11):1385-1396, 1995.

Peterson M, Meerdink G: Bites and stings of venomous animals. In Kirk RW, Bonagura JD, editors: *Current veterinary therapy,* ed 10, Philadelphia, 1989, Saunders.

POISONOUS PLANTS

See *Section 3, Toxic plants*

PRESCRIPTION DRUGS

See *Barbituates, Birth control pills, Tricyclic antidepressants*

PYRETHRINS AND PYRETHROIDS

Sources Many brands of insecticides contain pyrethrins or pyrethroids. Topical flea products may contain pyrethrin, allethrin, fenvalerate, resmethrin, sumethrin, and permethrin. Premise sprays may contain pyrethrins, permethrins, cypermethrin, resmethrin, tetramethrin, cyfluthrin, fenvalerate, tralomethrin, fluvalinate, pallethrin, and other pyrethroids or carbamates, organophosphates, and insect growth regulators.

Mechanism of action   Pyrethrins and pyrethroids are fat-soluble compounds that undergo rapid metabolism and excretion after dermal or oral absorption. Plasma esterases detoxify most compounds; because organophosphates inhibit plama esterase activity, simultaneous exposure to organophosphates may increase pyrethrin and pyrethroid toxicity. Synergists, such as piperonyl butoxide, inhibit cytochrome P-450 and impede metabolism of pyrethrins and pyrethroids. Pyrethrins and pyrethroids are neurotoxicants that reversibly prolong sodium conductance (type 1 and type 2 pyrethrins), which results in repetitive nerve firing. Type 2 pyrethrins also antagonize GABA, resulting in a strychnine-like effect. This is similar to that of organochlorine insecticides. Dermal absorption is poor compared with oral absorption. Cats are more sensitive to these compounds than dogs because of decreased glucuronide conjugation of the compounds. Overdosing small pets is easier than overdosing large pets because of the larger body surface area–to–weight ratio of smaller pets.

Clinical signs   Signs of pyrethrin, pyrethroid, or fenvalerate intoxication include depression, hypersalivation, muscle tremors, vomiting, ataxia, dyspnea, and anorexia. Hypothermia or hyperthermia may also be seen. Death rarely occurs. Differential diagnosis includes decompensated cardiomyopathy and thyroid or adrenal neoplasia. Cats occasionally exhibit ear flicking, paw shaking, and repeated contractions of superficial cutaneous muscles. These signs may be seen because of agitation or as a direct result of peripheral nerve stimulation.

Pyrethrin and pyrethroid toxicity can be differentiated from organophosphate and carbamate toxicity by the fact that the whole-blood cholinesterase value is depressed with organophosphates and organocarbamates but not by pyrethrins and pyrethroids. An atropine test, using 0.02 to 0.04 mg/kg atropine given IV, can assist in differentiation of organophosphate and organocarbamate (OP/OC) intoxication from pyrethrin and pyrethroid intoxication. If the pet responds to this dose of atropine (as by decreased salivation, mydriasis), organophosphate and organocarbamate intoxication is unlikely. Higher doses of atropine are usually needed to reverse signs caused by OP/OC poisonings. This low dose will usually control signs associated with pyrethrin and pyrethroid intoxication. Although this test can help differentiate, there is no *definitive* in-house test to confirm the suspected diagnosis. Toxic signs in cats are seen within 1 to 3 hours of exposure.

Treatment There is no antidote. It is fortunate that most pets do not develop severe signs; however, deaths have been reported from exposure to pyrethrins or pyrethroids. Copious bathing to remove the compound is needed. Maintenance of normal body temperature is important (hypothermia increases the toxicity). Extremely warm water is contraindicated because this may increase dermal perfusion and increase absorption. Emetics can be given within 1 to 2 hours after application to decrease GI absorption; emesis is contraindicated if the toxic product also contains petroleum distillates. Activated charcoal (which can reduce neurologic signs by decreasing enterohepatic circulation of the toxins) and a cathartic are given. Seizures are uncommon but can be controlled with diazepam or phenobarbital. Atropine is not antidotal but can be given incrementally in small doses to control hypersalivation. Most pets recover from pyrethrin intoxication within 24 to 48 hours; recovery from pyrethroid products may take longer. Animals not showing improvement within 24 hours should be reevaluated. Deaths do occur.

Signs

Depression
Hypersalivation
Muscle tremors
Vomiting
Ataxia
Dyspnea, bronchospasm
Anorexia
Hypothermia or hyperthermia
In cats, additionally may see:
  Ear flicking
  Paw shaking
  Contractions of superficial cutaneous muscles

EMERGENCY TREATMENT

Procedures

1. Secure the airway and ventilate as necessary (pp. 5, 9).
2. Administer supplemental oxygen (p. 7). Treat bronchospasm if present (p. 13).

3. Secure venous access. Collect blood and urine for laboratory testing.
4. Administer isotonic crystalloids as needed to support blood pressure and perfusion.
5. Control seizures (p. 24).
6. Treat hyperthermia if present (p. 25).

Decontaminate

- Induce emesis *only* if the ingestion was within the last 60 minutes, the patient shows no clinical signs, and the produce contains no petroleum distillates.
- Perform gastric lavage if the ingestion was within the last 2 to 4 hours.
- Give repeated doses of activated charcoal.
- Administer saline cathartic. Cathartics containing magnesium should be avoided.
- Consider whole bowel irrigation using CoLyte or GoLYTELY.

DERMAL EXPOSURE

- Wash *thoroughly* with warm (not hot) soapy water and shampoo or liquid handwashing (not electric dishwashing) compounds.
- Wear rubber gloves when bathing the patient
- Avoid chilling the patient.

Administer antidotes or other indicated supportive care

- There is no effective antidote.
- Anaphylaxis may indicate the need for epinephrine.
- Use atropine at (0.02 to 0.04 mg/kg IV, SQ, IM) to control parasympathetic signs; repeat as needed but avoid atropine intoxication. *Remember that atropine is NOT an antidote for pyrethrin and pyrethroid toxicity and is used only as needed to control parasympathetic signs.*
- Administer crystalloid fluids to maintain hydration and urine output.
- Muscle relaxants such as methocarbamol may be of benefit to the patient with excessive muscle activity.

Enhancement of elimination

There are no effective techniques of enhanced elimination.

Avoid

Phenothiazine derivatives are contraindicated.

Suggested Reading

Hansen SR, Villor D, Buck WB, Stemme KA: Pyrethrins and pyrethroids in dogs and cats, *Compend Cont Ed Pract Vet* 16(6):707-712, 1994.

Whittem T: Pyrethrin and pyrethroid insecticide intoxication in cats, *Compend Cont Ed Pract Vet* 17(4):489-494, 1995.

RATTLESNAKES

See *Snakebites* or *Pit vipers*

SASSAFRAS

Sources   Oil of sassafras, tea, insecticide (used externally), stimulant and diuretic (used internally)

Mechanism of action   Sassafras oil comes from the sassafras tree and contains 50% safrole, 10% pinene and phennadrene, and 6% to 8% *d*-camphor. The oil is toxic if taken internally: as little as 5 mL is toxic for an adult human, but a single herbal tea bag may be toxic for an animal (based on toxicity studies in laboratory animals).

Clinical signs　Signs include nausea, vomiting, mydriasis, cardiovascular collapse, and CNS depression. Cats would be especially sensitive to the phenolics in the oil. Safrole is hepatotoxic, hepatocarcinogenic, and a potent microsome enzyme inhibitor.

Signs

Nausea
Vomiting
Mydriasis
Cardiovascular collapse
CNS depression
Hepatotoxicity

Treatment　Treatment is supportive.

EMERGENCY TREATMENT

Procedures

1. Secure the airway and ventilate as necessary (pp. 5, 9).
2. Administer supplemental oxygen (p. 7).
3. Secure venous access. Collect blood and urine for laboratory testing.
4. Control seizures (p. 24).
5. Treat hyperthermia if present (p. 25).

Decontaminate

GI EXPOSURE (INGESTION)
- Induce emesis if recent ingestion and no signs are present (p. 50).
- Gastric lavage if signs are present after ingestion (p. 52).
- Adminster activated charcoal and a saline cathartic; repeat PRN q4-6h (p. 56).

DERMAL EXPOSURE
- Wash thoroughly with warm, soapy water. Wear rubber gloves when bathing the patient; avoid chilling.

Administer indicated supportive care

- There is no antidote.
- Administer fluids to support blood pressure or hydration and urine output (p. 58).
- Give supportive care for hepatotoxicity.

Suggested Reading

Poppenga R: Risks associated with herbal remedies. In Bonagura JD, Kirk RW, editors: *Current veterinary therapy*, ed 12, Philadelphia, 1995, Saunders.

SCORPION STINGS

Mechanism of action   Most scorpions common to the United States are relatively nontoxic. Their venom contains digestive enzymes that cause intense pain when injected. More dangerous scorpions (like *Centruroides exilicauda*) inject a venom that not only has hyaluronidase and phospholipase, but also includes a neurotoxin. This neurotoxin alters sodium-channel flow resulting in stimulation of the autonomic nervous system and neuromuscular junctions. *C. exilicauda* is found mostly in the arid regions of southwestern United States but has been found in many other states.

Clinical signs   Increased salivation, lacrimation, urination, and defecation (parasympathetic stimulation) are seen. Sympathetic signs include hypertension, mydriasis, hyperglycemia, and piloerection. Sympathetic or parasympathetic signs may occur. Skeletal muscle fasciculations may occur; death occurs because of hypertension, respiratory collapse, or cardiac dysrhythmias. Signs associated with scorpion poisoning must be differentiated from those caused by organophosphate poisoning, organocarbamate poisoning, respiratory distress, and idiopathic epilepsy.

Treatment   Treatment is supportive in most cases; as only mild analgesics are needed to control local pain from the sing. If the stinger is in the patient, it should be removed. The patient must be observed for the appearance of systemic signs listed above. When seen, treatment of the signs is aimed at correcting life-threatening dysrhythmias, muscle spasms, and hypertension. *Catecholamines should be avoided if possible because they may contribute to hypertension.* Corticosteroids and antihistamines are of no value in the routine treatment of scorpion stings but can be used if an allergic reaction occurs (corticosteroids can be used in shock as necessary; however, this would be extremely rare). Intravenous fluids are carefully used as necessary; pulmonary edema can occur if systemic hypertension is present.

Signs

Pain at the sting site
Salivation, lacrimation, urination, defecation (SLUD)
Hypertension
Mydriasis
Hyperglycemia
Piloerection
Skeletal muscle fasciculations
Death from hypertension, respiratory collapse, or cardiac arrhythmias.

EMERGENCY TREATMENT

Procedures

1. Secure the airway and ventilate as necessary (pp. 5, 9).
2. Administer supplemental oxygen (p. 7).
3. Secure venous access. Collect blood and urine for laboratory testing.
4. Administer isotonic crystalloids as needed to support blood pressure and perfusion.
5. Control seizures (p. 24).
6. Treat hyperthermia (p. 25), hypertension (p. 29), and cardiac dysrhythmias if present.

Decontaminate

- Wash wound thoroughly with warm, soapy water.

Administer antidotes or other indicated supportive care

- Scorpion antivenins have been manufactured, but because of the rarity of dangerous scorpion stings and the good results achieved with supportive care, this is not recommended in animal patients.
- Analgesia with aspirin (*dog:* 10 to 25 mg/kg PO q12h; *cat:* 10 to 20 mg/kg PO q48-72h) or butorphanol (*dog:* 0.1 to 0.2 mg/kg IV or 0.2 to 0.4 mg/kg IM, SC q4-12h; *cat:* 0.1 to 0.4 mg/kg IM, IV, SC q8-12h). *Avoid narcotic analgesics (morphine and meperidine) because they are synergistic with scorpion venom. Use of high doses of opiate derivatives has resulted in increased mortality in humans.*
- If muscle spasms are causing the patient pain, methocarbamol may be used.
- Administer fluids to maintain hydration and urine output.

Suggested Reading

Peterson M, Meerdink G: Bites and stings of venomous animals. In Kirk RW, Bonagura JD, editors: *Current veterinary therapy*, ed 10, Philadelphia, 1989, Saunders.

SMOKE INHALATION

Sources Small animals are most commonly affected by smoke after they have been trapped in a burning building, in a car, or even in areas overrun by fire (Oakland fire, Santa Barbara fire).

Mechanism of action Smoke inhalation may cause hypoxemia as a result of the displacement of oxygen from ambient air reducing the partial pressure of oxygen. This is quickly corrected by removal of the patient to an area with fresh air. Most commonly, patients suffer damage from thermal burns to the respiratory system or from the toxic substances found in the smoke.

Carbon monoxide is produced by combustion. This substance has an affinity for hemoglobin that is 240 times greater than that of oxygen. When carbon monoxide is combined with hemoglobin, it is known as carboxyhemoglobin. Carboxyhemoglobin levels of 10% or higher will cause confusion and dyspnea. Levels >60% (or sometimes less) are fatal.

Fumes from smoke combine with respiratory secretions to form toxic or noxious substances. These substances may cause damage to the respiratory system. Swelling and edema may result causing obstruction of the airways. Damage to alveolar epithelium may result in leakage of body fluids into the alveolar spaces (pulmonary edema). Pulmonary macrophages may be poisoned by toxic products, predisposing the patient to bacterial pneumonia. Inflammation, toxic substances, and hypoxia activate macrophages and neutrophils, which may result in release of mediators that predispose the patient to develop pulmonary edema or ARDS (acute or adult respiratory distress syndrome). Noxious products may cause bronchoconstriction resulting in dyspnea and hypoxemia.

The upper airway (nasal cavity, oral cavity, pharynx, larnyx, trachea, and mainstem bronchi) may be damaged by thermal injury or from toxic substances of smoke inhalation. Since this is the heat-dissipation system of our small animal patients, animals suffering smoke-inhalation damage are more prone to development of hyperthermia.

Clinical findings   Signs of smoke inhalation are directly related to the severity of the exposure. Mildly affected patients may present with minimal signs. More severe exposure will result in demonstration of dyspnea and tachypnea. Mucous membranes may be pale because of shock, pink or red because of carboxyhemoglobin formation or the hyperdynamic stage of shock, or cyanotic because of hypoxemia. The patient may have normal mentation or may be dull and confused as a result of hypoxemia or carboxyhemoglobinemia. The patient's cardiovascular status may be normal, or the patient may present in the compensated (rapid, bounding pulses, red or dark mucous membranes, rapid capillary-refill time) or decompensated (pale mucous membranes, hypothermia, tachycardia or bradycardia in terminal shock, weak pulses) stage of shock. Thermal burns are often observed on oral and nasal surfaces (as well as over the body). There is often a nasal discharge that may be serous, hemorrhagic, or purulent. Pulmonary edema (crackles) or bronchoconstriction (wheezes) may be present. Hypoxemia, hypercapnia, carbon monoxide poisoning, and acidemia may cause cerebral edema, stupor, or coma.

Laboratory findings

- Possible hemoconcentration
- Possible hypoalbuminemia
- Chemistry profile may not have any initial changes.
- Blood gases may reveal hypoxemia or acidosis; however, they do not reveal the presence or absence of carbon monoxide. Blood gas measurements are unaffected by the presence of carboxyhemoglobin.
- Oxygen saturation levels are falsely normal when determined by pulse oximetry because carboxyhemoglobin is "invisible" to this technologic method. Carboxyhemoglobin may be detected using direct oximetry or cooximetry.
- Electrolyte imbalances are often detected.

Radiographic Findings

- Chest radiographs are often normal initially. Pulmonary edema is radiographically evident after 16 to 24 hours.

EMERGENCY TREATMENT

Procedures

1. Establish an airway if necessary (p. 2).
2. Administer 80% to 100% oxygen for at least 30 minutes. It is best to assume that the patient suffers carbon monoxide poisoning and to administer oxygen. The half-life of carboxyhemoglobin approaches 300 minutes in room air but is decreased to about 30 minutes in 100% oxygen.
3. In all but the most minimally affected, it is advisable to ventilate the patient using intermittent positive pressure

ventilation (IPPV) with positive end-expiratory pressure (PEEP). The prophylactic use of IPPV and PEEP has been shown to reduce deaths (in human patients) related to respiratory failure that develops during resuscitation. The veterinarian should be mindful that use of IPPV and PEEP reduces venous return to the heart and therefore may decrease cardiac output requiring administration of positive inotropes (see below).

4. Evaluate for and treat cyanide poisoning if present (p. 120).
5. Administer bronchodilators if bronchoconstriction or bronchospasm is present (p. 13).
6. Establish IV access; preferably through intact (unburned) skin.
7. Administer crystalloid fluids at shock doses if shock is present (p. 17). *Caution is advised in the use of colloids during the first 12 hours in a patient who has suffered severe thermal burns. Use of colloids during the initial 12 hours is known to aggravate burn-wound edema.*
8. Administer analgesics.
9. Treat cerebral edema if necessary (p. 29).
10. Antibiotics are not indicated in the early stages of smoke inhalation.
11. Enteral or parenteral nutrition should be initiated early.

SNAKEBITES

See *Coral snakes, Pit vipers*

SOAPS

See also *Detergents, Builders, Acids and alkalis*

Mechanism of action Soaps not containing acids or alkalis have low oral toxicity. Essential oils, often used as fragrances, can be irritating to the GI tract.

Clinical signs   Nearly always, the only signs associated with ingestion of soap are vomiting and diarrhea. Some homemade soaps and laundry soaps have significant alkalinity and are therefore corrosive. In the cases of higher alkalinity soaps, oral and mucous membrane irritation and damage may be seen. Ptyalism is often seen owing to the animal's response to the taste or perhaps to the corrosive injury to the tongue and oropharynx.

Signs

Ptyalism
Vomiting
Diarrhea

EMERGENCY TREATMENT

Procedures

1.   Administer diluents such as water or milk.
2.   Administer activated charcoal.
3.   If extensive vomiting or diarrhea occurs, antiemetics and fluid therapy may be necessary to maintain perfusion, hydration, and electrolyte balance.

SODIUM PHOSPHATE ENEMAS

E L C A

Sources   Fleet enemas

Mechanism of action   Excessive amounts of sodium and phosphate contained in hypertonic sodium phosphate enemas are absorbed from the colon, leading to hypernatremia, hyperphosphatemia, increased osmolality, and a high anion-gap metabolic acidosis.

Clinical signs Neuromuscular dysfunction, caused by hypocalcemia and hypomagnesemia (which are secondary to hypernatremia and hyperphosphatemia), is manifested as tetanic convulsions. Hyperglycemia, secondary to hypertonicity and stress-induced catecholamine release, is often seen in cats.

Signs usually occur within 30 to 60 minutes after administration of the enema. Lethargy, ataxia, and tetany or convulsions can be seen. Occasionally, tachycardia with a weak pulse and hypothermia occur. Rarely, vomiting and bloody diarrhea are observed. Laboratory abnormalities are seen within 15 minutes to 4 hours after enema administration. Dehydration is possible, as are cardiac arrythmias and hypokalemia.

Treatment Many electrolyte and biochemical abnormalities are seen with sodium phosphate enema toxicity. If possible, electrolyte, calcium, phosphorus, blood urea nitrogen, glucose, and bicarbonate (or total CO_2) levels should be determined to direct therapy. If specific levels are not available on a stat. basis, treatment is symptomatic and supportive. Tetany is controlled with calcium gluconate given intravenously while an ECG or heart rate is monitored. Calcium administration should be slowed or stopped if bradycardia or Q-T interval shortening occurs. Magnesium sulfate or anticonvulsants can be used if calcium fails to resolve the signs. Isotonic crystalloid fluids are administered as needed to support blood pressure and perfusion. Hypotonic enemas (tap water with KCl and calcium added) can also be used in the treatment.

In cases of hypernatremia, the literature often recommends that fluids be given slowly to prevent fluid shifts that result in cerebral edema. In the case of hypertonic sodium phosphate enema toxicity this should not be a problem; the signs develop too rapidly after administration for the brain to develop "idiogenic osmoles." Keep in mind that if hypernatremia (or hyperosmolality) has been present for several hours the brain will begin to develop idiogenic osmoles that will protect the brain from shrinkage. These idiogenic osmoles will cause cerebral edema if the plasma sodium or osmolality is lowered too rapidly. Thus the clinician must decide: Is the hypernatremia acute and causing brain shrinkage, *or* is the hypernatremia long standing enough that idiogenic osmoles have been synthesized, thus creating the potential for formation of cerebral edema should the plasma sodium or osmolality be lowered too rapidly? One reference states that "If neurologic improvement is followed by deterioration, assume cerebral edema and treat with mannitol" (Atkins, 1986). We caution that deterioration may also be an indication of the acute effects of rapidly developing hypernatremia causing brain shrinkage, rupture of pia mater vessels, and central pontine myelinolysis. In this case, rapid administration of hypotonic fluids may be lifesaving. Again, it behooves the clinician to examine the patient for signs that indicate the source of the CNS deterioration.

Clinical signs

Neuromuscular dysfunction
Lethargy
Dehydration
Ataxia
Tetany or convulsions
Possible tachycardia
Possible weak pulses
Possible hypothermia
Possible cardiac dysrhythmia

RARELY
  Vomiting
  Bloody diarrhea

Laboratory findings

Signs of dehydration (increased packed cell volume and total protein [PCV-TP], prerenal azotemia, increased serum albumin)
Hypokalemia
Hypernatremia
Hyperphosphatemia
Hypocalcemia
Hypomagnesemia
High anion-gap metabolic acidosis
Hyperglycemia
Hyperosmolality

EMERGENCY TREATMENT

Procedures

1. Secure the airway and ventilate as necessary (pp. 5, 9).
2. Administer supplemental oxygen (p. 7).
3. Secure venous access. Collect blood for laboratory testing.
4. Control seizures (p. 24).
5. Administer isotonic crystalloids as needed to support blood pressure and perfusion.
6. Treat hypernatremia (p. 39).

Decontaminate

1. Remove toxins by induction of emesis (p. 50) or gastric lavage if exposure was by ingestion.
2. Administer activated charcoal.
3. Consider hypotonic (warm water) enemas.

Administer antidotes or other indicated supportive care

1. There are no specific antidotes.
2. Administer calcium for tetany.
3. Consider administration of magnesium sulfate if calcium administration fails to control tetany.

Enhancement of elimination

Hemodialysis, peritoneal dialysis

Suggested Reading

Atkins C: Hypertonic sodium phosphate enema intoxication. In Kirk RW, editor: *Current veterinary therapy,* ed 9, Philadelphia, 1986, Saunders.

Jorgensen LS, Center SA, Randolph JF, Brum D: Electrolyte abnormalities induced by hypertonic phosphate enemas in two cats, *J Am Vet Med Assoc* 187(12):1367-1368, 1985.

SPIDER BITES

Species   *Latrodectus* (female black and red widows) and *Loxosceles* (brown recluse).

Mechanism of action   *Latrodectus* spp. release a neurotoxin that is toxic to presynaptic nerve processes, which causes an increase of calcium ions. This locks open ion-exchange channels; thus the release of acetylcholine and norepinephrine is promoted. The toxicity of the bite is highest in autumn, lowest in spring. The amount of venom injected is variable; 15% of bites contain no venom.

Loxosceles spp. release a dermonecrotic toxin as well as several proteins that have direct toxic effects on erythrocytes.

Clinical signs   *Latrodectus* bites result in regional tenderness and numbness followed by hyperesthesia. Muscle pain (often severe) and fasciculations with cramping of the muscles of the chest, abdomen, lumbar area, and other large muscle groups occurs. Abdominal rigidity without tenderness is a classic sign of envenomation by the black widow spider. Spasmlike activity and possibly seizures can be noted. Respiration may be compromised because of abdominal cramping. Motor signs may abate within 10 to 20 hours after envenomation and may be followed by flaccid paralysis. Hypertension and tachycardia may be seen. Death is caused by respiratory or cardiovascular collapse. Cats are extremely sensitive to *Latrodectus* bites: severe pain, salivation, restlessness, and early and pronounced paralysis are seen. Death is common.

Loxosceles bites are initially not painful. If envenomation occurred, the cutaneous form (characterized by localized pain and erythema) is seen within 2 to 6 hours. A bleb or blister is seen within 12 hours of the bite; this lesion often evolves into the classic "bull's-eye" lesion (a dark necrotic center bordered by a white ischemic ring on an erythematous background). Dermal necrosis follows ischemia; focal ulceration occurs within 7 to 14 days. The viscerocutaneous form (characterized by fever, arthralgia, weakness, emesis,

convulsive seizures, hemolysis, hemoglobinuria, thrombocytopenia, and potentially acute renal failure) rarely occurs with *Loxosceles* bites but warrants careful monitoring.
Dermal healing is extremely slow, often taking from 8 weeks
to many months after the bite; permanent scarring often results.

Treatment   *Latrodectus* bites are treated with analgesics for
pain, calcium for control of muscular signs, antibiotics, and antivenin.

Loxosceles bites are treated with excision of the affected tissue
and antibiotics and observation for signs of the viscerocutaneous form of reaction.

Signs

Latrodectus bites

Salivation
Regional tenderness, numbness, hyperesthesia
Muscle pain (severe), fasciculations, cramping
Abdominal rigidity without tenderness
Spasmlike activity
Seizures
Respiratory distress
Paralysis
Tachycardia
Death

Loxosceles bites

Localized pain (mild to moderate)
Localized erythema
Bleb, vesicle initially, and then "bull's-eye" lesion
Dermal necrosis
Focal ulceration
Hyperthermia
Arthralgia
Weakness
Emesis
Convulsive seizures
Hemolysis, hemolytic anemia
Hemoglobinuria
Thrombocytopenia
Acute renal failure

EMERGENCY TREATMENT ▪

Procedures

1. Secure the airway and ventilate as necessary (pp. 5, 9).
2. Administer supplemental oxygen (p. 7).
3. Secure venous access. Collect blood and urine for laboratory testing.
4. Administer isotonic crystalloids as needed to support blood pressure and perfusion.
5. Control seizures (p. 24).
6. Treat hyperthermia if present (p. 25).

Administer antidotes or other indicated treatments

Latrodectus

1. If no systemic signs, aspirin may be useful for mild pain control at 10 to 25 mg/kg q12h (for dogs), or 10 to 20 mg/kg q48-72h (for cats). Systemic signs may take 24 to 72 hours to develop in mild envenomations, and so the animal should be hospitalized and observed closely.
2. Antivenin (Lyovac Antivenin, Merck Sharpe and Dohme, Equine) may be administered IV early in the treatment regimen when severe signs are present. One vial is usually sufficient regardless of the size of the patient. Pretreating the pet with diphenhydramine (1 mg/kg IV or IM) may help prevent allergic reactions.
3. For severe muscle cramping or fasciculations:
   a. Administer 10% calcium gluconate at 0.5 to 1.5 mL/kg IV slowly over 30 minutes (monitor ECG for Q-T interval prolongation or for bradycardia and dysrhythmias if no ECG present). The dose can be repeated in 4 to 6 hours if needed. If the pet is not free of fasciculations or cramping for more than 1.5 hours, further injections may not help.
   b. Methocarbamol may be used IV as needed for muscle cramping (up to 222.2 mg/kg PRN for dog; up to 44.4 mg/kg PRN for cat).
4. Control pain.

The prognosis is unknown for several days. It has been reported that complete recovery may take several months.

Loxosceles

1. Excise affected tissues, healing by primary intention. It may be prudent to delay excision until maximum lesion development has occurred.
2. Irrigate the area daily with warm water or Burow's solution. Additional débridement is performed as needed.
3. Broad-spectrum antibiotics are indicated if the wound becomes infected.
4. If available, hyperbaric oxygen at 1 to 2 atmospheres twice daily for 3 days is indicated.
5. Dapsone and colchicine have had limited use in people but has not been adequately evaluated in pets.
6. Corticosteroids can be used if systemic effects are seen.
7. Monitor for signs of intravascular hemolysis including anemia and icterus. Administer blood transfusion if warranted.
8. Administer crystalloid fluids to maintain perfusion, hydration, and urine output.

Avoid

Acidosis, especially in the presence of hemoglobinuria.

Suggested Reading

Bailey EM Jr, Garland T: Toxicologic emergencies. In Murtaugh RJ, Kaplan PM, editors: *Veterinary emergency and critical care medicine,* St. Louis, 1992, Mosby.

Peterson M, Meerdink G: Bites and stings of venomous animals. In Kirk RW, Bonagura JD, editors: *Current veterinary therapy,* ed 10, Philadelphia, 1989, Saunders.

STRYCHNINE

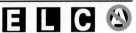

Sources   Pesticide, used to control gophers, moles, rats, coyotes, and other potential pests.

Mechanism of action Strychnine competitively and reversibly antagonizes glycine, an inhibitory neurotransmitter located in the brain and spinal cord. Although higher CNS centers experience inhibitory blockade, most of the signs noted are caused by antagonism of glycine released by Renshaw cells, which are located in the spinal cord. Renshaw cells are neurons that mediate inhibitory influences between the motoneurons of antagonistic muscle groups. The result is uninhibited simultaneous contraction of the muscle groups. Uncontrolled muscle contraction results in muscle injury, rhabdomyolysis, and hyperthermia. Respiratory muscles are contracted resulting in dyspnea, hypoxemia, and death if not treated.

Clinical signs Anxiety and restlessness is followed by onset of violent, tetanic muscle contractions with the more powerful muscle groups dominating. In most victims, this will be extensor dominance; however, it is interesting to note that the sloth, whose antigravity muscles are the flexors, demonstrates flexion as the dominant sign. These seizure-like contractions are induced by external stimuli such as touch or noise. Extensor dominance in dogs and cats results in a "saw-horse" stance. The contraction of facial muscles results in *risus sardonicus,* or the 'sardonic grin'. Tetanic contractions of respiratory muscles interferes with respiration resulting in dyspnea or apnea. Death occurs from asphyxia most commonly but may also be caused by exhaustion, acute renal failure (myoglobinuria), or sequelae of hypoxemia.

EMERGENCY TREATMENT

Procedures

1. Establish an airway and ventilate the patient if necessary.
2. Relax the muscle spasms.
   a. Induce anesthesia (for relaxation as well as decontamination procedures) using IV pentobarbital or other short-acting barbiturate.
   b. IV administration of diazepam and methocarbamol may relax some patients adequately but do not allow decontamination procedures.
3. Decontaminate the gut by gastric lavage (p. 52). Use of potassium permanganate (1:5000) or tannic acid solution

(1% to 2%) as the lavage solution is recommended by some.

4. Administer activated charcoal and a saline cathartic.
5. Treat hyperthermia (p. 25) and rhabdomyolysis (p. 26) as necessary.
6. Support blood pressure and hydration with crystalloids. Monitor electrolytes to determine whether replacement solutions (lactated Ringer's solution, saline) or maintainence solutions (Normosol-M, half-strength LRS in D_5W) are appropriate.
7. Keep the patient heavily sedated (diazepam, methocarbamol, barbiturates) and in a quiet, darkened room to minimize sensory input.
8. These patients may require treatment for 48 hours or longer. Symptomatic and supportive treatment must be maintained.

TOAD POISONING

Sources The tropical toad species responsible for poisoning small animal patients are *Bufo alvarius and Bufo marinus*. Dogs and cats (and other animals including humans) are poisoned by toxins produced in the parotid glands of these toads. Exposure is usually through oral exposure (mouthing the toad) but may be absorbed through wounds or broken skin.

Mechanism of action The venom contain bufagins, bufotoxins, and bufotenins, which are mostly responsible for the toxic effects. The secretions also contain epinephrine, cholesterol, ergosterol, and serotonin. Bufagins and bufotoxins exert a digitalis-like action that may result in ventricular fibrillation. Bufotenins exert an oxytocic action and a strong pressor action.

Clinical findings The venom is locally irritating; head shaking and hypersalivation are observed first. The exposed animal will often paw at its mouth and may retch or vomit profusely. In severe cases, the signs progress to cardiac dysrhythmias (indicated by cyanosis, weakness, collapse), tachypnea with increased depth of respiration, apparent blindness, seizures, collapse, and death within 30 to 60 minutes after exposure. Toxicity of the toad venom is variable. In certain areas (Florida mostly), the toads are reported to cause near 100% mortality in untreated dogs.

There are no consistent laboratory findings. Erythrocyte sedimentation rate will be increased, and PCV may be increased. Elevated blood glucose, BUN, potassium, and calcium have been reported.

The electrocardiogram will reveal abnormalities with progressive negative ventricular deflection and eventually ventricular fibrillation.

Diagnosis   There is no diagnostic test for poisoning by toad venom. Diagnosis is usually based on the history of exposure and physical findings.

EMERGENCY TREATMENT

Procedures

1. Secure the airway and ventilate as necessary (pp. 5, 9).
2. Administer supplemental oxygen (p. 7).
3. Secure venous access. Collect blood and urine for laboratory testing.
4. Administer isotonic crystalloids as needed to support blood pressure and perfusion.
5. Control seizures (p. 24).
6. Treat hyperthermia if present (p. 25).

Administer antidotes and other treatments

- Monitor ECG.
   a. Administer large doses of propranolol (1.5 to 5.0 mg/kg IV) with a repeat dose in 20 minutes if ECG does not normalize. NOTE: **These propranolol doses are for *Bufo* poisoning *only*.**
   b. If the patient has a preexisting heart disease or is a known asthmatic, administer propranolol IV in 0.25 to 0.5 mg/kg increments slowly while observing ECG. Discontinue infusion when ECG normalizes.

- Administer fluids to maintain hemodynamics or hydration as needed.
- Administer atropine (0.04 mg/kg IV) as necessary to control hypersalivation. It may also be useful to prevent asystole or bradycardia. Atropine is not antidotal.
- Lidocaine (*dogs:* 1 to 2 mg/kg IV followed by continuous infusion at 25 to 75 µg/kg/min; *cats:* 0.25 to 1 mg/kg IV bolus followed by 5 to 40 µg/kg/min IV infusion in cats) may be indicated for cardiac dysrhythmias.

Decontaminate

- Flush the mouth with copious amounts of water to remove the venom. It is advisable to anesthetize the patient, insert a cuffed endotracheal tube, and flush the mouth. This will allow more complete removal of the toxin.
- Although the venom is absorbed through the mucous membranes or broken skin, it is believed to enter the enterohepatic circulation. Therefore administration of multiple-dose activated charcoal is advised.
- Sorbitol cathartic is advised.

Suggested Reading

Baily EM Jr, Garland T: Toxicologic emergencies. In Murtaugh RJ, Kaplan PM, editors: *Veterinary emergency and critical care medicine,* St. Louis, 1992, Mosby.

TOLUENE AND TOLUOL

See *Organic solvents and fuels*

   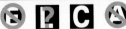

TRICHLOROETHANE AND TRICHLOROETHYLENE

See *Organic solvents and fuels*

   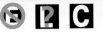

TRICYCLIC ANTIDEPRESSANTS

Sources   Tricyclic antidepressants (TCA) are often used in human medicine for treating depression and other conditions as well. These drugs are now finding their way into veterinary medicine. Examples include imipramine, desimipramine, trimipramine, amitriptyline, and doxepin. Proprietary names include Asendin, Elavil, Endep, Etrafon, Limbitrol, Ludiomil, Norpramin, Pamalor, Sinequan, Tofranil, Triavil, and Vivactil.

Ingestions of TCAs should be considered potentially lethal ingestions and should be treated as a medical emergency. Death may occur within 1 to 2 hours in animals who are not treated aggressively.

Mechanism of action   The tricyclic antidepressants potentiate the actions of biogenic amines (norepinephrine, serotonin, and dopamine) in the CNS by blocking reuptake at the nerve terminals. Tricyclics vary in the degree of potency and selectivity. That is, one TCA may block norepinephrine uptake very well but may have weak action against serotonin uptake, whereas another may have weak effects on norepinephrine and strong effects against serotonin or dopamine. TCAs also are known to act as antagonists at muscarinic cholinergic, alpha$_1$-adrenergic, and both H$_1$- and H$_2$-histaminergic receptor sites.

Clinical findings   Diagnosis is usually based on history of ingestion. Specific levels may be measured in clinical laboratories.

Signs

Vomiting
Disorientation, anxiety, aggression
Severe depression to semicomatose states
Seizures or status epilepticus
Hypothermia in depressed states, hyperthermia with status epilepticus
Ataxia, weakness, tremors
Shock (cardiogenic)
Death

ECG findings

Tachycardia or bradycardia is common
Prolonged QRS duration
Ventricular tachycardia or fibrillation
In humans, tricyclic antidepressant poisoning is strongly suspected in any patient presenting with lethargy, coma, or seizures accompanied by QRS interval prolongation.

Other tests of value

CBC count, electrolytes, glucose, BUN, CPK.
Urine analysis to check for myoglobin (rhabdomyolysis from exertion, seizures, or hyperthermia)
Arterial blood gases

EMERGENCY TREATMENT

Procedures

1. Secure the airway and ventilate the patient if necessary.
2. Treat coma (p. 29), hypotension (p. 17), and hypothermia (p. 30) if they exist.
3. Control seizures.
   - Administer diazepam first.
   - Phenobarbital should be administered concurrently with diazepam.
   - If diazepam and phenobarbital are not effective, induce anesthesia with pentothal or pentobarbital.
   - Consider neuromuscular blockade if seizures are difficult to control and hyperthermia is a problem. Administer pancuronium 0.03 to 0.06 mg/kg IV or vecuronium 10 to 20 µg/kg IV in the dog or 20 to 40 µg/kg in the cat). *These patients will not be able to breathe on their own and will require ventilation.*

Decontaminate

- *Do not* induce vomiting. The risk of rapid-onset seizures is too great.
- Perform gastric lavage.

- Administer activated charcoal. Repeat doses of activated charcoal have been reported to enhance elimination, but the data are not convincing.
- Administer cathartic.

Administer antidotes or other indicated supportive care

- Acidemia enhances TCA cardiotoxicity. Administer sodium bicarbonate (1 to 3 mEq/kg may be required) to maintain the plasma pH at 7.45 to 7.55. Monitor blood gases.
- Manage ventricular dysrhythmias with lidocaine. Quinidine sulfate, procainamide, and disopyramide are contraindicated.
- Beta-blockers (such as propranolol) may be useful in treating TCA cardiotoxicity and in controlling ventricular tachydysrhythmias.
- Routine nursing care is essential.
- Patients must be monitored closely for 12 hours after ingestion.
- Sudden death several days after apparent recovery has been reported in man.

Enhancement of elimination

Repeat doses of activated charcoal have been reported to enhance elimination, but the data are not convincing.

Avoid

Quinidine sulfate, procainamide, and disopyramide are contraindicated.

VITAMIN D RODENTICIDES

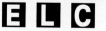

Sources Rodent baits such as Quintox, Rat-B-Gone, Mouse-B-Gone, or Rampage.

Mechanism of action   Vitamin D rodenticides contain cholecalciferol, which causes hypercalcemia by increasing intestinal absorption of calcium, bone resorption, and increased renal reabsorption of calcium. The half-life of cholecalciferol and its metabolite 25-hydroxycholecalciferol may be as long as 30 days with the duration of effects of several weeks.

Clinical signs   Signs are nonspecific and include anorexia and lethargy, depression, vomiting, constipation, and polyuria with polydipsia. More severe GI signs including hematemesis and bloody diarrhea are relatively common with mild to moderate cholecalciferol ingestions. Signs reported in cats include anorexia, depression, and renal pain. Shock, bradycardia, and other cardiac dysrhythmias have been reported. If hypercalcemia is severe, muscle twitching, seizures, and stupor may be seen. The LD_{50} for dogs is reportedly 88 mg/kg, but signs are seen at <10 mg/kg (as little as 2 to 3 mg/kg), and lethal toxicosis has been seen at 10 mg/kg. Hypercalcemia occurs within 12 to 24 hours of ingestion; hyperphosphatemia develops simultaneously. Azotemia can occur secondary to hypercalcemia and dehydration. The issue of secondary poisoning (poisoning of a pet after the accidental ingestion of a poisoned rodent) occasionally arises. With the rare exception of a puppy, kitten, small dog, or cat, the possibility of most pets being poisoned after the ingestion of a single poisoned rodent is remote.

Treatment   Treatment is aimed at decreasing serum calcium, preventing dehydration and renal failure, controlling seizures and cardiac arrhythmias, and correcting electrolyte imbalances. Diuretics (with avoidance of thiazides because they decrease renal calcium excretion) and corticosteroids are used to promote calciuresis; corticosteroids also decrease bone reabsorption and intestinal absorption of calcium. Calcitonin can be used in severe cases. Sodium bicarbonate may be needed to correct metabolic acidosis or possibly induce a mild alkalosis that favors shifting ionized (active) calcium to the unionized (inactive) form.

If ingestion occurred within 2 to 4 hours, induction of vomiting and administering activated charcoal may be the only treatment needed: recheck serum calcium phosphorus, BUN, and creatinine at 24, 48, and 72 hours and treat for hypercalcemia or azotemia if detected.

Signs

Anorexia, lethargy
Depression
Vomiting
Constipation
Polyuria, polydipsia
Muscle twitching
Seizures
Stupor
Hypercalcemia, hyperphosphatemia
Azotemia
Hematemesis
Bloody diarrhea

EMERGENCY TREATMENT ■

Procedures

1. Secure the airway and ventilate as necessary (pp. 5, 9).
2. Administer supplemental oxygen (p. 7).
3. Secure venous access. Collect blood and urine for laboratory testing. Administer 0.9% saline solution (saline decreases renal tubular reabsorption of calcium) intravenously at 2 to 3 times maintenance dose (initially 120 to 180 mL/kg/day and then 60 to 120 mL/kg/day, depending on the size of the pet). Supplement with KCl as needed (10 to 20 mEq/L). Fluids may be necessary 7 to 10 days or even longer depending on the degree of hypercalcemia and azotemia. The dose of fluid can be lowered as the hypercalcemia and azotemia are resolving; monitor urine output and avoid overhydration.
4. Control seizures (p. 24).
5. Treat hyperthermia if present (p. 25).

Decontaminate

GI EXPOSURE
- Induce emesis if recent ingestion (2 to 4 hours) and if signs are not present (p. 50).

- Perform gastric lavage if signs are present after ingestion (p. 52).
- Administer activated charcoal and a saline cathartic; repeat PRN q4-6h (pp. 54, 56).

Administer antidotes and other supportive care

- Furosemide (to promote calciuresis at 1 to 5 mg/kg 2 to 4 times per day for 2 to 4 weeks *after* fluid volume expansion; can be given PO (if no vomiting) or parenterally (preferred at least initially).
- Prednisolone or prednisone at 2 to 3 mg/kg PO, SC BID for 2 to 4 weeks.
- Calcitonin (Calcimar) at 4 to 6 IU/kg SC q2-12h (dogs only) for severe hypercalcemia (calcium >18 mg/dL). Calcitonin is expensive and may cause anorexia or vomiting as side effects; discontinue calcitonin if side effects are severe.
- Sodium bicarbonate q3-4h if severe metabolic acidosis (pH <7.05) (p. 139).
- Phosphate binders (aluminum hydroxide; Amphogel, Basagel) at 30 to 90 mg/kg PO q8-24h for 2 weeks) can be used for hyperphosphatemia.
- Feed a low calcium diet for 1 month; avoid vitamin-mineral supplements.
- Decrease exposure to sunlight to prevent skin conversion to active vitamin D.

Suggested Readings

Dorman D, Beasley V: Diagnosis of and therapy for cholecalciferol toxicosis. In Kirk RW, Bonagura JD, editors: *Current veterinary therapy*, ed 10, Philadelphia, 1989, Saunders.

Kruger JM, Osborne CA: Canine and feline hypercalcemic nephropathy, Part II: Detection, cure, and control, *Compend Cont Ed Pract Vet* 16(11):1445-1457, 1994.

VITAMIN K–ANTAGONIST RODENTICIDES

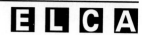

Uses   Rodenticide

Common products

FIRST-GENERATION HYDROXYCOUMARINS
(Warfarin, coumarin, etc.), D-Con, Ward 42, Rax, Rodex, Tox-Hid, Prolin, Ratron, Ratafin, Rat-A-Way, Lurat, Krunkill, Fumisol.

SECOND-GENERATION HYDROXYCOUMARINS
(Brodifacoum, bromadiolone, etc.), Talon, Havoc, Weather Block, Super Caid, Ratimus, Contrac.

INDANEDIONE ANTICOAGULANTS
Diphacinone, diphenadione, chlorphacinone, pindone, etc. (Valone, Promar, Ramik, Diphacin, Ciad Drat, Rozol, Pival, PMP).

Mechanism of action   Factors II, VII, IX, and X are produced in the liver in an inactive form. The final step of activation (a carboxylation step) before release as active clotting factors requires active vitamin K quinone as an essential cofactor. Vitamin K quinone is converted to an inactive form (vitamin K epoxide) by this step and is then reconverted to the active form by the vitamin K epoxide reductase system. Anticoagulant rodenticides inhibit the vitamin K epoxide reductase system, which renders the body unable to activate vitamin K. Stores of active vitamin K–dependent factors are depleted, resulting in prolongation of the extrinsic, intrinsic, and common coagulation pathways, leading to a coagulopathy. There is no effect on circulating factors; thus a lag time occurs before signs are seen.

Clinical signs   In general, repeated exposure to first-generation hydroxycoumarins is needed for severe toxicity. A single dose is all that is needed for second-generation hydroxycoumarins and indanediones to produce severe toxicity.

Half-life of warfarin, 14.5 hours

Half-life of second-generation hydroxycoumarins, 6 days
Half-life of indanediones, 4 to 5 days

Signs are related to bleeding and include depression, weakness, and pallor. Bleeding may be seen externally as petechia, ecchymosis, melena, epistaxis, hematemesis, hematuria, gingival bleeding, or bleeding excessively from small wounds. Bleeding may be internal (hemarthrosis, hemothorax, or hemoperitoneum). Intracranial bleeding causing CNS signs has been reported in dogs and cats. Fever is often present when bleeding has occurred into tissues or body cavities.

Abnormal coagulation tests include prolongation of the prothrombin time (PT), activated partial thromboplastin time (APTT), and proteins induced by vitamin K absence or antagonists (PIVKA). The PT is a useful test to monitor before and during treatment, though the PIVKA test (Thrombotest, Accurate Chemical & Scientific Corp., Westbury, NY; 516-333-2221) is more accurate and sensitive than the PT test.

There is always a concern about secondary poisoning (that is, a pet being poisoned after ingesting a rodent that died of an anticoagulant poison). With the rare exception of a puppy, kitten, small dog, or cat, secondary poisoning is extremely unlikely in most pets after the ingestion of one small poisoned rodent for first-generation rodenticides. Secondary poisoning is much more likely if poisons containing diphacinone or brodifacoum are involved. When in doubt, treat the pet and monitor clotting tests. Lactating animals may pass vitamin K antagonists to the young, and so nursing young should receive vitamin K therapy until coagulation parameters can be monitored.

Treatment   Vitamin K_1 is given as long as the anticoagulant is present in the body at toxic levels. The drug is given only PO or SQ, never IV (possible anaphylaxis) or IM (hematoma formation, anemia, shock, death). The dosage and length of treatment depends on whether the type of rodenticide is known (first- or second-generation or indanedione) and, if known, what class of compound it is. Fresh blood, fresh plasma, or fresh frozen plasma is administered as needed. The animal should be prevented from possibly injuring itself and causing a bleeding diathesis.

Signs

Anorexia
Cough
Depression
Weakness
Pallor
Melena
Epistaxis
Hematemesis
Hematuria
Gingival bleeding
Excessive bleeding from small wounds
Hemothorax, hemoperitoneum
Increased PT, APTT, PIVKA

EMERGENCY TREATMENT

Procedures

1. Secure the airway and ventilate as necessary (pp. 5, 9).
2. Administer supplemental oxygen (p. 7).
3. Secure venous access. Collect blood for laboratory testing.
4. Administer fresh whole blood, fresh plasma, or fresh frozen plasma as needed to support blood pressure and perfusion.
   - If shock is present, blood or blood products are best, but administration of crystalloids may be lifesaving. Caution is advised in overhydration or dilution of blood when using crystalloids. Give only to improve hemodynamic parameters.
   - Colloids such as hetastarch and dextran may rapidly improve hemodynamic parameters but are known to have anticoagulant complications; they should be avoided if possible.
   - Gelatins (such as Vetaplasma, SmithKline Beecham, Philadelphia, Pa.) may be useful in the treatment of shock. As above, it should be used only to improve hemodynamic parameters so that they are minimally acceptable. If administered to normalize blood

pressure, it may induce bleeding tendencies through increased pressure.

5. Perform therapeutic thoracocentesis if a large volume of blood within the chest is interfering with respiration. Use strict caution because this procedure may restart the bleeding.

6. Look for evidence of hemopericardium and perform emergency pericardiocentesis if indicated.

Decontaminate

- Induce emesis *only* if the ingestion was within the last 60 minutes and the patient shows no clinical signs.
- Perform gastric lavage if the ingestion was within the last 2 to 4 hours.
- Give repeated doses of activated charcoal.
- Administer saline or osmotic cathartic.

Administer antidotes or other indicated supportive care

Vitamin K_1 is antidotal. The oral form is reported to be superior to the injectable form. It is rapidly absorbed from the gastrointestinal tract and transported directly to the liver where it is utilized. The injectable form of vitamin K_1 is indicated when there are contraindications to the oral form (emesis, activated charcoal administration, etc.).

Vitamin K_1 should be administered at a dose of 1 to 5 mg/kg q24h for 1 to 3 weeks. (One of us [RWG] prefers to administer vitamin K_1 0.5 to 2.5 mg/kg q12h, but the literature reports single daily dosing to be effective.) The coagulation status of the patient should be checked after cessation of the vitamin K_1. If the one-stage prothrombin time (OSPT) is used, it should be checked 48 to 72 hours after the last dose of vitamin K. If the test is normal, it should be repeated in another 48 to 72 hours. If either test results in prolonged time, the patient should receive another 1 to 3 weeks of vitamin K_1 therapy. The coagulation status should be checked again after any subsequent course of therapy as recommended above.

If the PIVKA test is used to montior coagulation status, it is recommended that it be performed on day 1 and day 3 after vitamin K therapy. If the test shows decreased activity (decreased coagulation), the vitamin K therapy should be reinstituted for 1 to 3 weeks.

Enhancement of elimination

There are no known effective techniques

Avoid

Trauma, overhydration, or hypertension; anything that may result in more bleeding tendency. Phenothiazines, corticosteroids, sulfonamide drugs, phenylbutazone, aspirin, aminophylline, furosemide (Lasix), and many other drugs may worsen the effects of vitamin K–antagonist rodenticides and should be avoided.

Suggested Reading

Felice LJ, Murphy MJ: CVT update: anticoagulant rodenticides. In Bonagura JD, Kirk RW, editors: *Current veterinary therapy,* ed 12, Philadelphia, 1995, Saunders.

Mount ME, Woody BJ, Murphy MJ: The anticoagulant rodenticides. In Kirk RW, editor: *Current veterinary therapy,* ed 9, Philadelphia, 1986, Saunders.

Mount ME: Proteins induced by vitamin K absence or antagonists (PIVKA). In Kirk RW, editor: *Current veterinary therapy,* ed 9, Philadelphia, 1986, Saunders.

Murphy MJ, Gerken DF: The anticoagulant rodenticides. In Kirk RW, Bonagura JD, editors: *Current veterinary therapy,* ed 10, Philadelphia, 1989, Saunders.

VITAMINS

Sources   Vitamin supplements

Mechanism of action   Acute overdosage of vitamin supplements is uncommon unless the preparation contains iron (see *Iron,* p. 158).

XYLENE AND XYLOL

See *Organic solvents and fuels*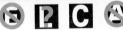

ZINC

Sources Pennies minted after 1982 (some pennies minted in 1982 did contain higher levels also), a zinc oxide ointment used in veterinary hospitals (Desitin), and metallic hardware of transport cages are the three most commmon sources of zinc. Other sources of zinc that have been reported in zinc toxicoses include drinking water from galvanized metal containers, zinc pieces from board games, certain paints, other types of hardware (nails, staples), an ointment containing zinc undecylenate (Desenex), sun-block preparations containing zinc oxide, and some fertilizers.

Mechanism of action It is known that zinc oxide is a gastric mucosal irritant. Systemic toxicosis depends on the rate of absorption of zinc from the gastrointestinal system. The acid pH of the stomach is ideal for gradual release of zinc from the above sources. Once leeched from the ingested material, zinc is absorbed and transported to various organs bound to protein. The mechanism of toxicity has not been fully elucidated. Zinc is believed to interfere with certain enzymes and may be able to cause direct damage to cell membranes and organelles. Chronic zinc toxicosis interferes with absorption and utilization of copper and iron.

Clinical signs Signs of zinc intoxication are usually related to the gastrointestinal tract. Vomiting, diarrhea, anorexia, and generalized depression are common. These signs are seen most consistently and may occur with short-term exposure or smaller amount of ingestion. More severe signs are likely to be found with long-term exposure or if large quantities of zinc are ingested. Severe signs include severe intravascular hemolytic anemia, hemoglobinuria, hematuria, prehepatic jaundice, weakness, and death. Signs associated with sepsis and multiple organ failure may become evident.

Diagnosis Laboratory findings include:

1. Regenerative anemia with hemolysis or hemoglobinemia. Increased numbers of nucleated red blood cells, polychromasia, basophilic stipling, target cells, and an inflammatory leukon are commonly reported.
2. Increased alkaline phosphatase.
3. Hyperbilirubinemia.
4. Increased serum alanine aminotransferase.
5. Increased BUN and azotemia.
6. Increased serum creatinine.

Acute renal failure has been reported in dogs with acute zinc toxicosis. Findings include azotemia, hypercreatinemia, hyperphosphatemia, and granular casts.

The diagnosis of zinc ingestion is usually based on history of exposure to zinc in a patient showing gastrointestinal signs or signs of anemia. A complete blood cell count indicating intravascular hemolytic anemia and radiographic evidence of metallic foreign bodies in the GI tract are adjunctive tests indicating possible zinc toxicosis. Laboratory analysis of serum, tissue (kidney, liver, pancreas), or urine zinc concentration will reveal increased levels of zinc. Samples must be carefully collected because blood tubes, syringes, and plastic containers have been found to contain zinc stearate, which will contribute to the analyzed levels. *Special vacuum tubes are available for analysis of serum or blood trace metals.* It is recommended that the laboratory be contacted for proper handling of samples.

EMERGENCY TREATMENT ■

Procedures

Stabilize the patient.

1. If anemia is causing signs of hypoxia, administer supplemental oxygen. Transfuse packed red blood cells, stored whole blood, or fresh whole blood, preferably after

crossmatching has been completed. Stroma-free hemo-globin solutions (such as oxyglobin, not yet approved by the FDA) are near marketing in veterinary medicine. These may be used without blood typing and cross-matching if available.

2. Administer intravenous crystalloids (lactated Ringer's so-lution, Normosol-R) to treat hypovolemia, shock, or de-hydration (p. 17). Implant a urethral catheter to monitor urine production. Fluids should be administered to maintain urine production >1 mL/kg/hour to minimize chances of acute renal failure.

3. If signs of acute renal failure exist, treat acute renal failure with furosemide, mannitol, and dopamine as needed.

4. If evidence of disseminated intravascular coagulopathy (DIC) exists (thrombocytopenia, increased levels of fibrin split products, decreased levels of antithrombin III, ap-pearance of schistocytes or spherocytes on a blood smear), therapy should include cryoprecipitate, fresh plasma, fresh frozen plasma, or fresh whole blood. The use of heparin in DIC is controversial. It is contraindi-cated in the actively bleeding patient. Heparin is effective only if adequate levels of antithrombin III are available. There may be an advantage to injecting heparin into the products named above and allowing incubation for 30 minutes before infusing into the patient.

5. Chelation therapy should be begun with CaEDTA as soon as fluid deficits are corrected. CaEDTA is nephro-toxic. Do not administer to a dehydrated patient. The optimum dose for CaEDTA has not been worked out for animal species. It has been used in dogs at 25 mg/kg ad-ministered SC q6h. CaEDTA should be diluted in D_5W to minimize local irritation at the site of injection.

Succimer (Chemet, McNeil Consumer Products Co., Fort Washington, PA 19034) has recently been made available in the USA. Succimer is believed to be less toxic than dimercaprol, calcium EDTA, or penicillamine. It is unknown as of this writing whether succimer will effectively chelate zinc in dogs and cats.

6. Since an acid environment will enhance zinc release and absorption, it may be of value to minimize stomach acid production using the H_2-blockers cimetidine (*dog* 4 to 10 mg/kg IV, IM, PO q8-12h; *cat* 2.5 to 5 mg/kg IV, PO q8-

12h), ranitidine (*dog* 1 to 2 mg/kg IV, SC, PO q8-12h; *cat* 0.5 mg/kg IV q12h), or famotidine (*dog* 0.5 to 1.0 mg/kg PO, IV q12-24h), or omeprazole.

7. If a metallic foreign body can be seen radiographically, it should be removed endoscopically or surgically as soon as possible to prevent further zinc absorption.

Suggested Reading

Ramsey DT, Casteel SW, Fagella AM, et al: Use of orally administered succimer (*meso*-2,3-dimercaptosuccinic acid) for treatment of lead poisoning in dogs, *J Am Vet Med Assoc* 208(3):371-375, 1996.

■ SECTION THREE

TOXIC PLANTS

Main entries are not listed in this cross-reference list unless functioning also as common terms. For them consult directly the next part of this section.

"Spp." is 'species', the plural of singular *species*.

Acacia; see *Acacia dealbata*
Acalypha; see *Acalypha*
Aconite; see *Aconitum*
Adam-and-Eve plant; see *Arum*
Adelfa; see *Nerium*
Algerian ivy; see *Hedera helix*
Allamanda; see *Allamanda cathartica*
Aloe; see *Aloe*
Amaryllis; see *Amaryllis* or *Hippeastrum*
American allspice; see *Calycanthus*
American ivy; see *Parthenocissus quinquefolia*
Anemone; see *Anemone*
Anthurium; see *Anthurium*
Anturio; see *Anthurium*
Apple; see *Malus sylvestris*
Apricot; see *Prunus*
April fool; see *Anemone*
Arum lily; see *Zantedeschia*
Asthma flower; see *Lobelia*
Autumn crocus; see *Colchicum autumnale*
Azalea; see *Rhododendron*
Baneberry; see *Actaea*
Barbados lily; see *Amaryllis* or *Hippeastrum*
Barbados nut; see *Jatropha*
Barbados pride; see *Caesalpinia*
Bead vine; see *Arbrus precatorius*
Bean tree; see *Laburnum anagyroides*
Bear's foot; see *Aconitum*
Beauty of the night; see *Mirabilis*
Beaver poison; see *Cicuta*
Beefsteak plant; see *Acalypha*
Belladonna; see *Atropa belladonna*
Belladonna lily; see *Amaryllis* or *Hippeastrum*
Berlander lobelia; see *Lobelia*
Bird-of-paradise bush; see *Caesalpinia*
Bird-of-paradise flower; see *Strelitzia reginae*
Bitter almond; see *Prunus*

Black calla; see *Arum*
Black-eyed Susan; see *Abutilon hybridum*
Black locust; see *Robinia*
Black nightshade; see *Atropa belladonna* and *Solanum*
Black walnut; see *Juglans*
Bleeding heart; see *Dicentra*
Blue cardinal flower; see *Lobelia*
Blue cohosh; see *Caulophyllum thalictroides*
Blue ginseng; see *Caulophyllum thalictroides*
Blue star; see *Ipomoea tricolor*
Blueberry root; see *Caulophyllum thalictroides*
Bluebonnets; see *Lupinus*
Bog laurel; see *Kalmia*
Bog onion; see *Arisaema*
Boneset; see *Eupatorium*
Bongay; see *Aesculus*
Brown dragon; see *Arisaema*
Bubby-blossoms; see *Calycanthus*
Bubbybush; see *Calycanthus*
Buckeye; see *Aesculus*
Buckthorn; see *Rhamnus*
Buffalo burr; see *Solanum*
Bull flower; see *Caltha*
Bull nettle; see *Solanum*
Burn bean; see *Sophora*
Burroweed; see *Isocoma*
Buttercup; see *Ranunculus*
Bushman's poison; see *Acokanthera*
Cactus; see *Lophophora*
Caladium; see *Arum*
Caley pea; see *Lathyrus*
Calfkill; see *Kalmia*
Calico bush; see *Kalmia*
California false-hellebore; see *Veratrum*
California fern; see *Conium*
California rose bay; see *Rhododendron*
Calla lily; see *Zantedeschia*
Calycanth; see *Calycanthus*
Canary ivy; see *Hedera helix*
Candelabra cactus; see *Euphorbia*
Candlenut; see *Aleurites*
Candleberry; see *Aleurites*
Cape belladonna; see *Amaryllis* or *Hippeastrum*

Caper spurge; see *Euphorbia*
Cardinal flower; see *Lobelia*
Carolina allspice; see *Calycanthus*
Carolina horse nettle; see *Solanum*
Carolina (yellow) jasmine; see *Gelsemium sempervirens*
Carolina (yellow) jessamine; see *Gelsemium sempervirens*
Cashes; see *Conium*
Castor oil plant, castorbean; see *Ricinus communis*
Cat's-eyes; see *Anemone*
Ceriman; see *Monstera*
Chenille plant; see *Acalypha*
Cherry (Carolina cherry, sour cherry, sweet cherry, laurel cherry); see *Prunus*
Children's bane; see *Cicuta*
China tree, Chinaball tree, Chinaberry; see *Melia azedarach*
Chinawood oil tree; see *Aleurites*
Chinese inkberry; see *Cestrum*
Christ-thorn; see *Euphorbia*
Chokecherry (black western chokecherry, southwestern chokecherry, western chokecherry); see *Prunus*
Climbing lily; see *Gloriosa*
Cloverbloom; see *Baptisia*
Clustered fishtail palm; see *Caryota*
Coffeeberry; see *Rhamnus*
Cohosh; see *Actaea*
Common tansy; see *Tanacetum*
Conquerors; see *Aesculus*
Copperleaf; see *Acalypha*
Cordatum; see *Philodendron*
Coral bead plant; see *Abutilon hybridum*
Coral bean; see *Sophora*
Coral plant; see *Jatropha*
Corn lily; see *Veratrum*
Country walnut; see *Aleurites*
Cowslip; see *Caltha*
Crab's-eye vine; see *Abutilon hybridum*
Crazyweed; see *Astragalus* or *Oxytropis*
Crocus; see *Colchicum autumnale*
Croton; see *Croton*
Crown flower; see *Calotropis*
Crown of thorns; see *Euphorbia*
Cuckoopint; see *Arum*
Cuckoo plant; see *Arisaema*

Cutleaf philodendron; see *Monstera*
Cypress spurge; see *Euphorbia*
Daffodil; see *Narcissus*
Dasheen; see *Colocasias*
Datura; see *Datura*
Day lily; see *Hemerocallis*
Day-blooming jasmine; see *Cestrum*
Day-blooming jessamine; see *Cestrum*
Deadly nightshade; see *Atropa belladonna* or *Solanum*
Death camas; see *Zygadenus*
Death-of-man; see *Cicuta*
Delphinium; see *Delphinium*
Devil's-apple; see *Datura* and *Solanum*
Devil's ivy; see *Monstera*
Devil's trumpet; see *Datura*
Digitalis; see *Digitalis*
Dogbane; see *Apocynum*
Dog parsley; see *Aethusa cynapium*
Dog poison; see *Aethusa cynapium*
Doll's-eyes; see *Actaea*
Dragon arum; see *Arisaema*
Dragon tail; see *Arisaema*
Dragon's-head; see *Arisaema*
Dumbcane; see *Dieffenbachia*
Dutchman's-breeches; see *Dicentra*
Dwarf bay; see *Daphne*
Dwarf laurel; see *Kalmia*
Dwarf poinciana; see *Caesalpinia*
Easter lily; see *Lilium*
Elder, elderberry; see *Sambucus*
Elephant's ear; see *Colocasia* or *Alocasia*
Emory milk vetch; see *Astragalus*
English ivy; see *Hedera helix*
European bittersweet see *Solanum*
European hemlock; see *Conium*
Everlasting pea; see *Lathyrus*
Eyebright (only when Indian tobacco); see *Lobelia*
Fairy bells, fairy cap, fairy glove, fairy thimbles; see *Digitalis*
Fall crocus; see *Colchicum autumnale*
False hellebore; see *Veratrum*
False indigo; see *Baptisia*
False parsley; see *Aethusa cynapium*
False sago palm; see *Cycas revoluta*

February daphne; see *Daphne*
Female water dragon; see *Calla palustris*
Fire dragon; see *Acalypha*
Firethorn; see *Pyracantha*
Fish poison; see *Aesculus*
Fishtail palm; see *Caryota*
Flamingo flower; see *Anthurium*
Flamingo lily; see *Anthurium*
Flat pea; see *Lathyrus*
Flat-topped spurge; see *Euphorbia*
Flax olive; see *Daphne*
Fleur-de-lis; see *Iris*
Flowering spurge; see *Euphorbia*
Flying saucers; see *Ipomoea tricolor*
Folk's-glove; see *Digitalis*
Fool's cicely; see *Aethusa cynapium*
Fool's parsley; see *Aethusa cynapium*
Foothill death camas; see *Zygadenus*
Four-o'clock; see *Mirabilis*
Foxglove; see *Digitalis*
Foxtail; see *Acalypha*
Friar's cap; see *Aconitum*
Friar's cowl; see *Aconitum*
Frijolillo; see *Sophora*
Fruit salad plant; see *Monstera*
Gag weed; see *Lobelia*
Garden hyacinth; see *Hyacinthus*
Garden monkshood; see *Aconitum*
Gloriosa lily; see *Gloriosa*
Glory lily; see *Gloriosa*
Giant milkweed; see *Calotropis*
Golden pothos; see *Epiprenum*
Graceful nightshade; see *Solanum*
Grassy death camas; see *Zygadenus*
Great blue lobelia; see *Lobelia*
Great laurel; see *Rhododendron*
Great lobelia; see *Lobelia*
Green dragon; see *Arisaema*
Golden chain; see *Laburnum anagyroides*
Goldenrod; see *Isocoma*
Goosefoot; see *Chenopodium*
Gosling; see *Anemone*
Hairy nightshade; see *Solanum*

Hairy spurge; see *Euphorbia*
Hartshorn plant; see *Anemone*
Heavenly blue; see *Ipomoea tricolor*
Helmet flower; see *Aconitum*
Hemp dogbane; see *Apocynum*
Herb bonnet; see *Conium*
Herb Christopher; see *Actaea*
High belia; see *Lobelia*
Hog physic; see *Lobelia*
Holly; see *Ilex*
Horse blob; see *Caltha*
Horse chestnut; see *Aesculus*
Horse fleaweed; see *Baptisia*
Horsehead; see *Philodendron*
Horse nettle; see *Solanum*
Horsefly; see *Baptisia*
Horsefly weed; see *Baptisia*
Hurricane plant; see *Monstera*
Hyacinth; see *Hyacinthus*
Hydrangea; see *Hydrangea*
Indian apple; see *Datura*
Indian hemp; see *Apocynum*
Indian licorice vine; see *Abutilon hybridum*
Indian pink; see *Lobelia*
Indian-tree spurge; see *Euphorbia*
Indian tobacco; see *Lobelia*
Indian walnut; see *Aleurites*
Inkweed; see *Phytolacca*
Iris; see *Iris*
Irish potato; see *Solanum*
Italian arum; see *Arum*
Ivy; see *Hedera helix*
Ivy bush; see *Kalmia*
Jack-in-the-pulpit; see *Arisaema*
Jacob's coat; see *Acalypha*
Jaggary palm; see *Caryota*
Jamaican walnut; see *Aleurites*
Jamestown weed; see *Datura*
Japan oil tree; see *Aleurites*
Japanese andromeda; see *Pieris*
Japanese aucuba; see *Aucuba japonica*
Japanese laurel; see *Aucuba japonica*
Japanese privet; see *Ligustra*

Japanese show lily; see *Lilium*
Jatropha; see *Jatropha*
Jerusalem cherry; see *Solanum*
Jimmyweed; see *Isocoma*
Jimsonweed; see *Datura*
Jonquil; see *Narcissus*
Kansas thistle; see *Solanum*
Kill-cow; see *Conium*
Kingcup; see *Caltha*
Laburnum; see *Laburnum anagyroides*
Lady laurel; see *Daphne*
Lady's-thimbles; see *Digitalis*
Lambert's crazyweed; see *Oxytropis*
Lambkill; see *Kalmia*
Lamb's-quarters; see *Chenopodium*
Lantana; see *Lantana*
Larkspur; see *Delphinium*
Leafy spurge; see *Euphorbia*
Lesser hemlock; see *Aethusa cynapium*
Licorice vine; see *Abutilon hybridum*
Lily; see *Gloriosa, Hemerocallis, Lilium, Ornithogalum, Urginea*
Lily of the field; see *Anemone*
Lily of the valley; see *Convallaria majalis*
Lion's beard; see *Anemone*
Lion's-mouth; see *Digitalis*
Lirio; see *Amaryllis* or *Hippeastrum*
Lobelia; see *Lobelia*
Locoweed; see *Astragalus, Oxytropis*
Locust; see *Robinia*
Lousiana belia; see *Lobelia*
Love apple; see *Solanum*
Love apple; see *Lycopersicon esculentum*
Love bean; see *Arbrus precatorius*
Lucky bean; see *Arbrus precatorius*
Lupine (many types including Big Bend lupine, Douglas
    spurred lupine, low lupine, silvery or silky lupine, loose
    flower lupine, Washington lupine); see *Lupinus*
Mad apple; see *Datura*
Madeira ivy; see *Hedera helix*
Marble queen; see *Epiprenum*
Marvel of Peru; see *Mirabilis*
Match-me-if-you-can; see *Acalypha*
May blob; see *Caltha*

Meadow bright; see *Caltha*
Meadow death camas; see *Zygadenus*
Meadow saffron; see *Colchicum autumnale*
Memory root; see *Arisaema*
Mescal, mescal buttons; see *Lophophora*
Mescal bean; see *Sophora*
Mexican breadfruit; see *Monstera*
Mexican elderberry; see *Sambucus*
Mezereon, mezereum; see *Daphne*
Milkbush; see *Euphorbia*
Milk spurge; see *Euphorbia*
Milkvetch; see *Astragalus*
Mimosa; see *Acacia dealbata*
Mistletoe; see *Phoradendron* or *Viscum album*
Monkey-fiddle; see *Euphorbia*
Monkshood; see *Aconitum*
Monstera; see *Monstera*
Moonflower; see *Datura*
Morning glory; see *Ipomoea tricolor*
Mother-in-law; see *Monstera*
Mountain laurel; see *Kalmia*
Mountain fetterbush; see *Pieris*
Mu oil tree; see *Aleurites*
Mu tree; see *Aleurites*
Mulberry; see *Morus*
Mushrooms; see p. 184; also *Agaricus, Amanita, Boletus,*
    Chlorophyllum, Clitocybe,Conocybe, Copelandia, Coprinus,
    Galerina, Gymnopilus,Gyromitra, Inocybe, Lactarius, Lepiota,
    Panaeolus, Psilocybe, Russula
Musquash poison, musquash root; see *Cicuta*
Mustard; see *Brassica*
Mysteria; see *Colchicum autumnale*
Naked lady; see *Colchicum autumnale*
Naked lady lily; see *Amaryllis* or *Hippeastrum*
Natal cherry; see *Solanum*
Nebraska fern; see *Conium*
Necklacepod sophora; see *Sophora*
Necklaceweed; see *Actaea*
Nettle; see *Urtica*
Night-blooming jasmine; see *Cestrum*
Night-blooming jessamine; see *Cestrum*
Nightcaps; see *Anemone*
Nightshade; see *Atropa belladonna* or *Solanum*

Nimble weed; see *Anemone*
Nut Falls death camas; see *Zygadenus*
Oleander; see *Nerium*
Otaheite walnut; see *Aleurites*
Pacific yew; see *Taxus*
Pale laurel; see *Kalmia*
Palma christi; see *Ricinus communis*
Panela; see *Philodendron*
Papoose root; see *Caulophyllum thalictroides*
Pasqueflower; see *Anemone*
Passionflower; see *Lycopersicon esculentum*
Passion fruit; see *Lycopersicon esculentum*
Peach; see *Prunus*
Pearly gates; see *Ipomoea tricolor*
Penciltree; see *Euphorbia*
Petty spurge; see *Euphorbia*
Pepper turnip; see *Arisaema*
Peyote; see *Lophophora*
Philodendron; see *Philodendron* or *Monstera*
Philippine medusa; see *Acalypha*
Physic nut; see *Jatropha*
Pie plant; see *Rheum rhaponticum*
Pigeonberry; see *Rhamnus*
Pigtail plant; see *Anthurium*
Pineapple shrub; see *Calycanthus*
Pink-lady; see *Amaryllis* or *Hippeastrum*
Plum (common plum, wild plum); see *Prunus*
Poinsettia; see *Euphorbia*
Poison bush; see *Acokanthera*
Poison hemlock; see *Conium*
Poison ivy, poison oak; see *Rhus* and *Toxicodendron*
Poison parsley; see *Conium*
Poison tree; see *Acokanthera*
Poison vetch; see *Astragalus*
Poisonweed; see *Delphinium*
Pokeberry, pokeweed, poke salad see *Phytolacca*
Popdock; see *Digitalis*
Pothos; see *Epiprenum*
Prairie berry; see *Solanum*
Prairie crocus; see *Anemone*
Prairie dogbane; see *Apocynum*
Prairie hen's flower; see *Anemone*
Prairie indigo; see *Baptisia*

Prairie smoke; see *Anemone*
Prayer bead; see *Arbrus precatorius*
Prayer bean; see *Arbrus precatorius*
Prickly poppy; see *Argemone*
Priests pentle; see *Arisaema*
Privet; see *Ligustra*
Puke weed; see *Lobelia*
Purple nightshade; see *Solanum*
Pyracantha; see *Pyracantha*
Rabbit flower; see *Digitalis*
Rattlebush, rattleweed; see *Baptisia*
Rayless goldenrod; see *Isocoma*
Red baneberry; see *Actaea*
Red bead vine; see *Arbrus precatorius*
Red bean; see *Sophora*
Red emerald; see *Philodendron*
Red-hot cattail; see *Acalypha*
Red lobelia; see *Lobelia*
Red mulberry; see *Morus*
Red princess; see *Philodendron*
Red squill; see *Urginea*
Red-stemmed peavine; see *Astragalus*
Resurrection lily; see *Amaryllis* or *Hippeastrum*
Rhododendron; see *Rhododendron*
Rhubarb; see *Rheum rhaponticum*
Richweed; see *Eupatorium*
Rosary pea; see *Arbrus precatorius*
Rose bay; see *Rhododendron*
Rose laurel; see *Nerium*
Rosenlorbeer; see *Nerium*
Rubrum lily; see *Lilium*
Sacred datura; see *Datura*
Sago palm; see *Cycas revoluta*
Sandbriar, sand brier; see *Solanum*
Scarlet lobelia; see *Lobelia*
Seminole bread; see *Arbrus precatorius*
Sheepkill; see *Kalmia*
Shoofly; see *Baptisia*
Silver bush; see *Sophora*
Silver wattle; see *Acacia dealbata*
Silverleaf nightshade; see *Solanum*
Singletary pea; see *Lathyrus*
Scoke; see *Phytolacca*

Skoke; see *Phytolacca*
Skunk cabbage; see *Symplocarpus* and *Veratrum*
Sleeping nightshade; see *Atropa belladonna*
Small hemlock; see *Aethusa cynapium*
Snakeberry; see *Actaea*
Snakeroot; see *Eupatorium*
Snakeweed; see *Conium*
Snow-on-the-mountain; see *Euphorbia*
Soldier's buttons; see *Caltha*
Soldier's-cap; see *Aconitum*
Solomon's lily; see *Arum*
Spicebush; see *Calycanthus*
Spotted cowbane; see *Cicuta*
Spotted hemlock; see *Conium*
Spotted parsley; see *Conium*
Spotted spurge; see *Euphorbia*
Spreading dogbane; see *Apocynum*
Spurge olive; see *Daphne*
Squaw root; see *Caulophyllum thalictroides*
Squill; see *Urginea*
Squirrel corn; see *Dicentra*
Staggerweed; see *Delphinium*
Star-of-Bethlehem (lily); see *Ornithogalum*
Starchwort; see *Arisaema*
Stinging nettle; see *Urtica*
Stinkweed; see *Datura*
Strawberry bush; see *Calycanthus*
Summer skies; see *Ipomoea tricolor*
Sun spurge; see *Euphorbia*
Sweet Betty; see *Calycanthus*
Sweet pea; see *Lathyrus*
Sweet shrub; see *Calycanthus*
Swiss cheese plant; see *Monstera*
Tailflower; see *Anthurium*
Tansy; see *Tanacetum*
Tapiro; see *Sambucus*
Taro; see *Colocasia*
Taro vine; see *Epiprenum*
Texas buckeye; see *Aesculus*
Texas croton; see *Croton*
Texas loco; see *Astragalus*
Texas mountain laurel (not to be confused with *Kalmia*); see *Sophora*

Texas thistle; see *Solanum*
Thimbleweed; see *Anemone*
Thimbles; see *Digitalis*
Thoroughwort; see *Eupatorium*
Tiger lily; see *Lilium*
Timber milk vetch; see *Astragalus*
Thornapple; see *Argemone*
Three-leaved Indian turnip; see *Arisaema*
Throatwort; see *Digitalis*
Tobacco (including burley tobacco, coyote tobacco, desert tobacco, tree tobacco, wild tobacco); see *Nicotiana*; see also *Nicotine*, p. 191
Toddy fishtail palm; see *Caryota*
Tolguacha; see *Datura*
Tomato; see *Lycopersicon esculentum*
Toothed spurge; see *Euphorbia*
Treadsalve; see *Solanum*
Trompillo; see *Solanum*
Trumpet flower; see *Gelsemium sempervirens*
Tuber anemone; see *Anemone*
Tufted fishtail palm; see *Caryota*
Tung nut; see *Aleurites*
Tung oil tree; see *Aleurites*
Turk's cap; see *Aconitum*
Umbrella tree; see *Melia azedarach*
Variegated philodendron; see *Epiprenum*
Virginia creeper; see *Parthenocissus quinquefolia*
Wake-robin; see *Arisaema*
Walnut; see *Juglans*
Water arum; see *Calla palustris*
Water dragon; see *Calla palustris*
Water hemlock; see *Cicuta*
Water lobelia; see *Lobelia*
Waxleaf privet; see *Ligustra*
Weather plant or vine; see *Abutilon hybridum*
Wedding bells; see *Ipomoea tricolor*
Western azalea; see *Rhododendron*
Western baneberry; see *Actaea*
Western bleedingheart; see *Dicentra*
Western hellebore; see *Veratrum*
Western monkshood; see *Aconitum*
White laurel; see *Rhododendron*
White loco(weed); see *Oxytropis*

White mulberry; see *Morus*
White potato; see *Solanum*
White sanicle; see *Eupatorium*
White snakeroot; see *Eupatorium*
Wicky; see *Kalmia*
Wild bleedingheart; see *Dicentra*
Wild calla; see *Calla palustris*
Wild corn; see *Veratrum*
Wild crocus; see *Anemone*
Wild indigo; see *Baptisia*
Wild licorice or vine; see *Abutilon hybridum*
Wild monkshood; see *Aconitum*
Wild tobacco (only as Indian tobacco); see *Lobelia*
Wild winter pea; see *Lathyrus*
Windflower; see *Anemone*
Wine palm; see *Caryota*
Winter fern; see *Conium*
Wintersweet; see *Acokanthera*
Wisteria (Japanese wisteria, Chinese wisteria); see *Wisteria*
Witch's thimbles; see *Digitalis*
Wode whistle; see *Conium*
Wolfsbane; see *Aconitum*
Wonder bulb; see *Colchicum autumnale*
Woodbine; see *Parthenocissus quinquefolia*
Woolly locoweed; see *Astragalus*
Yellow allamanda; see *Allamanda cathartica*
Yellow ginseng; see *Caulophyllum thalictroides*
Yellow jasmine; see *Gelsemium sempervirens*
Yellow jessamine; see *Gelsemium sempervirens*
Yellow monkshood; see *Aconitum*
Yew (American yew, English yew, ground hemlock,
    Japanese yew, Pacific yew, western yew); see *Taxus*

Some of the poisonous plants hereafter listed have recommendations for "symptomatic and supportive" treatment. This nonspecific phrase was encountered in numerous references. Section One was written to address this wide-ranging recommendation. Therefore refer to Section One for more specific and supportive treatment recommendations.

Acacia dealbata

Common name(s)   Acacia, mimosa, silver wattle.

Toxin(s)   None known.

Toxic part(s)   None known.

Signs   Has been known to cause grazing animals to lose control of their muscles after long-term consumption. Has been reported to cause rashes.

Treatment   Since no cases of small animal poisoning were found, no specific treatment can be suggested.

Acalypha spp.

Common name(s)   Acalypha, chenille plant, red-hot cattail, foxtail, philippine medusa, Jacob's coat, copperleaf, fire dragon, beefsteak plant, match-me-if-you-can.

Toxin(s)   Diterpenes.

Toxic part(s)   Latex.

Signs   Causes nausea and vomiting. GI upset. Rashes.

Treatment   Symptomatic and supportive (see Section One).

Acokanthera spp.

Common name(s)   Bushman's poison, poison bush, poison tree, wintersweet.

Toxin(s)   Cardiac glycoside (resembles ouabain).

Toxic part(s) Distributed throughout the plant in varying amounts. The seeds contain the highest concentration, the wood, stems, and leaves contain less, and the fruit contains the least.

Signs Pain, cramping, pawing at the mouth, diarrhea. Cardiac dysrhythmias, conduction defects, and hyperkalemia may be seen in a clinical work-up.

Treatment Induce emesis (p. 50) or perform gastric lavage (p. 52) if ingestion was recent and the patient is not showing systemic signs. Administer activated charcoal and a cathartic (p. 56). Repeat in 3 to 4 hours. Treat hyperkalemia (p. 41) if detected. Monitor ECG and treat dysrhythmias by generally accepted means. If bradycardia is unresponsive to atropine, consider cardiac pacing. Dialysis and diuresis are not effective in enhancing elimination.

Aconitum spp.

Common name(s) Aconite, friar's cap, friar's-cowl, soldier's-cap, turk's cap, helmet flower, monkshood (garden m., yellow m., western m., wild m.), wolfsbane, bear's foot.

Toxin(s) Alkaloids including aconitine.

Toxic part(s) All, including vase water.

Signs The alkaloid aconitine disrupts heart nerve impulses at low doses and inhibits them at higher doses. Causes irritation to mucous membranes of the mouth when ingested. Salivating, nausea, and vomiting are common. Some animals may appear nearly or completely blind. People report blurred vision. These signs are followed by cardiac dysrhythmias and death.

Treatment Treatment is supportive (see Section One). Treat dysrhythmias as necessary. Usually refractory to treatment. Bradycardia is treated with atropine. Ventricular dysrhythmias have been treated with phenytoin.

Actaea spp.

Common name(s)   Baneberry, cohosh, doll's-eyes, herb Christopher, necklaceweed, red baneberry, snakeberry, western baneberry.

Toxin(s)   Unknown.

Toxic part(s)   Berries and roots.

Signs   Intense mucous membrane irritation and pain (which usually limits amount ingested). Salivation, vomiting (hemorrhagic), diarrhea, cramping, and abdominal pain. Renal damage is possible. CNS signs include dizziness, ataxia, confusion, apparent hallucinations, syncope, and possible convulsions.

Treatment   The irritating nature of the toxin normally prohibits ingesting enough toxin to cause systemic signs. If signs are present, gastric and enteric emptying will probably already have occurred. If not, induction of emesis (p. 50) or gastric lavage (p. 52) are appropriate followed by activated charcoal. (It has not been shown scientifically that activated charcoal is effective in the treatment of *Actaea* spp. poisoning but will cause no harm and may help.) Appropriate fluid therapy is essential to prevent perfusion or hydration problems. Electrolyte imbalances should be corrected as needed. Renal function must be monitored to detect renal damage.

Aesculus spp.

Common name(s)   Horse chestnut, buckeye, bongay, conquerors, fish poison, Texas buckeye.

Toxin(s)   Possibly several, including saponins, narcotic alkaloids, or glycosides.

Toxic part(s)   Nuts, twigs, flowers, possibly leaves.

Signs   Causes gastroenteritis, fluid loss, and electrolyte imbalances. Dilated pupils and mental dullness may be seen. In severe poisonings, tremors followed by paralysis, convulsions, coma, and death may be seen.

Treatment   Symptomatic and supportive (see Section One). Gastric and enteric emptying is usually unnecesary because the patient is usually vomiting and has diarrhea. If the ingestion was witnessed and the patient is not showing signs, induction of emesis or gastric emptying with lavage is appropriate. Administration of a cathartic is indicated. Balance fluid and electrolyte needs.

Aethusa cynapium

Common name(s)   Fool's parsley, dog parsley, dog poison, false parsley, fool's cicely, lesser hemlock, small hemlock.

Toxin(s)   Aethusin, related to cicutoxin.

Toxic part(s)   Whole plant.

Signs   Most commonly only nausea and vomiting seen. Severe signs could include convulsions, respiratory arrest, and death, but concentration is usually too low to cause these signs.

EMERGENCY TREATMENT

Procedures

1. Secure the airway and ventilate if needed (pp. 5, 9).
2. Administer supplemental oxygen (p. 7).
3. Secure venous access. Collect blood and urine for laboratory testing.
4. Administer isotonic crystalloids as needed to support blood pressure and perfusion.
5. Control seizures (p. 24).

Decontaminate

- Induce emesis *only* if the ingestion was within the last 60 minutes and the patient shows no clinical signs.
- Perform gastric lavage if the ingestion was within the last 2 to 4 hours.
- Give repeated doses of activated charcoal.
- Administer saline cathartic. Magnesium-containing solutions should be avoided.
- Consider whole bowel irrigation using CoLyte or GoLytely.
- Monitor and correct electrolyte imbalances.

Agaricus spp.

See *Mushrooms*, p. 184.

Aleurites spp.

Common name(s) Japan oil tree, tung nut, tung oil tree, Chinawood oil tree, candlenut, candleberry, country walnut, Jamaican walnut, Indian walnut, Otaheite walnut, *mu* tree* (*A. montana*), *mu* oil tree.

Toxin(s) A derivative of phorbol, an irritant.

Toxic part(s) Whole plant.

Signs Signs are related to gastroenteritis, fluid loss, or electrolyte imbalances.

Treatment Induce emesis or perform gastric lavage if necessary. Administer activated charcoal and cathartic if necessary (not usually necessary because these patients most commonly

---

*EDITOR'S NOTE: "*Mu*" originally was an English misnomer for Mandarin Chinese *mu*[4] 'tree' + English *tree*. In China a "mu tree" is commonly a *shih*[2]-*li*[4] tree, a 'rock-chestnut tree'!

have vomiting and diarrhea from the toxin). Administer fluids to support blood pressure, perfusion, and hydration. Correct electrolyte imbalances. Administer analgesic medication if abdominal pain is noted.

Allamanda cathartica

Common name(s)   Allamanda, yellow allamanda.

Toxin(s)   Unknown.

Toxic part(s)   Whole plant.

Signs   Usually a mild catharsis; however, persistent diarrhea may be seen.

Treatment   Usually none is necessary.

Allium spp.

See *Onion and garlic toxicity*, p. 197.

Alocasia spp.

Common name(s)   Elephant's ear (preferable genus name is *Colocasia*).

Toxin(s)   Calcium oxalate and possibly other irritant proteins.

Toxic part(s)   Leaves and stems.

Signs   Oral pain, edema of the mouth and oropharynx, rarely swelling will interfere with swallowing or breathing.

Treatment   Usually none necessary. The irritant nature of the toxin usluly prevents serious ingestion in animals. Treatment of the oral pain and swelling is symptomatic (see Section One). Rarely the swelling may require that the airway be secured.

Aloe spp.

Common name(s)   Aloe.

Toxin(s)   Barbaloin is found in the latex under the skin.

Toxic part(s)   Latex under the skin of the plant.

Signs   Usually a pronounced catharsis is seen after ingestion. If the patient has alkaline urine, the toxin may cause it to turn red. Nephritis may be caused by large ingestions.

Treatment   Rarely necessary. If anything, fluids may be required to replace losses from the purgative action.

Amanita spp.

See *Mushrooms,* p. 184.

Amaryllis spp.

Common name(s)   Amaryllis, Barbados lily, belladonna lily, cape belladonna, *lirio,* naked lady lily, pink-lady, resurrection lily. (See also *Hippeastrum* spp.)

Toxin(s)   Lycorine (an emetic) and small amounts of alkaloids.

Toxic part(s)   Bulbs.

Signs   Related to gastroenteritis—usually mild vomiting, diarrhea.

Treatment   Rarely necessary. Fluid replacement may be required in patients more severely affected.

Anemone spp.

Common name(s)   Pasqueflower, anemone, April fool, cat's-eyes, gosling, hartshorn plant, lily of the field, lion's beard, nightcaps, nimble weed, prairie crocus, prairie hen's flower, prairie smoke, thimbleweed, tuber anemone, wild crocus, windflower.

Toxin(s)   Protoanemonin.

Toxic part(s)   Whole plant.

Signs   The toxin is quite irritating to mucous membranes. Blisters are commonly seen after the plant is chewed. Ingestion is rare. If ingested, signs of severe, hemorrhagic gastroenteritis are seen and may lead to shock. Convulsions and death are possible.

Treatment   Usually only symptomatic for oral vesicles or ulceration (see Section One). Rarely, gastric emptying may be required if large ingestions are witnessed. Activated charcoal and a cathartic are administered after gastric emptying. Fluids are administered to support blood pressure, perfusion, and hydration as necessary. Seizures are controlled by generally accepted means (p. 24). Analgesics may be indicated.

Anthurium spp.

Common name(s)   Anthurium, *anturio,* flamingo flower, flamingo lily, pigtail plant, tailflower.

Toxin(s)   Calcium oxalate and possibly irritant proteins.

Toxic part(s)   Leaves and plants.

Signs Pain and swelling of the oral cavity. Acute inflammation of the oropharynx accompanied by salivation, pawing at the mouth, and drooling. Edema of the lips, tongue, and throat may be seen.

Treatment Usually none required. Occasionally analgesics may be required. Swelling may be treated with cool compresses. It is unknown if diuretics or glucocorticosteroid would help with the inflammation. Rarely the swelling will interfere with respiration. If necessary, secure the airway (p. 2).

Apocynum spp.

Common name(s) Dogbane, hemp dogbane, Indian hemp, prairie dogbane, spreading dogbane.

Toxin(s) Cardiac glycosides.

Toxic part(s) Entire plant.

Signs Most of today's literature is based on a report that may have confused the dogbanes with *Nerium oleander,* because both genera belong to the *Apocynaceae* family. Signs in animals are said to be cold extremities, hyperthermia, hypothermia, mydriasis, sore mouth, anorexia, gastric distress, tachycardia (or bradycardia), and death.

Treatment Treatment is symptomatic and supportive (see Section One). Digoxin immune Fab (ovine) (Digibind, Glaxo Wellcome, Inc., Research Triangle Park, N.C.) has been reported to be of value in treating animals poisoned by ingesting oleander. Human poison control centers do not recommend it for cases of dogbane ingestion.

Arbrus precatorius

Common name(s) Bead or red bead vine, black-eyed Susan, coral bead plant, crab's-eye vine, Indian or wild licorice or licorice vine, love bean, lucky bean, rosary pea, prayer bead, prayer bean, Seminole bread, weather plant or vine.

Toxin(s)   Abrin, which inhibits protein synthesis in cells of the intestinal wall.

Toxic part(s)   The seed is the toxic part. If it is swallowed whole, it will usually pass without release of the toxic principle.

Signs   Nausea, vomiting, diarrhea (sometimes hemorrhagic), hypovolemia, electrolyte disturbances.

Treatment   The effects may not be seen until many hours to days after ingestion. Gastric or enteric emptying is unrewarding in patients who are showing signs. Treatment is supportive. Administer fluids to support hydration and perfusion. Electrolytes must be determined and imbalances corrected.

Argemone spp.

Common name(s)   Prickly poppy, thornapple.

Toxin(s)   Toxic alkaloids including protopine, berberine, sanguinarine, and dihydrosanguinarine.

Toxic part(s)   Mostly the seeds or oil from the seeds.

Signs   Small animals are unlikely to be poisoned by this plant. The alkaloids will cause gastrointestinal disturbances if ingested.

Treatment   Treatment is symptomatic and supportive (see Section One).

Arisaema spp.

Common name(s)   Green dragon, dragon arum, dragon tail, dragon's-head (*A. draconitium;* do not confuse with the mint *Dracocephalum*), Jack-in-the-pulpit, bog onion, brown dragon, cuckoo plant, memory root, pepper turnip, priests pentle (*A. triphyllum*), starchwort, three-leaved Indian turnip, wake-robin.

Toxin(s)   Calcium oxalate and possibly irritant proteins.

Toxic part(s)   Whole plant.

Signs   Pain and swelling of the oral cavity. Acute inflammation of the oropharynx accompanied by salivation, pawing at the mouth, and drooling. Edema of the lips, tongue, and throat may be seen.

Treatment   Usually none required. Analgesics may be required. Swelling may be treated with cool compresses. It is unknown if diuretics or glucocorticosteroid would help with the inflammation. Rarely, the swelling will interfere with respiration. If necessary, secure the airway (p. 2).

Arum spp.

Common name(s)   Adam-and-Eve plant, black calla, caladium, cuckoopint, Italian arum, Solomon's lily.

Toxin(s)   Calcium oxalate and possibly irritant proteins.

Toxic part(s)   Whole plant.

Signs   Pain and swelling of the oral cavity. Acute inflammation of the oropharynx accompanied by salivation, pawing at the mouth, and drooling. Edema of the lips, tongue, and throat may be seen.

Treatment   Usually none required. Analgesics may be required. Swelling may be treated with cool compresses. It is unknown if diuretics or glucocorticosteroid would help with the inflammation. Rarely, swelling of the tongue, glottis, or pharynx will interfere with respiration. If necessary, secure the airway (p. 2).

Astragalus spp.

Common name(s)   Crazyweed, emory milk vetch, locoweed, milk vetch, poison vetch, red-stemmed peavine, Texas loco, timber milk vetch, woolly locoweed. (See also *Oxytropis* spp.)

Toxin(s)   Several alkaloids, methemoglobin formation.

Toxic part(s)   Leaves.

Signs   Poisoning of dogs and cats would be unlikely with this plant. It has been known to cause serious loss in cattle, sheep, and other range animals. Humans have also been reported to have been poisoned. Signs reported in humans are related to selenium accumulation. Reported signs include pallor, garlicky odor on the breath, gastrointestinal disturbances, nausea, vomiting, tightness in the chest, drowsiness, and brain damage.

Treatment   Treatment is supportive and symptomatic (see Section One). If methemoglobinemia is detected, it is treated as follows:
1.   Ascorbic acid 20 to 30 mg/kg PO or 20 mg/kg IV slowly
2.   Methylene blue
   Dogs   3 to 4 mg/kg IV slowly if ascorbic acid has not been of benefit.
   Cats   1.5 mg/kg has been reported to be beneficial to cats with nitrite-induced methemoglobinemia. Given in the absence of methemoglobinemia, methylene blue may cause Heinz body formation.

Atropa belladonna

Common name(s)   Deadly nightshade, belladonna, black nightshade, nightshade, sleeping nightshade.

Toxin(s)   Atropine and other belladonna alkaloids.

Toxic part(s)   Whole plant.

Signs   Ingestion causes atropine-like signs—dry mouth, repeated swallowing efforts, dysphagia, tachycardia, mydriasis, and urinary retention.

Treatment   If ingestion was recent, gastric emptying by induction of emesis or lavage is appropriate. Administer activated charcoal and a cathartic. Human literature recommends slow IV administration of physostigmine to effect, that is, until symptoms abate or until cholinergic signs appear. Since belladonna alkaloids have a longer half-life than physostigmine has, repeated doses of physostigmine may be required.

Aucuba japonica

Common name(s)   Japanese aucuba, Japanese laurel.

Toxin(s)   Aucubin, a glycoside.

Toxic part(s)   Whole plant.

Signs   Moderate signs of GI upset including nausea, vomiting, and rarely diarrhea.

Treatment   Rarely necessary. Supportive for fluid loss and electrolyte imbalance (see Section One).

Baptisia spp.

Common name(s)   Wild indigo, cloverbloom, false indigo (when not *Amorpha*), horse fleaweed, horsefly, horsefly weed, prairie indigo, rattlebush, rattleweed, shoofly.

Toxin(s)   Alkaloids including cytisine.

Toxic part(s)   Whole plant.

Signs Rare. Nausea, possibly vomiting. The toxin theoretically could cause hypoventilation and respiratory arrest.

Treatment If emesis has not occurred, gastric emptying is advised. Activated charcoal and cathartic are administered. If respiratory depression is significant, secure the airway and ventilate the patient. If constipation or urinary retention are noted, they may respond to administration of bethanechol.

Boletus spp.

See *Mushrooms*, p. 184.

Brassica spp.

Common name(s) Mustard.

Toxin(s) Mustard oils including isothiocyanate and beta-phenyl isothiocyanate.

Toxic part(s) Mostly the roots and the seeds.

Signs The toxins are very irritating to the eyes and mucous membranes. Ingestion may cause gastrointestinal distress, nausea, vomiting, and diarrhea (sometimes bloody). If the toxin should gain access to the eye, permanent blindness may result. Contact with the skin will cause blistering and burning with intense pruritus and self-mutilation.

Treatment Treatment involves gastrointestinal decontamination including induction of emesis (p. 50) or gastric lavage as necessary. Activated charcoal is recommended. Dermal exposure is treated by bathing the affected area with a mild shampoo and copious rinsing. Mustard oil in the eye should be treated by copious irrigation of the eye with water or saline. Gastrointestinal disturbances (vomiting, diarrhea) may result in hypovolemia, electrolyte imbalances, and dehydration, which require assessment and treatment.

Caesalpinia spp.

Common name(s) Bird-of-paradise bush (see *Strelitzia reginae* for the bird-of-paradise flower), Barbados pride, dwarf poinciana.

Toxin(s) Tannins.

Toxic part(s) Seeds (roasting the seed renders them edible).

Signs GI signs including vomiting and diarrhea.

Treatment Rarely indicated. Recovery is usually seen within 24 hours. Fluid therapy may be indicated in cases where losses exceed intake.

Calla palustris

Common name(s) Water arum, female water dragon, water dragon, wild calla.

Toxin(s) Calcium oxalate and possibly irritant proteins.

Toxic part(s) Whole plant, especially the roots.

Signs Pain and swelling of the oral cavity. Acute inflammation of the oropharynx accompanied by salivation, pawing at the mouth, and drooling. Edema of the lips, tongue, and throat may be seen.

Treatment Usually none required. Analgesics may be required. Swelling may be treated with cool compresses. It is unknown if diuretics or glucocorticosteroid would help with the inflammation. Rarely the swelling will interfere with respiration. If necessary, secure the airway (p. 2).

Calotropis spp.

Common name(s) Crown flower, giant milkweed.

Toxin(s) Cardiac glycoside, vesicant (may induce allergic dermatitis rather than direct effect).

Toxic part(s) The whole plant contains the glycoside. The latex contains the vesicant.

Signs Acrid taste usually limits ingestion. Exposure of the skin or mucous membranes to the latex may result in vesicle formation. Keratoconjunctivitis will result if the cornea is exposed. Ingestion of significant quantities will result in ECG abnormalities.

Treatment Wash the exposed tissue with plenty of warm water and soap. Flush the eyes with sterile saline or water for 15 minutes. If cardiac abnormalities are seen, manage according to ECG assessment.

Caltha spp.

Common name(s) Bull flower, cowslip, kingcup, horse blob, May blob, meadow bright, soldier's buttons.

Toxin(s) Protoanemonin.

Toxic part(s) Whole mature plant (immature plants are boiled and eaten as greens).

Signs The toxin is quite irritating to mucous membranes. Blisters are commonly seen after the plant is chewed. Ingestion is rare. If ingested, signs of severe, hemorrhagic gastroenteritis are seen.

Treatment Usually only symptomatic for oral vesicles or ulceration (see Section One). Rarely, gastric emptying may be required if large ingestions are witnessed. Activated charcoal and a cathartic are administered after gastric emptying. Fluids are administered to support blood pressure, perfusion, and hydration as necessary. Analgesics may be indicated.

Calycanthus spp.

Common name(s) American allspice, Carolina allspice, calycanth, pineapple shrub, spicebush, strawberry bush, strawberry shrub, sweet shrub, sweet Bettie, bubby-blossoms, bubbybush.

Toxin(s) Calycanthin, other alkaloids.

Toxic part(s) Seeds.

Signs No case reports were found in the literature. Reports of animals given the alkaloids indicate that the animals suffered strychnine-like convulsions, myocardial depression, and hypotension.

Treatment No convincing recommendations were found in the literature. Treatment would be supportive and symptomatic (see Section One).

Caryota spp.

Common name(s) Clustered fishtail palm, fishtail palm, jaggary palm, toddy fishtail palm, tufted fishtail palm, wine palm.

Toxin(s) Calcium oxalate and possibly irritant proteins.

Toxic part(s) Whole plant, especially the roots.

Signs Pain and swelling of the oral cavity. Acute inflammation of the oropharynx accompanied by salivation, pawing at the mouth, and drooling. Edema of the lips, tongue, and throat may be seen.

Treatment Usually none required. Analgesics may be required. Swelling may be treated with cool compresses. It is unknown if diuretics or glucocorticosteroid would help with the inflammation. Rarely the swelling will interfere with respiration. If necessary, secure the airway (p. 2).

Caulophyllum thalictroides

Common name(s) Blue cohosh, blueberry root, papoose root, squaw root, blue ginseng, yellow ginseng.

Toxin(s) Saponins, *N*-methycytisine, which is a nicotine-like alkaloid.

Toxic part(s) Berries and roots.

Signs Usually limited to gastroenteritis.

Treatment Rarely necessary; fluid replacement for excessive losses.

Cestrum spp.

Common name(s) Day-blooming jessamine (jasmine), night-blooming jessamine (jasmine), Chinese inkberry.

Toxin(s) Solanine (a cholinesterase-inhibiting compound) predominates in unripe berries, whereas tropane alkaloids (which are like atropine) are prevalent in the ripe berry. Saponins, alkaloids, and traces of nicotine are also found in plants. *Cestrum diurnum* contains 1,25-dihydroxyvitamin D glucoside.

Toxic part(s) Fruit, leaves, and sap are poisonous.

Signs Both solanine and tropane may mimic atropine poisoning (mydriasis, tachycardia, xerostomia, dyspnea, ileus, urinary retention, CNS stimulation followed by depression, paralysis, seizures). If solanine predominates, mild to severe gastrointestinal signs may predominate. Normal to increased borborygmi may indicate predominance of solanine, whereas lack of bowel sounds may hint at an atropine-like toxin.

Treatment   Rarely, fluid therapy to replace losses. In cases where atropine-like signs are life threatening, physostigmine may be carefully administered (CAUTION: physostigmine may cause asystole). Begin with 0.02 mg/kg administered IV over 5 minutes. If delerium or coma is abolished, use repeated doses as needed. If no effect is noted or gastrointestinal signs predominate, consider cautious administration of atropine and observe for signs of improvement. Tachydysrhythmias that do not respond to physostigmine may respond to administration of propranolol. If *Cestrum diurnum* is the plant involved, monitor for evidence of hypercalcemia and treat accordingly. (See Vitamin D rodenticides, p. 255.)

Chenopodium spp.

Common name(s)   Lamb's-quarters, goosefoot.

Toxin(s)   Nitrates and oxalic acid.

Toxic part(s)   Whole plant.

Signs   No reports of cases involving dogs and cats were found. Poisoning has been reported in humans and geese, but evidence of poisoning was not detected when the plants were fed to swine.

Treatment   No studies have been done to determine efficacy of treatment protocols. Treatment is symptomatic and supportive (see Section One).

Chlorophyllum spp.

See *Mushrooms*, p. 184.

Cicuta spp.

Common name(s) Beaver poison, children's bane, death-of-man, musquash poison, musquash root, spotted cowbane, water hemlock.

Toxin(s) Cicutoxin.

Toxic part(s) Entire plant.

Signs Reports of small animal cases of cicutoxin poisoning are lacking. Poisoning of livestock and humans are reported most often. Signs include frothing at the mouth, tremors, convulsions, mydriasis, violent gastrointestinal disturbances, collapse, paralysis, respiratory failure, and death. The signs progress rapidly.

Treatment There is no known treatment. If the victim lives >2 hours, it will likely survive. Treatment is symptomatic and supportive (see Section One).

Clitocybe spp.

See *Mushrooms*, p. 184.

Cnidocolus

See *Urtica* spp.

Colchicum autumnale

Common name(s) Autumn crocus, crocus, fall crocus, meadow saffron, mysteria, naked lady, wonder bulb.

Toxin(s)   The alkaloid colchicine and related compounds.

Toxic part(s)   Entire plant, especially bulbs.

Signs   Salivation, nausea, vomiting, diarrhea, respiratory depression, muscle weakness, collapse, shock, and death. Renal failure is also possible in some patients surviving the initial signs.

Treatment   Gastric emptying (emesis or lavage) followed by activated charcoal. Cathartics are recommended but usually not necessary because of the purgative action of the toxin. Fluids are administered as necessary to maintain blood pressure, perfusion, and hydration. Urine output should be monitored for signs of acute renal failure. The ECG should be monitored and dysrhythmias treated by conventional means. Electrolyte imbalances should be corrected.

Colocasia spp.

Common name(s)   Elephant's ear, elephant ear (see also *Alocasia*), dasheen, taro.

Toxin(s)   Calcium oxalate and possibly other irritant proteins.

Toxic part(s)   Leaves and stems.

Signs   Oral pain, edema of the mouth and oropharynx; rarely swelling will interfere with swallowing or breathing.

Treatment   Usually none necessary. The irritant nature of the toxin usually prevents serious ingestion in animals. Treatment of the oral pain and swelling is symptomatic (see Section One). Rarely the swelling may block the airway, requiring immediate action to secure the airway.

Conium spp.

Common name(s)   California fern, cashes, European hemlock, herb bonnet, kill-cow, Nebraska fern, poison hemlock, poison parsley, snakeweed, spotted hemlock, spotted parsley, winter fern, wode whistle.

Toxin(s)   Coniine and other alkaloids.

Toxic part(s)   Roots and seeds are most toxic, but the entire plant is toxic.

Signs   Reports of small animal toxicosis are lacking. Signs in livestock and humans are similar to nicotine poisoning. Signs include hypersalivation, abdominal pain, burning sensation of the mouth and mucous membranes, weakness, paralysis, bradycardia, mydriasis, weak pulses, frequent urination, collapse, and death from respiratory paralysis.

Treatment   Specific treatment regimens are lacking for small animal ingestion. Routine gastrointestinal decontamination (emesis, gastric lavage, activated charcoal, cathartics) and symptomatic and supportive treatment are recommended (see Section One).

Conocybe spp., Copelandia spp., Coprinus spp.

See *Mushrooms*, p. 184.

Convallaria majalis

Common name(s)   Lily of the valley.

Toxin(s)   Cardiac glycosides, including convallotoxin.

Toxic part(s)   Whole plant.

Signs   Vomiting, anorexia, nausea, diarrhea, ataxia, cardiac dysrhythmias, weakness, confusion, collapse, and death.

Treatment   In the case of a witnessed ingestion, the animal should be made to vomit (see Emesis induction, p. 50) followed by administration of activated charcoal. Treat as for digitalis overdose. The use of Digibind (p. 291) may be considered in patients suffering life-threatening signs of poisoning, although the efficacy of this product has not been proved in poisoning by this plant.

Croton spp.

Common name(s)   Croton, Texas croton.

Toxin(s)   Oil of croton.

Toxic part(s)   Seeds.

Signs   Burning sensation in the mouth is reported by humans. Animals may paw at the mouth, salivate, and vomit. Tachycardia, diarrhea (sometimes bloody), coma, and death may result.

Treatment   The oil is very potent in the dog. Witnessed ingestions of the seeds should be followed by immediate induction of emesis. If emesis does not occur, gastric lavage is indicated, followed by administration of activated charcoal. Other treatment regimens are symptomatic and supportive (see Section One).

Cycas revoluta

Common name(s)   False sago palm, sago palm. (There appears to be some confusion in naming these plants. Some sources list the false sago palm as *Cycas revoluta,* whereas others list it as the "true" sago palm.)

Toxin(s)   Cycasin, macrozamin, and possibly others.

Toxic part(s)   Seeds have caused poisoning in dogs. Other parts of the plants may be toxic, including the root ball.

Signs   Signs develop in 12 hours after ingestion. Gastrointestinal signs (vomiting, anorexia, abdominal discomfort) are followed by signs of acute hepatotoxicity. Polydipsia, ascites, icterus, and cirrhosis may be found. Bruising, epistaxis, hemoptysis, melena, hematochezia, and hemarthrosis may be seen as a result of a developing coagulopathy. The coagulopathy is characterized by thrombocytopenia, prolongation of PT, activated clotting time, and activated PTT. Laboratory analysis will often reveal elevated bilirubin levels, elevated liver enzymes (although these may not be dramatic), hypoproteinemia, hyponatremia, hypocalcemia, hypokalemia, azotemia, and a metabolic alkalosis. Urine analysis may reveal glucosuria, bilirubinuria, hematuria, and crystals or casts in the sediment.

Treatment   The prognosis for cycad poisoning is generally poor. Treatment is symptomatic and supportive (see Section One). Witnessed ingestions indicate the need for immediate induction of emesis or gastric lavage, followed by administration of activated charcoal and a cathartic.

Daphne spp.

Common name(s)   Dwarf bay, February daphne, flax olive, lady laurel, mezereon, mezereum, spurge laurel, spurge olive.

Toxin(s)   Mezereinic acid anhydride (an irritant) and daphnin.

Toxic part(s)   The entire plant is toxic.

Signs   Dermal exposure may cause systemic signs. Experimentally, dried bark of Daphne was fed to dogs and produced a fatal syndrome. Systemic signs include gastroenteritis (perhaps bloody), weakness, collapse, shock, coma, and death. Convulsions may be seen. Nonlethal ingestions may result in acute renal failure. Dermal exposure will cause vesicle formation.

Treatment Dermal exposure should be treated with aggressive bathing and rinsing. The caregiver must take care to avoid exposure of himself or herself to the plant. Ingestion should be treated with gastrointestinal emptying followed by activated charcoal and cathartic administration. Fluids are administered to support blood pressure, perfusion, and hydration. Urine production should be monitored. Attention should be paid to electrolyte levels and imbalances corrected.

Datura spp.

Common name(s) Datura, devil's-apple (when not *Podophyllum* or *Mandragora* or *Solanum*), devil's trumpet, Indian apple (*D. metaloides;* when not *Podophyllum*), Jamestown weed, Jimsonweed, mad apple, moonflower, sacred datura (*D. metaloides*), stinkweed, *tolguacha*.

Toxin(s) Atropine, hyoscyamine, and scopolamine.

Toxic part(s) Entire plant, especially the seeds.

Signs Signs relate to parasympatholytic action of the alkaloids; the syndrome resembles atropine poisoning (mydriasis, tachycardia, xerostomia, dyspnea, ileus, urinary retention, CNS stimulation followed by depression, paralysis, seizures).

Treatment Rarely, fluid therapy to replace losses. In cases where atropine-like signs are life threatening, physostigmine may be carefully administered (CAUTION: physostigmine may cause asystole). Begin with 0.02 mg/kg administered IV over 5 minutes. If delirium or coma is abolished, use repeated doses as needed. Tachydysrhythmias that do not respond to physostigmine may respond to administration of propranolol.

Delphinium spp.

Common name(s) Larkspur, delphinium, poisonweed (when not a lupine), staggerweed (when not a *Dicentra* or a *Stachys*).

Toxin(s) Several alkaloids, one of which has curare-like (neuromuscular blockade) effects.

Toxic part(s) The whole plant is toxic.

Signs No reports of cases involving dogs and cats have been found. Poisoning has been reported in humans, cattle, horses, and sheep. Signs include muscular weakness, hyperexcitability, confusion, salivating followed by dry mouth, bloating, constipation, vomiting or regurgitation, collapse, convulsions, coma, and death. Sudden death may be seen if significant quantities are ingested.

Treatment No studies have been done to determine efficacy of treatment protocols. Treatment is symptomatic and supportive (see Section One). Physostigmine is reported to be effective in larkspur poisoning. Carefully administer 0.04 to 0.08 mg/kg IV slowly to effect. Repeat dosing may be required.

Dicentra spp.

Common name(s) Bleedingheart, Dutchman's-breeches, squirrel corn, staggerweed (but see also *Delphinium*), western bleedingheart, wild bleedingheart.

Toxin(s) Protopine, an isoquinoline alkaloid.

Toxic part(s) Whole plant.

Signs Acute onset after ingestion of the plant. Trembling, hyperexcitability, salivation, and vomiting are seen within minutes. Signs can progress to recumbency, opisthotonos, and seizures. Death occurs rarely. This is not a common small animal poisoning but is more likely in ruminants.

Treatment If ingestion is noted, gastric emptying through induction of emesis (p.50) or gastric lavage is indicated. Most animals recover without treatment. Treatment is symptomatic and supportive (see Section One).

Dieffenbachia spp.

Common name(s)   Dumbcane.

Toxin(s)   Calcium oxalate crystals, which the plant, using special contractile cells, actually propels into the tissue of the patient. Recently, research has disclosed that proteolytic enzymes are also contained by these plants. Such enzymes trigger the release of histamines and kinins in the body and contribute to clinical signs.

Toxic part(s)   Entire plant.

Signs   Immediate pain in the mouth on chewing the plant. The animal may recoil from the plant, begin to salivate heavily, and shake its head vigorously. A change of voice may be noted by owners. The tissues of the mouth and throat will swell, rarely causing obstruction of the airway. Dyspnea or painful respirations may be noted. Nausea, vomiting, and diarrhea may be seen. Discussion of rare cardiac dysrhythmias, mydriasis, coma, and death resulting from ingestion of dumbcanes (and other members of the family *Araceae*) are found in the literature.

Treatment   Symptomatic and supportive (see Section One). Rinse the mouth with water or milk. The calcium in the milk may precipitate soluble oxalates. Antihistamines may be useful. Fluids and electrolytes may be necessary in patients who have severe fluid losses or hypotension.

Digitalis spp.

Common name(s)   Digitalis, fairy bells, fairy cap, fairy glove, fairy thimbles, folk's-glove, foxglove, lady's thimbles, lion's-mouth, popdock, rabbit flower, thimbles, throatwort, witch's thimbles.

Toxin(s)   Numerous, including cardiac and steroid glycosides.

Toxic part(s)   The entire plant as well as water from vases containing foxglove plants.

Signs   Abdominal pain, nausea, vomiting, salivation, and local irritation of the mucous membranes are noted soon after ingestion. Pulses may be slow and strong (early with moderate digitalis-like intoxication) or rapid and weak (later). Cardiac conduction disturbances are seen on ECG and may be severe enough to contribute to signs including ataxia, hypotension, shock, collapse, and death. Pupils may be dilated. Delirium may be followed by coma. Hyperkalemia, hypocalcemia, and hypoglycemia may be seen on laboratory analysis.

Treatment   The gastrointestinal tract should be decontaminated. Induction of emesis (p. 50) or gastric lavage should be performed as needed, followed by administration of activated charcoal. Cathartics should also be used if necessary. Treat as for digitalis overdose. Digibind (Glaxo Wellcome, Research Triangle Pk., NC 27709) has been used successfully in treating digitalis overdose in humans and dogs. Research has revealed that Digibind given at a dose of 60 mg/kg IV resulted in survival (from oleander, which contains cardiac glycoside toxins similar to those from *Digitalis* spp.) and conversion to normal sinus rhythm. Repeat injections may be necessary. In humans, digitalis-like intoxications may be treated with temporary cardiac pacing by use of a transvenous pacemaker. This option should be explored. A call to a pacemaker company may bring a representative who can offer a temporary, external pacemaker. The technique to implant the leads and set up the pacemaker is not difficult.

Serum potassium should be monitored. The patient should be treated for hypokalemia (p. 42) or hyperkalemia (p. 41) if necessary. Cardiac dysrhythmias may be treated with phenytoin.

Epiprenum spp.

Common name(s)   Devil's ivy, golden pothos, marble queen, pothos, taro vine, variegated philodendron

Toxin(s)   Calcium oxalate and perhaps proteolytic enzymes.

Toxic part(s)   Probably the entire plant including the roots.

Signs   Pain and swelling of the oral cavity. Acute inflammation of the oropharynx accompanied by salivation, pawing at the mouth, and drooling. Edema of the lips, tongue, and throat may be seen.

Treatment   Usually none required. Rinse the mouth copiously with water or milk. Give the animal milk or other source of calcium. The calcium may precipitate soluble oxalates. Antihistamines may be helpful. Analgesics may be required. Swelling may be treated with cool compresses. It is unknown if diuretics or glucocorticosteroid would help with the inflammation. Rarely, swelling of the tongue, glottis, or pharynx will interfere with respiration. If necessary, secure the airway (p. 2).

Eupatorium spp.

Common name(s)   Boneset, richweed, snakeroot, thoroughwort, white sanicle, white snakeroot.

Toxin(s)   Tremetol and certain glycosides.

Toxic part(s)   Entire plant.

Signs   Poisoning is likely only in dogs and cats fed raw milk from a cow grazing on these plants. No reports have been found in the literature, though other species have been poisoned including cows, horses, sheep, goats, and humans. This syndrome is not acute, and recovery from nonlethal ingestions usually extends over several days to weeks. Weakness, nausea, vomiting, tremors, liver damage, dyspnea-tachypnea, collapse, convulsions, coma, and death have been described.

Treatment   No studies have been done to determine treatment. Recommendations at this time would be for routine decontamination (gastric emptying, activated charcoal, and a cathartic) and symptomatic support (see Section One).

Euphorbia spp.

Common name(s) Candelabra cactus, caper spurge, Christ-thorn (*E. milli*; do not confuse with *Paliuris* or *Ziziphus*), crown of thorns, cypress spurge, flat-topped spurge, flowering spurge, leafy spurge, hairy spurge, Indian-tree spurge, milkbush, milk spurge, monkey-fiddle, penciltree, petty spurge, poinsettia, snow-on-the-mountain, spotted spurge, sun spurge, toothed spurge.

Toxin(s) Phorbol esters.

Toxic part(s) Leaves, stems, and sap.

Signs Severe irritation of the oropharynx and esophagus. Coughing, choking, retching, and pawing at the mouth may be noted. Vomiting, diarrhea, temporary blindness, and intestinal cramping may also be seen. Syncope has been reported to occur in humans.

Treatment There are no antidotes. Treatment is symptomatic and supportive (see Section One). Gastric emptying via induction of emesis or gastric lavage followed by activated charcoal and a cathartic is indicated. Fluid and electrolyte needs must be attended to.

The poinsettia has long been believed by the public to be highly toxic. Research fails to comfirm this because lethal toxicosis could not be produced in rats. The Illinois Animal Poison Control Center reports that ingestion rarely causes a problem. When entire plants were eaten, the animals may have significant vomiting and diarrhea requiring fluid and electrolyte therapy.

Galerina spp.

See *Mushrooms*, p. 184.

Gelsemium sempervirens

Common name(s)   Carolina jessamine (jasmine), Carolina yellow jessamine (jasmine), trumpet flower, yellow jessamine.

Toxin(s)   Gelsemine and gelseminine—alkaloids related to strychnine.

Toxic part(s)   Entire plant including nectar. Honey made from nectar may be toxic.

Signs   No cases of poisoning in dogs or cats have been found. Signs in humans and livestock include intense muscle cramps, weakness, convulsions, hypoventilation, and paralysis of motor nerves. Death is from respiratory paralysis.

Treatment   No studies have been done to determine specific treatment. Decontamination and treatment is symptomatic and supportive, except that induction of emesis should not be recommended because of the possibility of rapid onset of seizures (see Section One).

Gloriosa spp.

Common name(s)   Climbing lily, gloriosa lily, glory lily, lily.

Toxin(s)   Colchicine and other alkaloids.

Toxic part(s)   The entire plant including root stock.

Signs   No reports of cases involving dogs and cats have been found. Poisoning has been reported in humans. Signs reported included numbness of the lip, tongue, and throat; gastrointestinal distress; difficulty breathing; collapse; shock; convulsions; and death.

Treatment   No studies have been done to determine efficacy of treatment protocols. Treatment is symptomatic and supportive (see Section One).

Gymnopilus spp.

See *Mushrooms*, p. 184.

Gyromitra spp.

See *Mushrooms,* p. 184.

Hedera helix

Common name(s)   Algerian ivy, Canary ivy, English ivy, ivy, Madeira ivy.

Toxin(s)   A saponin called hederagenin by one reference but hederin by another.

Toxic part(s)   The entire plant is toxic.

Signs   Reports of poisoning of children are found in the literature. Signs include nausea, vomiting, diarrhea, excitement, difficulty in breathing, and convulsions (rarely).

Treatment   Treatment is symptomatic and supportive (see Section One).

Hemerocallis spp.

Common name(s)   Day lily.

Toxin(s)   Unknown.

Toxic part(s)   The entire plant is toxic to cats.

Signs   Cats are reported to be sensitive to an unknown toxin found in these lily species. Ingestion of this toxin results in non-specific signs followed by acute renal failure (usually anuric) within 24 to 48 hours. It is unknown whether dogs or birds are sensitive to the toxin found in these plants.

Treatment   There is no specific antidote. If a dog or cat is witnessed ingesting *Hemerocallis*, immediate induction of emesis or gastric lavage is indicated followed by administration of activated charcoal and cathartic. Fluid diuresis is indicated. Urine production should be maintained at at least 2 mL/kg/hour in the cat and 3 mL/kg/hour in the dog. If aggressive treatment is begun early enough to maintain renal tubular flow, the recovery rate is satisfactory. If, however, the renal failure syndrome develops, mortality is high. Dialysis has been reported to be successful in patients (at least one reported) even after the renal failure became apparent.

Hippeastrum spp.

Common name(s)   Amaryllis, Barbados lily, belladonna lily, cape belladonna, *lirio,* naked lady lily, pink-lady, resurrection lily. (See also *Amaryllis*)

Toxin(s)   Lycorine (an emetic) and small amounts of alkaloids.

Toxic part(s)   Bulbs.

Signs   Related to gastroenteritis—usually mild vomiting, diarrhea.

Treatment   Rarely necessary. Fluid replacement may be required in patients more severely affected.

Hyacinthus spp.

Common name(s)   Hyacinth, garden hyacinth.

Toxin(s)   Confusion seems to exist on the toxicity of *Hyacinthus*. One reference reports the toxic principal as calcium oxalate crystals, whereas another lists alkaloids that cause gastrointestinal distress as the toxin.

Toxic part(s)   Bulbs are most toxic.

Signs   Signs listed include only gastrointestinal distress, nausea, vomiting. If calcium oxalate crystals were the toxin, one would expect signs similar to those seen with exposure to plants of the *Araceae* family.

Treatment   Gastrointestinal decontamination including emesis, lavage, and activated charcoal would be indicated. If signs of oral irritation and pain exist, allowing the pet to drink milk may cause precipitation of soluble oxalates.

Hydrangea spp.

Common name(s)   Hydrangea.

Toxin(s)   The plant is known to contain a cyanogenic glycoside called "hydrangin" (or "umbelliferone"), but signs of poisoning rarely mimic cyanide poisoning.

Toxic part(s)   The entire plant is toxic.

Signs   Poisoning of dogs and cats is rare. Signs may include gastrointestinal signs (vomiting, diarrhea, bloody diarrhea, colic) or, rarely, signs of cyanide poisoning (tachypnea, respiratory distress, cherry-red blood).

Treatment   Witnessed ingestions should be treated with gastric emptying and activated charcoal. Treatment for gastrointestinal signs are symptomatic and supportive (see Section One).

Ilex spp.

Common name(s)   Holly.

Toxin(s)   Most references list ilicin as the toxin; however, others attribute toxicity to theobromine and caffeine.

Toxic part(s)   Leaves and berries.

Signs   Gastrointestinal distress and CNS depression have been reported. Poisoning by ingestion of holly is rare.

Treatment   Symptomatic and supportive (see Section One).

Inocybe spp.

See *Mushrooms*, p. 184.

Ipomoea tricolor

Common name(s)   Blue star, flying saucers, heavenly blue, morning glory, pearly gates, summer skies, wedding bells.

Toxin(s)   LSD and related compounds.

Toxic part(s)   Seeds.

Signs   These are hallucinogenic compounds and as such cause bizarre behavior in animals. Animals may appear confused, ataxic, vocalize, frantic, restless, or disoriented. Nausea, vomiting, diarrhea, and hypotension have been seen. Mydriasis has been reported.

Treatment   Gastroenteric emptying (emesis or gastric lavage if indicated) is followed by administration of activated charcoal. Seizures are controlled by administration of diazepam or barbiturates if needed. Phenothiazine tranquilizers may be of benefit but are known to lower the seizure threshold; therefore the caregiver must be aware that administration may precipitate seizure activity.

Iris spp.

Common name(s)   Iris, fleur-de-lis.

Toxin(s)   Irisin.

Toxic part(s)   Leaves and root stock, rhizomes.

Signs   No reports of poisoning of dogs and cats have been found. Signs reported in humans include a burning sensation, congestion, nausea, vomiting, diarrhea, and abdominal cramps; possible blindness.

Treatment   Treatment is symptomatic and supportive (see Section One).

Isocoma spp.

Common name(s)   Burroweed, goldenrod, jimmyweed, rayless goldenrod.

Toxin(s)   Tremetol.

Toxic part(s)   Whole plant.

Signs   No reports of cases involving dogs and cats were found. Poisoning has been reported in humans who drank milk from cows that were eating these plants. Signs reported in poisoned humans included gastrointestinal distress, vomiting, constipation, weakness, tremors, liver damage, anuric or oliguric renal failure, seizures, coma, and death.

Treatment   No studies that determine efficacy of treatment protocols have been found. Treatment would be symptomatic and supportive (see Section One).

Jatropha spp.

Common name(s)   Barbados nut, coral plant, jatropha, physic nut.

Toxin(s)   The sap contains the toxalbumin curcin, a phytotoxin.

Toxic part(s)   The entire plant, especially the seeds.

Signs   Reports of poisoning in humans are common, but animal toxicity reports are lacking. Gastrointestinal distress, nausea, vomiting, diarrhea, colic, muscle cramps, drowsiness, coma, and rarely death. Recovery from nonlethal ingestion is usually complete after 24 hours.

Treatment   Treatment protocols are not found in the literature. Routine decontamination and symptomatic support are indicated (see Section One).

Juglans spp.

Common name(s)   Black walnut.

Toxin(s)   Juglone (5-hydroxynaphthoquinone) was previously identified as the toxin, but this is no longer believed to be the toxic agent.

Toxic part(s)   Hulls, sawdust from the black walnut tree.

Signs   Signs reported in the literature (for canines) include vomiting and seizures. Not all samples of black walnut hulls or shavings are toxic.

Speculating: perhaps the convulsions seen in the dog are related to the growth of a fungus that produces penitrem A (p. 21). The growth of this neurotoxin-producing fungus in nuts is a common occurrence in California, so commonly associated with walnuts that it was called "walnut poisoning" for many years before the toxin (penitrem A) was identified.

Treatment (See *Penitrem A*, p. 211.) The stomach should be emptied and activated charcoal administered with a cathartic. Abnormal muscle activity (tremors, tonic-clonic spasms) may be controlled with diazepam and methocarbamol. Phenothiazine tranquilizers are known to lower the seizure threshold but have been used (anecdotally) without any apparent harm in cases of ingestions of tremorogenic substances such as penitrem A.

Kalmia

Common name(s) Bog laurel, calfkill, calico bush, dwarf laurel, ivy bush, lambkill, mountain laurel, pale laurel, sheepkill, wicky.

Toxin(s) Andromedotoxin.

Toxic part(s) The entire plant is toxic.

Signs Cats have been poisoned by these plants. Some believe that secondary poisoning may result in carnivores eating the flesh of animals that ingested *Kalmia*. Signs include epiphora, ptyalism, and nasal discharge. Neurologic signs including lateral recumbency with limb paddling, intermittent "running fits," opisthotonos, and paralysis of the limbs. Death may result.

Treatment Routine gastrointestinal decontamination (emesis or gastric lavage followed by activated charcoal and a cathartic if necessary) is recommended. Multiple doses of activated charcoal are advised at 2- to 3-hour intervals. Bradycardia may be treatable with atropine if necessary. Fluids are given to support blood pressure, perfusion, and hydration. Monitor electrolytes and correct imbalances. Monitor ECG for cardiac dysrhythmias, and treat by previously accepted means.

Laburnum anagyroides

Common name(s)   Bean tree, golden chain, laburnum.

Toxin(s)   Cytisine.

Toxic part(s)   Pods and seeds are highly toxic, but other parts of the plant also contain the toxin.

Signs   Cytisine is similar to nicotine and the signs noted are similar. Excitement, incoordination, salivation, nausea, vomiting, diarrhea, urination, and lacrimation may be seen. Mydriasis may be noted. Convulsions, tremors, muscular twitches, and paresis or paralysis may be followed by tachycardia, collapse, coma, and death.

Treatment   See *Nicotine*, p. 191.

Lactarius spp.

See *Mushrooms*, p. 184.

Lantana spp.

Common name(s)   Lantana.

Toxin(s)   Lantanin or lantadene A.

Toxic part(s)   The entire plant.

Signs   Photosensitization has been seen in animals. Poisoning has been reported in humans, with signs that include gastrointestinal distress, bloody diarrhea, muscular weakness, jaundice, collapse, and even death.

Treatment   No studies have been done to determine efficacy of treatment protocols. Treatment is symptomatic and supportive (see Section One). Remove the animal from the source of the plant if chronic dermatitis or photosensitization occurs.

Laportea spp.

See *Urtica* spp.

Lathyrus spp.

Common name(s)   Caley pea, everlasting pea, flat pea, singletary pea, sweet pea, wild winter pea.

Toxin(s)   Amine-bearing compounds.

Toxic part(s)   The whole plant, especially the seeds.

Signs   Reports of sweet pea poisoning in the small animal patient are not reported. The plant is known to be toxic to livestock and humans and is listed here for completeness. Signs reported in livestock and humans include permanent paralysis, bone deformities, cardiovascular collapse, pain, lameness, hyperexcitability, convulsions, and death.

Treatment   Specific treatment advice cannot be recommended because this intoxication has not been studied. Treatment is therefore said to be "symptomatic and supportive" (see Section One).

Lepiota spp.

See *Mushrooms*, p. 184.

Ligustra spp.

Common name(s)   Japanese privet, privet, waxleaf privet.

Toxin(s)   Unknown alkaloids.

Toxic part(s)   Mostly the berries and leaves.

Signs   Gastrointestinal signs including nausea, vomiting, diarrhea, collapse, convulsions, acute renal failure, hypothermia, and death. Small animal poisonings have not been reported. Only cases involving humans (children primarily) and livestock have been reported.

Treatment   Treatment is symptomatic and supportive (see Section One). Witnessed ingestion should be treated by immediate induction of emesis or gastric lavage followed by administration of activated charcoal and a cathartic (if necessary).

Lilium spp.

Common name(s)   Easter lily, Japanese show lily, rubrum lily, tiger lily.

Toxin(s)   Unknown.

Toxic part(s)   The entire plant is toxic to cats.

Signs   Cats are reported to be sensitive to an unknown toxin found in these lily species. Ingestion of this toxin results in non-specific signs followed by acute renal failure (usually anuric) within 24 to 48 hours. It is unknown whether dogs or birds are sensitive to the toxin found in these plants.

Treatment   There is no specific antidote. If a dog or cat is witnessed ingesting *Lilium*, immediate induction of emesis or gastric lavage is indicated, followed by administration of activated charcoal and a cathartic. Fluid diuresis is indicated. Urine production should be maintained at at least 2 mL/kg/hour in the cat and 3 mL/kg/hour in the dog. If aggressive treatment is begun early enough to maintain renal tubular flow, the recovery rate is satisfactory. If, however, the renal failure syndrome develops, mortality is high. Dialysis has been reported to be successful in patients (at least one reported) even after the renal failure became apparent.

Lobelia spp.

Common name(s)   Asthma flower, Berlander lobelia, blue cardinal flower, cardinal flower, eyebright (when equatable to Indian tobacco and when not *Euphrasia*), gag weed, great blue lobelia, great lobelia, high belia, hog physic, Indian pink, Indian tobacco, lobelia, Lousiana belia, puke weed, red lobelia, scarlet lobelia, water lobelia, wild tobacco (only when equatable to Indian tobacco).

Toxin(s)   Lobeline, lobelamine, and other alkaloids that are similar to nicotine.

Toxic part(s)   Whole plant.

Signs   Lobeline has been used as an emetic, respiratory stimulant, and expectorant. Signs most often noted include nausea, vomiting, weakness, mydriasis, pain, hypothermia, salivation, diarrhea, anorexia, cardiovascular collapse, shock, and death. Poisoning of dogs and cats is unlikely because this plant is not usually eaten by these species.

Treatment   There is no specific treatment. Treatment is symptomatic and supportive (see Section One).

Lophophora spp.

Common name(s) Cactus, mescal, mescal buttons, peyote.

Toxin(s) Mescaline and other alkaloids.

Toxic part(s) The entire plant.

Signs Signs reported in humans include hallucinations, anxiety, tremors, and delirium. Also reported have been headache, vomiting, diarrhea, cramps (stomach), dizziness, euphoria, depression, and forgetfulness. The effects are similar to those of LSD.

Treatment Perform gastrointestinal decontamination (emesis, gastric lavage) followed by activated charcoal. Other treatment is symptomatic and supportive (see Section One).

Lupineus spp.

Common name(s) Bluebonnets, lupine (many types including Big Bend lupine, Douglas spurred lupine, low lupine, silvery or silky lupine, loose flower lupine, Washington lupine).

Toxin(s) Lupinine and other toxic alkaloids

Toxic part(s) All of the plant is toxic, but the pods and seeds are most toxic.

Signs No cases of poisoning involving dogs or cats have been found. Human exposure is rare. Lupine causes more deaths in range livestock than any other single plant in the states of Montana, Idaho, and Utah.

Treatment No specific treatment has been reported. Treatment would therefore be symptomatic and supportive (see Section One).

Lycopersicon esculentum

Common name(s)   Tomato, love apple, passionflower, passion fruit.

Toxin(s)   Solanine.

Toxic part(s)   Leaves, vines, sprouts, and green fruit.

Signs   Reports of poisoning in the small animal patient are lacking. Humans poisoned by ingestion of toxin report headache, stomach pain, vomiting, diarrhea, hypothermia, cardiovascular collapse, and respiratory depression.

Treatment   Treatment is symptomatic and supportive (see Section One). The stomach should be emptied by induction of emesis (p. 50) or gastric lavage (p. 52) followed by administration of activated charcoal and a cathartic if necessary. Fluids are given to support blood pressure, perfusion, and hydration as necessary. Electrolytes should be monitored and imbalances corrected.

Malus sylvestris

Common name(s)   Apple.

Toxin(s)   Cyanogenic compound.

Toxic part(s)   Seeds, possibly leaves.

Signs   Cyanide poisoning (p. 120). Signs include cherry-red mucous membranes, tachypnea, tachycardia, nausea, vomiting, shock, convulsions, and death. Signs progress rapidly. There is often a characteristic odor of almonds on the breath or in the stomach contents.

EMERGENCY TREATMENT

See *Cyanide—emergency treatment, p. 120.*

Procedures

1. Secure the airway and ventilate if needed (p. 6).
2. Administer supplemental oxygen (p. 7).
3. Secure venous access. Collect blood and urine for laboratory testing.
4. Administer isotonic crystalloids as needed to support blood pressure and perfusion.
5. Control seizures (p. 24).
6. Treat hyperthermia if present (p. 29).

Decontaminate

1. If a known cyanide-containing substance was ingested within the last 15 minutes and no signs are present, induce vomiting.
2. If a known cyanide-containing substance was ingested within the last 15 to 60 minutes and no signs are present, perform gastric lavage.
3. Although cyanide is generally not adsorbed by activated charcoal, administration of activated charcoal may be of value if the toxin was ingested.

Administer antidotes and other supportive care

- 1.65 mL/kg 25% sodium thiosulfate IV.
- *Only if the diagnosis of cyanide is certain* should sodium nitrite be administered IV at 16 mg/kg. This drug may cause nitrite-induced methemoglobinemia, which could be fatal if cyanide poisoning is not present.
- Hydroxocobalamin is an investigational drug that shows much promise in the treatment of cyanide toxicosis. It is currently not available in the United States.

Melia azedarach

Common name(s)   Chinaberry, china tree, Chinaball tree, umbrella tree.

Toxin(s)   Narcotic resinoid or alkaloid.

Toxic part(s)   Fruit, flowers, and bark.

Signs   Nausea, vomiting, miosis, euphoria, depression, hypoventilation or respiratory depression, coma, death.

Treatment   Symptomatic and supportive (see Section One). It is unknown whether narcotic antagonists would work to reverse signs.

Mirabilis spp.

Common name(s)   Four-o'clock, marvel of Peru, beauty of the night.

Toxin(s)   Trigonelline.

Toxic part(s)   Roots and seeds.

Signs   No reports of poisoning of dogs and cats have been found. Signs reported in humans include nausea, vomiting, abdominal cramps, diarrhea, and irritation of the mucous membranes.

Treatment   Usually self-limiting in children. Treatment is not normally necessary.

Monstera spp.

Common name(s)   Ceriman, cutleaf philodendron, fruit salad plant, hurricane plant, Mexican breadfruit, monstera, mother-in-law, Swiss cheese plant.

Toxin(s)   Calcium oxalate.

Toxic part(s)   Probably the entire plant including the roots.

Signs   Pain and swelling of the oral cavity. Acute inflammation of the oropharynx accompanied by salivation, pawing at the mouth, and drooling. Edema of the lips, tongue, and throat may be seen.

Treatment   Usually none required. Rinse the mouth copiously with water or milk. Give the animal milk or other source of calcium. The calcium may precipitate soluble oxalates. Antihistamines may be helpful. Analgesics may be required. Swelling may be treated with cool compresses. It is unknown if diuretics or glucocorticosteroid would help with the inflammation. Rarely, swelling of the tongue, glottis, or pharynx will interfere with respiration. If necessary, secure the airway (p. 2).

Morus spp.

Common name(s)   Mulberry, red mulberry, white mulberry.

Toxin(s)   Unreported toxins that cause CNS disturbances and possibly hallucinations.

Toxic part(s)   Green berries, sap.

Signs   No cases of intoxication of dogs and cats have been found. Birds may be affected. Humans who ingest the toxin report hallucinations, CNS stimulation, and often gastrointestinal disturbances.

Treatment   There is no specific treatment; treatment is symptomatic and supportive (see Section One).

Narcissus spp.

Common name(s)   Daffodil, jonquil.

Toxin(s)   Alkaloids including narcissine, narcipoietin, and lycorine.

Toxic part(s) Entire plant; however, the alkaloids are concentrated in the bulbs.

Signs Gastrointestinal distress including vomiting, cramping, and diarrhea. Rarely, tremors or convulsions are seen. Hypotension and death may occur in severe cases.

Treatment Gastric emptying is usually initiated by the alkaloids. If vomiting has not occurred, induce vomiting or perform gastric lavage (if ingestion was recent). Administer activated charcoal and a cathartic if necessary. Control seizures by generally accepted means (p. 24). Fluids and electrolytes may be indicated.

Nerium spp.

Common name(s) Oleander, rose laurel, *adelfa, Rosenlorbeer.*

Toxin(s) Several cardiac glycosides similar to digitalis.

Toxic part(s) The entire plant including leaves, stems, and roots.

Signs Abdominal pain, nausea, vomiting, salivation, and local irritation of the mucous membranes are noted soon after ingestion. Pulses may be slow and strong (early with moderate digitalis-like intoxication) or rapid and weak (later). Cardiac conduction disturbances are seen on ECG and may be severe enough to contribute to signs including ataxia, hypotension, shock, collapse, and death. Pupils may be dilated. Delirium may be followed by coma. Hyperkalemia, hypocalcemia, and hypoglycemia may be seen on laboratory analysis.

Treatment The gastrointestinal tract should be decontaminated. Induction of emesis (p. 50) or gastric lavage should be performed as needed, followed by administration of activated charcoal. Cathartics should also be used if necessary.

Treat as for digitalis overdose. Digibind (Glaxo Wellcome, Research Triangle Pk., NC 27709) has been used successfully in treating oleander toxicosis in humans and dogs. Research has revealed that Digibind given at a dose of 60 mg/kg IV resulted in survival and conversion to normal sinus rhythm. Repeat injections may be necessary. In humans, digitalis-like intoxications may be treated with temporary cardiac pacing using a transvenous pacemaker. This option should be explored. A call to a pacemaker company may bring a representative who can offer a temporary external pacemaker. The technique to implant the leads and set up the pacemaker is not difficult.

Serum potassium should be monitored. The patient should be treated for hypokalemia (p. 42) or hyperkalemia (p. 41) if necessary. Cardiac dysrhythmias may be treated with phenytoin.

Nicotiana spp.

Common name(s) Tobacco.

Toxin(s) Nicotine and other alkaloids.

Toxic part(s) The entire plant.

Signs and treatment See *Nicotine*, p. 191.

Ornithogalum spp.

Common name(s) Star-of-Bethlehem (belonging to the lily family).

Toxin(s) Poisonous alkaloids.

Toxic part(s) Bulbs, leaves, and flowers.

Signs   Reports of poisoning in small animals are lacking. This plant has been responsible for poisoning in children, and so one should assume that it would be toxic to dogs and cats. Children experience nausea, vomiting, and diarrhea. Deaths have been reported.

Treatment   The stomach should be emptied by induction of emesis (p. 50) or gastric lavage (p. 52) followed by administration of activated charcoal and a cathartic if necessary. Fluids are given to support blood pressure, perfusion, and hydration as necessary. Electrolytes should be monitored and imbalances corrected. Additional treatment is symptomatic and supportive (see Section One).

Oxytropis spp.

Common name(s)   Crazyweed, Lambert's crazyweed, locoweed, white loco. (See also *Astragalus*).

Toxin(s)   Several alkaloids, methemoglobin formation.

Toxic part(s)   Leaves.

Signs   Poisoning of dogs and cats would be unlikely with this plant. It has been known to cause serious loss in cattle, sheep, or other range animals. Humans have also been reported to have been poisoned. Signs reported in humans are related to selenium accumulation. Reported signs include pallor, garlicky odor on breath, gastrointestinal disturbances, nausea, vomiting, tightness in the chest, drowsiness, and brain damage.

Treatment   Treatment is supportive and symptomatic (see Section One).

Panaeolus spp.

See *Mushrooms*, p. 184.

Parthenocissus quinquefolia

Common name(s)   American ivy, Virginia creeper, woodbine.

Toxin(s)   Oxalic acid.

Toxic part(s)   The berries are known to be toxic. The leaves are probably toxic.

Signs   No reports of small animal poisoning have been found. Children who have eaten the berries have gastrointestinal disturbances including nausea, vomiting, and diarrhea (which may be bloody). Headache, drowsiness, stupor, muscle cramps, acute renal failure, and death have been reported in humans.

Treatment   The stomach should be emptied by induction of emesis (p. 50) or gastric lavage (p. 52) followed by administration of activated charcoal and a cathartic if necessary. Fluids are given to support blood pressure, perfusion, and hydration as necessary. Electrolytes should be monitored and imbalances corrected.

Philodendron spp.

Common name(s)   Cordatum, horsehead, philodendron, red emerald, red princess.

Toxin(s)   Oxalates. May also initiate histamine release in the body.

Toxic part(s)   Probably the entire plant including the roots.

Signs   Pain and swelling of the oral cavity. Acute inflammation of the oropharynx accompanied by salivation, pawing at the mouth, and drooling. Edema of the lips, tongue, and throat may be seen.

Treatment Usually none required. Rinse the mouth copiously with water or milk. Give the animal milk or other source of calcium. The calcium may precipitate soluble oxalates. Antihistamines may be helpful. Analgesics may be required. Swelling may be treated with cool compresses. It is unknown if diuretics or glucocorticosteroid would help with the inflammation. Rarely, swelling of the tongue, glottis, or pharynx will interfere with respiration. If necessary, secure the airway (p. 2).

Phoradendron spp.

Common name(s) Mistletoe (see also *Viscum album*).

Toxin(s) Phoratoxin, a lectin that inhibits cellular protein synthesis, plus other toxic amines.

Toxic part(s) The entire plant, especially the berries.

Signs Signs may be delayed several hours after ingestion. Gastrointestinal upset, nausea, vomiting, and diarrhea are commonly seen. Animals may be hypothermic, polyuric, bradycardic or tachycardic, and demonstrate mydriasis. CNS signs may include delirium, ataxia, seizures, and coma or hyperactivity. Patients may experience dyspnea. Cardiovascular collapse, shock, and death are seen later in the severe intoxication.

Treatment Gastroenteric emptying is accomplished by induction of emesis or gastric lavage if appropriate. Administration of charcoal with a cathartic is recommended. If CNS signs are noted, it is best to avoid cathartics that contain magnesium. Bradycardia is usually responsive to administration of atropine. Cardiac effects of the toxin are treated symptomatically. Indicated symptomatic support includes fluid and electrolyte therapy to correct imbalances.

Phytolacca spp.

Common name(s) Pokeweed, pokeberry, poke salad, inkweed, scoke (standard spelling), skoke (a recent misspelling).

Toxin(s) A bitter glycoside and a glycoprotein.

Toxic part(s) The entire plant.

Signs The plant is bitter to the taste, and it is unlikely that a dog or cat will eat it. Toxicities have been reported in humans and livestock. Gastrointestinal disturbances, salivation, tremors, convulsions, and death have been reported. Boiling the leaves and roots destroys the toxin making *Phytolacca* fit for consumption.

Treatment Treatment is symptomatic and supportive (see Section One). Ingestion should be treated by usual gastrointestinal decontamination and administration of activated charcoal.

Pieris spp.

Common name(s) Japanese andromeda, mountain fetterbush.

Toxin(s) Andromedotoxin.

Toxic part(s) Leaves, flowers, and nectar. Honey made from the nectar may also contain toxin.

Signs The toxin disrupts normal channels in the cellular membranes allowing an influx of sodium into cells. This action on the heart muscle cells may mimic digitalis intoxication (disruption of Na^+/K^+-ATPase allowing influx of sodium), though the mechanism is different. Signs include gastrointestinal disturbances that begin within 6 hours of ingestion. Salivation, nausea, and vomiting are seen. Epiphora, bradycardia, weakness, collapse, stupor, coma, convulsions, and death may result.

Treatment Routine gastrointestinal decontamination (emesis or gastric lavage followed by activated charcoal and a cathartic if necessary) is recommended. Multiple doses of activated charcoal are advised at two to three intervals. Bradycardia may be treatable with atropine if necessary. Fluids are given to support blood pressure, perfusion, and hydration. Monitor electrolytes and correct imbalances. Monitor ECG for cardiac dysrhythmias and treat by previously accepted means.

Prunus spp.

Common name(s) Apricot, bitter almond, cherry (Carolina cherry, sour cherry, sweet cherry, laurel cherry), chokecherry (black western chokecherry, southwestern chokecherry, western chokecherry), peach, plum (common plum, wild plum).

Toxin(s) Cyanogenic compound (amygdalin most commonly).

Toxic part(s) Seeds, possibly leaves. All of the chokecherry plant including the bark contains toxin.

Signs Cyanide poisoning (p. 120). Signs include cherry-red mucous membranes, tachypnea, tachycardia, nausea, vomiting, shock, convulsions, and death. Signs progress rapidly. There is often a characteristic odor of almonds on the breath or in the stomach contents.

EMERGENCY TREATMENT

See *Cyanide*, p. 120.

Procedures
1. Secure the airway and ventilate if needed (p. 6).
2. Administer supplemental oxygen (p. 7).
3. Secure venous access. Collect blood and urine for laboratory testing.

4. Administer isotonic crystalloids as needed to support blood pressure and perfusion.
5. Control seizures (p. 24).
6. Treat hyperthermia if present (p. 25).

Decontaminate

1. If a known cyanide-containing substance was ingested within the last 15 minutes and no signs are present, induce vomiting.
2. If a known cyanide-containing substance was ingested within the last 15 to 60 minutes and no signs are present, perform gastric lavage.
3. Although cyanide is generally not adsorbed by activated charcoal, administration of activated charcoal may be of value if the toxin was ingested.

Administer antidotes and other supportive care

- 1.65 mL/kg 25% sodium thiosulfate IV.
- *Only if the diagnosis of cyanide is certain* should sodium nitrite be administered IV at 16 mg/kg. This drug may cause nitrite-induced methemoglobinemia, which could be fatal if cyanide poisoning is not present.
- Hydroxocobalamin is an investigational drug that shows much promise in the treatment of cyanide toxicosis. It is currently not available in the United States.

Psilocybe

See *Mushrooms* p. 184.

Pyracantha spp.

Common name(s) Most commonly known as pyracantha but has been called firethorn.

Toxin(s) None known.

Toxic part(s) The berries were believed for many years to be toxic. Studies have shown them to be safe for ingestion (at least in small quantity).

Signs None.

Treatment None necessary. This plant is included because it has long been thought of as a poisonous plant.

Ranunculus spp.

Common name(s) Buttercup.

Toxin(s) Protoanemonin.

Toxic part(s) Whole mature plant (immature plants are boiled and eaten as greens).

Signs The toxin is quite irritating to mucous membranes. Blisters are commonly seen after the plant is chewed. Ingestion is rare. If ingested, signs of severe, hemorrhagic gastroenteritis are seen.

Treatment Usually only symptomatic for oral vesicles or ulceration. Rarely, gastric emptying may be required if large ingestions are witnessed. Activated charcoal and a cathartic are administered after gastric emptying. Fluids are administered to support blood pressure, perfusion, and hydration as necessary. Analgesics may be indicated.

Rhamnus spp.

Common name(s) Buckthorn, coffeeberry, pigeonberry.

Toxin(s) Glycosides, which are strong laxatives.

Toxic part(s) Bark, berries (fruit), and leaves.

Signs   Mild to severe gastrointestinal distress, cramping, diarrhea.

Treatment   Fluid therapy to support blood pressure, perfusion, and hydration as needed. Electrolyte imbalances may be corrected if detected. It is unknown if activated charcoal is effective, but administration is probably indicated.

Rheum rhaponticum

Common name(s)   Rhubarb, pie plant.

Toxin(s)   Oxalic acid, calcium oxalate, potassium oxalate, and possibly other toxins.

Toxic part(s)   The leaf blades are highly toxic. The stems are nontoxic.

Signs   No cases of small animal poisoning have been found in the literature; however, this plant is considered to be nontoxic by the general public and is included here for educational purposes. Severe poisoning of livestock and humans has occurred from eating small amounts of the leaf blades (raw or cooked). Swine poisoned by the toxin develop staggering, ptyalism, and gastrointestinal disturbances and die in convulsions. In humans, symptoms reported include nausea, vomiting, diarrhea, severe abdominal cramps, weakness, labored breathing, muscle tremors, internal bleeding, epistaxis, electrolyte imbalances (especially a refractory hypokalemia), convulsions, acute renal failure, and death. Hypocalcemia may induce tetanic spasms.

Treatment   If ingestion of a leaf is witnessed, the animal should be fed milk (to precipitate insoluble calcium oxalate) and then induced to vomit. If presented to the veterinarian, oral administration of milk, calcium gluconate, calcium lactate, or calcium hydroxide should be followed by gastric lavage and administration of activated charcoal and a cathartic. Intravenous fluids are administered to support blood pressure and perfusion and hydration. Electrolytes must be monitored and imbalances corrected. Be watchful for hypocalcemia.

Rhododendron spp.

Common name(s)   Azalea, California rose bay, great laurel, rhododendron, rose bay, western azalea, white laurel.

Toxin(s)   A glycoside known as either andromedotoxin or grayanotoxin.

Toxic part(s)   The entire plant.

Signs   The toxin disrupts normal channels in the cellular membranes allowing an influx of sodium into cells. This action on the heart muscle cells may mimic digitalis intoxication (disruption of Na^+/K^+-ATPase allowing influx of sodium), though the mechanism is different. Signs include gastrointestinal disturbances that begin within 6 hours of ingestion. Salivation, nausea, and vomiting are seen. Epiphora, bradycardia, weakness, collapse, stupor, coma, convulsions, and death may result.

Treatment   Routine gastrointestinal decontamination (emesis or gastric lavage followed by activated charcoal and a cathartic if necessary) is recommended. Multiple doses of activated charcoal are advised at two to three intervals. Bradycardia may be treatable with atropine if necessary. Fluids are given to support blood pressure, perfusion, and hydration. Monitor electrolytes and correct imbalances. Monitor ECG for cardiac dysrhythmias and treat by previously accepted means.

Rhus or *Toxicodendron*

Rhus toxicodendron or *Rhus radicans* (both names for poison ivy) is often classified in the separate genus *Toxicodendron*, p. 347.

Ricinus communis

Common name(s) Castorbean, castor oil plant, palma christi.

Toxin(s) Ricin, an extremely potent phytotoxin.

Toxic part(s) Whole plant but particularly the seeds.

Signs Very low doses may cause acute anaphylaxis-like re-action, collapse, and death. Sometimes burning of the mouth, vomiting, diarrhea, cramps, muscular twitching, convulsions, and possibly renal failure are noted.

Treatment If ingestion is witnessed, immediate induction of vomiting is indicated. If vomiting does not clear the ingested material, gastric lavage followed by activated charcoal and a cathartic must be performed. Symptomatic support would in-clude fluids and electrolytes while one monitors for onset of renal failure.

Robinia spp.

Common name(s) Black locust, locust.

Toxin(s) Robin (a phytotoxin) and robitin (a glycoside).

Toxic part(s) Bark, leaves, and seeds.

Signs No cases of poisoning involving dogs or cats have been found. Human exposure to the poison results in nausea, vom-iting, weakness, diarrhea, depression, collapse, shock, and death.

Treatment Treatment is symptomatic and supportive (see Section One).

Russula spp.

See *Mushrooms*, p. 184.

Sambucus spp.

Common name(s) Elder, elderberry, Mexican elderberry.

Toxin(s) Bitter alkaloid and perhaps a cyanogenic glycoside.

Toxic part(s) Leaves, flowers, bark, stems, and roots. Unripe berries (especially the red ones) are also toxic. (It should be noted that one resource reports that the flowers are harmless.) No cases of poisoning in the dog or cat have been found.

Signs The alkaloid causes nausea, vomiting, and diarrhea. CNS signs including dizziness, stupor, ataxia, and collapse may be seen if cyanide poisoning is a problem.

Treatment Gastric emptying (emesis or lavage) is followed by administration of activated charcoal and a cathartic (if necessary). Fluids and electrolytes may be necessary if fluid losses from vomiting or diarrhea are substantial.

Solanum spp.

Common name(s) Black nightshade (when not *Atropa*), buffalo burr, bull nettle, Carolina horse nettle, deadly nightshade (when not *Atropa*), devil's-apple (when not *Datura*, *Podophyllum*, or *Mandragora*), European bittersweet, graceful nightshade, hairy nightshade, horse nettle, Irish potato, Jerusalem cherry, Kansas thistle, love apple (*S. capsicoides*; do not confuse with *Lycopersicon*), natal cherry, nightshade, prairie berry, purple nightshade, sandbriar (sand brier), silverleaf nightshade, Texas thistle (when not *Centaurea* or *Hymenocallis*), treadsalve, trompillo, white potato.

Toxin(s) Solanine—a gastrointestinal irritant with cholinesterase-inhibiting abilities—is found in many species. Atropine-like alkaloids (making choice of therapy difficult), saponins, and other toxins are found in varying quantities. *S. nigrum* is known to have an alkaloid (solanocapsine) that produces profound bradycardia.

Toxic part(s) The entire plant including tubers and ripened and unripe fruit. Spoiled Irish, or white, potatoes, sprouts on the potatoes, and unripe berries from the plant are toxic.

Signs Signs are variable depending on the toxic principle that predominates. Toxins that inhibit cholinesterase and those with atropine-like characteristics cause similar signs: mydriasis, tachycardia, xerostomia, dyspnea, ileus, urinary retention, CNS stimulation followed by depression, paralysis, seizures, coma, and death). If solanine (a cholinesterase inhibitor) predominates, mild to severe gastrointestinal signs (irritation of the oral cavity, nausea, vomiting and diarrhea that is often bloody) may predominate. Normal to increased borborygmi may indicate predominance of solanine, whereas lack of bowel sounds may hint at an atropine-like toxin. Hemolysis and renal failure have been reported.

Treatment Fluid therapy to replace losses. In cases where atropine-like signs are life threatening, physostigmine may be carefully administered (CAUTION: physostigmine may cause asystole; listen for bowel sounds—see note above). Begin with 0.02 mg/kg administered IV over 5 minutes. If delirium or coma is abolished, use repeated doses as needed. If no effect is noted or if gastrointestinal signs predominate, consider cautious administration of intravenous atropine and observe for signs of improvement. Tachydysrhythmias that do not respond to physostigmine may respond to administration of propranolol.

Sophora spp.

Common name(s)   Burn bean, coral bean, frijolillo, mescal bean, necklacepod sophora, red bean (when not *Dysoxylum*), silver bush (for this genus only), silky sophora, Texas mountain laurel (not to be confused with the *Kalmia* spp.).

Toxin(s)   Cytisine, sophorine, and other toxic alkaloids.

Toxic part(s)   The whole plant is toxic, especially the seeds.

Signs   Poisoning of the small animal species is possible but not likely. Signs reported in other animals (including humans) include mucous membrane irritation, salivation, nervousness, tremors, exercise-induced rigidity of rear limbs, nausea, vomiting, diarrhea, excitement, delirium, hallucinations, paralysis, coma, and death from respiratory paralysis.

Treatment   There is no specific treatment. If gastric emptying is appropriate, induce emesis or lavage the stomach (pp. 50, 52). Administer activated charcoal. Treat as for nicotine toxicosis (p. 191).

Strelitzia reginae

Common name(s)   Bird-of-paradise flower.

Toxin(s)   Unknown irritant.

Toxic part(s)   Seeds and seedpods.

Signs   Ingestion of seeds or seedpods may cause gastrointestinal distress. Nausea, vomiting, and diarrhea may be seen.

Treatment   Fluids and electrolyte imbalances are rarely seen. Replacement fluids and electrolytes would be indicated if imbalances are detected.

Symplocarpus spp. (also *Lysichiton* spp.)

Common name(s)   Skunk cabbage.

Toxin(s)   Calcium oxalate and an unidentified protein.

Toxic part(s)   Leaves, whole plant.

Signs   Pain and swelling of the oral cavity. Acute inflammation of the oropharynx accompanied by salivation, pawing at the mouth, and drooling. Edema of the lips, tongue, and throat may be seen.

Treatment   Usually none required. Rinse the mouth copiously with water or milk. Give the animal milk or other source of calcium. The calcium may precipitate soluble oxalates. Antihistamines may be helpful. Analgesics may be required. Swelling may be treated with cool compresses. It is unknown if diuretics or glucocorticosteroid would help with the inflammation. Rarely, swelling of the tongue, glottis, or pharynx will interfere with respiration. If necessary, secure the airway (p. 2).

Tanacetum spp.

Common name(s)   Common tansy, tansy.

Toxin(s)   Tanacetin or oil of tansy.

Toxic part(s)   Leaves, stems, and flowers.

Signs   No reports of small animal poisoning were found. Signs reported in humans include dermatitis, nausea, vomiting, diarrhea, tremors, frothing at the mouth, mydriasis, cardiovascular collapse, acute renal failure, and death.

Treatment   Treatment is symptomatic and supportive (see Section One). The stomach should be emptied by induction of emesis (p. 50) or gastric lavage (p. 52) followed by administration of activated charcoal and a cathartic if necessary. Fluids are given to support blood pressure, perfusion, and hydration as necessary. Electrolytes should be monitored and imbalances corrected.

Taxus spp.

Common name(s)   American yew, English yew, ground hemlock, Japanese yew, Pacific yew, western yew, yew.

Toxin(s)   Taxines.

Toxic part(s)   Wood, bark, leaves, and seeds.

Signs   Signs may be rapid or delayed after ingestion. The animal is noted to tremble, become nauseated, and show signs of gastroenteritis (including vomiting and diarrhea) and collapse. Dogs may have tetanic seizures (reported but not reproduced experimentally). Ataxia, dyspnea, and mydriasis may be seen. If significant quantities of the toxin are ingested, the patient will suffer acute cardiac failure asystole (taxine interferes with the conduction system of the heart) and death.

Treatment   There are no specific antidotes. If ingestion is witnessed, immediate induction of emesis (p. 50) is indicated. If emesis is contraindicated (dogs may have seizures if taxine has been absorbed), gastric lavage should be accomplished. Administration of activated charcoal and a cathartic is indicated. If dyspnea should develop, secure the airway and ventilate the patient if necessary. Atropine is indicated; it is much more effective in countering the effects of taxine if given early. Administer fluids to support blood pressure and perfusion and to maintain hydration and urine production. Administer symptomatic support as indicated (see Section One).

Toxicodendron spp. (or *Rhus* spp.)

Common name(s)   Poison ivy, poison oak.

Toxin(s)   Urushiol is an oil resin found in the sap that is a known irritant to most tissues.

Toxic part(s)   Sap, found in the entire plant, including pollen.

Signs   Most frequent signs are of dermatitis after dermatologic exposure. If the plant is ingested (which is unlikely in small animal patients), signs of gastrointestinal irritation are seen. Mucous membranes may be reddened and irritated. Vomiting and diarrhea may be mild or severe enough to cause acute dehydration, hypovolemia, electrolyte imbalances, collapse, and death.

Treatment   Dermatologic exposure should be treated by prolonged bathing and rinsing (at least 10 minutes). Ingestion should be treated by gastric lavage and activated charcoal administration. Fluid and electrolyte imbalances should be corrected.

Urginea spp.

Common name(s)   Red squill, squill (a member of the lily family).

Toxin(s)   A cardiac glycoside (scilliroside).

Toxic part(s)   The bulb is used to make rat poisons.

Signs   The poison from this lily is distasteful to animals, and they readily vomit it up after ingestion. The rat is unable to vomit, and so this toxin is made much more deadly. The toxin causes signs similar to digitalis intoxication. Signs from mild gastrointestinal disturbances to severe cardiovascular collapse, cardiac dysrhythmias, and death are seen.

Treatment The toxin usually is eliminated from small animals when they vomit shortly after ingestion. If the animal does not vomit, routine gastrointestinal decontamination is recommended. The stomach should be emptied by induction of emesis (p. 50) or gastric lavage (p. 52) followed by administration of activated charcoal and a cathartic if necessary. Fluids are given to support blood pressure, perfusion, and hydration as necessary. Electrolytes should be monitored and imbalances corrected.

Digibind (Glaxo Wellcome, Research Triangle Pk., NC 27709) has been used successfully in treating digitalis and oleander toxicosis in humans and dogs. Whether this would be efficacious in squill poisoning has not been studied. In humans, digitalis-like intoxications may be treated with temporary cardiac pacing using a transvenous pacemaker. This option should be explored. A call to a pacemaker company may bring a representative who can offer a temporary, external pacemaker. The technique to implant the leads and set up the pacemaker is not difficult.

Serum potassium should be monitored. The patient should be treated for hypokalemia (p. 42) or hyperkalemia (p. 41) if necessary.

The ECG should be monitored. Cardiac dysrhythmias may be treated with phenytoin or other acceptable antidysrhythmic drugs.

Urtica spp.

Common name(s) Nettle, stinging nettle.

Toxin(s) Acetylcholine, histamine, formic acid, serotonin, and possibly others.

Toxic part(s) Stinging hairs found on the plant.

Signs Symptoms include salivation, burning sensation in the mouth and nose, muscle weakness, and tremors. Most commonly, dogs return from a run in a field containing the stinging nettle and a short time later become weak. Most reports indicate that rear-limb paresis or paralysis is noted initially. Signs may progress and rarely result in death.

Treatment   Atropine is antidotal (dosages up to 2 mg per dog may be needed). Antihistamines may be useful, but efficacy is unproved; mild sedation or analgesia is helpful if oral cavity pain is excessive. General nursing care and flushing of the oral cavity are indicated.

Veratrum spp.

Common name(s)   California false hellebore, corn lily, false hellebore, skunk cabbage (properly for *Symplocarpus*), western hellebore, wild corn.

Toxin(s)   Numerous glycoalkaloids, toxic alkaloids, and teratogenic alkaloids.

Toxic part(s)   The entire plant is toxic.

Signs   Reports of canine or feline poisonings were not found. Humans, goats, sheep, and cows have been poisoned by these plants. Signs include salivation, nausea, vomiting, abdominal cramps, hypotension, hypoventilation, generalized muscle weakness, collapse, shock, convulsions, and death. Teratogenic alkaloids produce numerous birth defects including cleft lip, "monkey face," anophthalmia, cleft palate, and fetal death.

Treatment   No studies have been done to determine treatment protocols. Recommended treatment is symptomatic and supportive (see Section One). Administer oxygen if ventilation is noted. Secure the airway and ventilate the patient if necessary. Control seizures with diazepam or barbiturates. Fluids, inotropic drugs, and chronotropic drugs may be necessary for cardiovascular support. Decontamination efforts are routine (gastroenteric emptying, lavage, whole bowel irrigation, activated charcoal).

Viscum album

Common name(s)   Mistletoe (see also *Phoradendron*).

Toxin(s)   Viscumin and viscotoxin and possibly others.

Toxic part(s)   The entire plant, especially the berries.

Signs   Signs may be delayed several hours after ingestion. Gastrointestinal upset, nausea, vomiting, and diarrhea are commonly seen. Animals may be hypothermic, polyuric, bradycardic or tachycardic, and demonstrate mydriasis. CNS signs may include delirium, ataxia, seizures, and coma or hyperactivity. Patients may experience dyspnea. Hemolysis may occur. Cardiovascular collapse, shock, and death are seen later in the severe intoxication.

Treatment   Gastroenteric emptying is accomplished by induction of emesis or gastric lavage if appropriate. Administration of charcoal with a cathertic is recommended. If CNS signs are noted, it is best to avoid cathartics that contain magnesium. Bradycardia is usually responsive to administration of atropine. Cardiac effects of the toxin are treated symptomatically. Indicated symptomatic support includes fluid and electrolyte therapy to correct imbalances (see Section One). Blood transfusion may be required if hemolysis is severe. Fluid diuresis is indicated if hemolysis is severe and hemoglobinuria is noted.

Wisteria spp.

Common name(s)   Wisteria, Japanese wisteria, Chinese wisteria.

Toxin(s)   A toxic resin and glycoside.

Toxic part(s)   Pods and seeds.

Signs   Reports of small animal poisonings are lacking. Signs in children include nausea, vomiting, and other gastrointestinal signs. Signs may be severe enough to cause acute dehydration, hypovolemia, shock, and collapse.

Treatment   The stomach should be emptied by induction of emesis (p. 50) or gastric lavage (p. 52) followed by administration of activated charcoal and a cathartic if necessary. Fluids are given to support blood pressure, perfusion, and hydration as necessary. Electrolytes should be monitored and imbalances corrected.

Zantedeschia spp.

Common name(s)   Arum lily, calla lily.

Toxin(s)   Oxalates.

Toxic part(s)   Probably the entire plant including the roots.

Signs   Pain and swelling of the oral cavity. Acute inflammation of the oropharynx accompanied by salivation, pawing at the mouth, and drooling. Edema of the lips, tongue, and throat may be seen.

Treatment   Usually none required. Rinse the mouth copiously with water or milk. Give the animal milk or other source of calcium. The calcium may precipitate soluble oxalates. Antihistamines may be helpful. Analgesics may be required. Swelling may be treated with cool compresses. It is unknown if diruetics or glucocorticosteroid would help with the inflammation. Rarely, swelling of the tongue, glottis, or pharynx will interfere with respiration. If necessary, secure the airway (p. 2).

Zygadenus spp.

Common name(s)   Death camas, foothill death camas, grassy death camas, meadow death camas, Nut Falls death camas.

Toxin(s)   Alkaloids.

Toxic part(s)   The whole plant, especially the seeds and bulb. One resource reported that the leaves are more toxic than the bulb.

Signs   Gastrointestinal signs including salivation, vomiting, and abdominal pain are seen first. Often the vomiting will rid the animal of the toxic substance and avoid serious poisoning. Animals that do not vomit will suffer tachypnea, tachycardia, stiffened gait, muscle weakness, staggering, incoordination, convulsions, shock, collapse, and death. It is unlikely that a dog or cat would eat the toxic plant.

Treatment   Gastric emptying is indicated. Activated charcoal is indicated. Seizures are controlled by generally accepted means (p. 24). Treatment is symptomatic and supportive (see Section One).

Acetylcysteine (Mucomyst)

Use   Acetaminophen poisoning, experimental arsenic poisoning

Dose   *Dog*   280 mg/kg PO loading dose; then 140 mg/kg PO q4h for 3 days

         Cat   140 to 240 mg/kg PO; then 70 mg/kg PO q6h for 3 days

Acetylcysteine may be given intravenously if the patient is vomiting. It is recommended that the solution be administered at the lower dose, diluted with D_5W and given through a 0.2 µm filter over 15 to 30 minutes.

Acetylpromazine (acepromazine)

Use   Tranquilization, amphetamine toxicosis

Dose   0.05 to 0.25 mg/kg IV, IM, SC
         Rarely doses up to 1 mg/kg are recommended.
         Use higher doses with caution.
         Recent reports indicate the Boxer may be hypersensitive to acetylpromazine. The drug is not recommended for use in this breed.

Use   Hypertension

Dose   0.05 to 0.1 mg/kg IV q1h PRN

Acetylsalicylic acid

Use   Antiinflammatory agent, analgesia, antipyretic, antithrombotic

Dose   *Dog*   10 to 25 mg/kg PO q12h
         Cat   10 to 20 mg/kg PO q48-72h

Activated charcoal

Use   Gastrointestinal adsorbent

Dose   2 g/kg of body weight (1 g/5 mL of water: give 10 mL of slurry/kg PO)

Albuterol (Ventolin, Proventil)

Use   Bronchodilatation

Dose   *Dog*   0.02 to 0.04 mg/kg PO q8-24h

Allopurinol (Zyloprim)

Use   Xanthine oxidase inhibition

Dose   10 mg/kg q8-24h

Aluminum hydroxide (Amphogel, Basagel)

Use   Phosphate binder

Dose   30 to 90 mg/kg q8-24h PO with meals

Aminophylline

Use   Bronchodilatation

Dose   *Dog* 9 to 11 mg/kg PO, IM, or IV slowly q6-8h
          Cat 4 to 8 mg/kg IM, SC PO q12h

Amlodipine

Use   Hypertension, calcium-channel blocker

Dose   *Cat* 0.625 mg PO q24h

Ammonium chloride

Use   Urine acidification

Dose   *Dog* 100 to 200 mg/kg/day PO divided q8-12h
          Cat 20 mg/kg PO q12h

Amphetamine sulfate

Use   CNS stimulant for certain depressant toxicoses

Dose   *Dog* 1 to 4 mg/kg SC PRN
          Cat 5 mg PO q24h for 4 days

Amrinone (Inocor)

Use   Low-output heart failure

Dose   *Dog* 0.75 mg/kg IV over 2 to 3 minutes followed by 5
          to 10 µg/kg/min IV

Apomorphine

Use   Induction of vomiting

Dose   *Dog* 0.04 mg/kg IV or 0.08 mg/kg IM, SC
It is also known to be effective to place a tablet or part of a tablet
in the conjunctival sac.

Ascorbic acid

Use   Copper-induced hepatotoxicity

Dose   *Dog*   25 mg/kg PO

Use   Reduction of methemoglobin

Dose   30 mg/kg PO, SC q6h
20 mg/kg IV slowly q8h

Use   Urine acidification

Dose   *Dog*   100 to 500 mg PO q8-24h
Cat   100 mg/kg PO q8-24h

Atipamezole (Antisedan)

Use   Alpha$_2$-adrenergic receptor antagonist, amitraz intoxication

Dose   50 µg/kg IM q3-4h
Atipamizole is approved in the USA for use in dogs only.

Atenolol (Tenormin)

Use   Hypertension

Dose   *Cat*   5 mg PO q12-24h

Atracurium besylate (Tracrium)

Use   Paralyzing agent

Dose   *Dog*   0.1 to 0.25 mg/kg IV

Atropine sulfate

Use   Atropine response test, preanesthetic

Dose   0.02 to 0.04 mg/kg IV

Use   Cholinergic toxins

Dose   0.2 to 2.0 mg/kg; give $1/4$ of the dose IV and the rest SC or IM

Use   Preanesthesia, antisialogogue

Dose   0.02 to 0.04 mg/kg IM, SC

Use   Sinus block, AV block, bradycardia

Dose   0.02 to 0.04 mg/kg IV, IM, SC, PO q6-8h

BAL; *see* Dimercaprol

Bisacodyl

Use   Laxative, stool softener

Dose *Dog* 5 to 20 mg PO q24h
     Cat 5 mg PO q24h

Bismuth (Pepto-Bismol)

Use Gastrointestinal protectant

Dose *Dog* 0.25 to 2.00 mL/kg PO q6-8h

Buprenorphine (Buprinex)

Use Analgesia

Dose *Dog* 0.005 to 0.02 mg/kg (5 to 20 µg/kg) IM, SC q4-8hr
     Cat 0.005 to 0.010 mg/kg (5 to 10 µg/kg) IM, q12h

Butorphanol tartrate

Use Analgesia

Dose *Dog* 0.1 to 0.2 mg/kg IV or 0.2 to 0.4 mg/kg SC, IM q4-12h
     Cat 0.1 to 0.4 mg/kg IM, IV, SC q8-12h

Calcitonin (Calcimar)

Use Hypercalcemia

Dose *Dog* 4 to 6 IU/kg SC, IM q2-12h

Calcium carbonate (Tums)

Use Hypocalcemia

Dose 100 to 150 mg/kg PO divided q8-12h

Calcium chloride 10%

Use Hypocalcemia, hyperkalemia

Dose 0.1 to 0.3 mL/kg IV over 10 to 30 minutes. Monitor ECG for bradycardia.

Calcium EDTA (Versenate)

Use Lead poisoning

Dose 25 mg/kg SC q6h for 5 days = total dose. Make solution of 1 g of Versenate/100 mL of D_5W, divide total quantity of milliliters of solution into 20 aliquots, and give 1 aliquot SC q6h.

Calcium gluconate

Use Hypocalcemia, hyperkalemia

Dose 0.25 to 1.5 mL/kg IV slowly over 5 to 30 minutes while watching for bradycardia.

Calcium lactate (Calphosan)

Use Hypocalcemia

Dose 130 to 200 mg/kg PO q8h

Captopril

Use Angiotensin-converting enzyme inhibitor, hypertension

Dose *Dog* 0.5 to 2 mg/kg PO q8-12h
Cat 2 mg PO q8-12h

Castor oil

Use Cathartic

Dose *Dog* 8 to 30 mL PO
Cat 4 to 10 mL PO

Chlorothiazide

Use Diuretic, pulmonary edema, hypertension

Dose 20 to 40 mg/kg PO q12h

Chlorpromazine

Use Muscle relaxation

Dose 1 to 2 mg/kg IM q12h PRN (dosages up to 15 mg/kg have been reported)

Use Antiemetic

Dose 0.05 mg/kg IV q4h

Cholestyramine

Use Ion-binding resin

Dose *Dog* 200 to 300 mg/kg PO q12h

Cimetadine

Use H_2-receptor blockade

Dose *Dog* 4 to 10 mg/kg IV, IM, PO q6-12h
Cat 2.5 to 5 mg/kg IV, PO q8-12h

Dantrolene

Use Malignant hyperthermia

Dose 1 to 10 mg/kg IV has been suggested.

Use Adjunctive therapy for black widow spider bite

Dose 1 mg/kg IV followed by 1 mg/kg PO q4h
The safety of dantrolene has not been established, and approval by the FDA has not been granted for use in animals.

Deferoxamine, desferoxamine (Desferal)

Use Iron chelator for iron toxicosis

Dose Empirical at this time. FDA approval for use in animals has not been granted. 15 mg/kg/hour IV has been suggested as the dose for iron toxicosis.

Dexamethasone sodium phosphate

Use Cerebral edema

Dose 2 to 3 mg/kg IV followed by 1 mg/kg SC q6-8h in tapering doses

Use Shock

Dose 2 to 8 mg/kg IV slowly

Dextran 40

Use Shock

Dose 10 to 20 mL/kg IV

Dextran 70

Use Shock

Dose 10 to 20 mL/kg IV

Dextrose 50%

Use Hypoglycemia

Dose 2.0 mL/kg PO or 0.25 to 2.0 mL/kg IV slowly
CAUTION: 50% dextrose is hyperosmotic and must be diluted 1:1 with sterile water or sterile saline before administration through a peripheral vein. It may be administered in a large central vein without dilution.

Diazepam

Use Anticonvulsant

Dose 0.5 to 1.0 mg/kg IV in increments of 5 to 20 mg to effect. It may also be administered rectally at a dose of 1 to 4 mg/kg in increments of 5 to 20 mg to effect for a rapid response.

CAUTION: Diazepam has been reported to be associated with causing severe hepatopathy in cats.

Diazoxide

Use Hypertension

Dose *Dog* 5 to 13 mg/kg PO q12h

Digoxin immune FAB (Digibind)

Use Digitalis/digoxin overdose, oleander poisoning

Dose Unknown at this time. Each 40 mg vial of Digibind will bind 0.6 mg of digoxin or digitoxin in humans. Researchers used 60 mg/kg IV in one research project involving experimental treatment of oleander intoxication.

Diltiazem

Use Hypertension accompanied by tachycardia

Dose *Dog* 0.75 to 1.5 mg/kg PO q8h
Cat 3.5 to 7.0 mg PO q8h

Dimenhydrinate

Use Antiemetic

Dose *Dog* 25 to 50 mg PO q8-24h
Cat 12.5 mg PO q8-24h
NOTE: This is not per kilogram but a total dose.

Dimercaprol (BAL)

Use Arsenic toxicosis

Dose 3 to 4 mg/kg IM q8h until recovery. In severe exposures, dose may be increased to 6 or 7 mg/kg IM q8h on the first day.

Use Lead poisoning

Dose 2.5 mg/kg IM q4h on days 1 and 2, q8h on day 3, and then q12h. The dose may be increased to 5 mg/kg on day 1 only in acute, severe cases.

Dioctyl sulfosuccinate

Use Stool softener

Dose *Small dogs and cats* 25 mg PO q12-24h
Larger dogs 50 to 100 mg PO q12-24h

Diphenhydramine HCl

Use H$_1$-receptor blockade

Dose 0.5 to 2.2 mg/kg IV slowly, IM

Use Organophosphate toxicosis

Dose 1 to 4 mg/kg q8h IM, PO

Diphenylthiocarbazone

Use Thallium toxicosis

Dose 50 to 70 mg/kg PO q8h

Dobutamine HCl

Use Inotropic agent

Dose *Dog* 2 to 40 µg/kg/min IV infusion
Cat 2.5 to 15 µg/kg/min IV infusion
May cause seizures in cats.

Dopamine HCl

Use Inotropic support

Dose 5 to 20 µg/kg/min IV infusion

Use Renal vasodilator, acute renal failure

Dose 1 to 3 µg/kg/min IV infusion

Doxapram HCl

Use Respiratory stimulant

Dose 1 to 10 mg/kg IV to effect; repeat q15-30min PRN

Edrophonium chloride

Use Diagnosis of myasthenia gravis, treatment of curare poisoning

Dose *Dog* 0.1 to 0.2 mg/kg IV (maximum 5 mg)
Cat No dosage for cats has been determined.

Enalapril

Use Hypertension

Dose *Dog* 0.25 to 1.00 mg/kg PO q12-24h
Cat 0.25 to 0.5 mg/kg PO q12-24h

Ephedrine

Use Bronchodilator

Dose *Dog* 5 to 15 mg/kg PO q8-12h
     Cat 2 to 4 mg/kg PO q8-12h

Epinephrine

Use Anaphylaxis

Dose 0.01 mg/kg IV, IM

Use Cardiac arrest

Dose *Low dose* 0.01 mg/kg IV, or 0.02 mg/kg intratracheally
     High dose 0.2 mg/kg IV, or 0.4 mg/kg intratracheally

Use Bronchodilator

Dose 0.02 mg/kg IV, IM

Use Vasopressor

Dose 0.01 to 0.3 µg/kg/min IV infusion
NOTE: A 1:1000 solution of epinephrine contains 1 mg/mL.
     A 1:10,000 solution contains 0.1 mg/mL.

Ethacrynic acid

Use Loop diuretic similar to furosemide

Dose 0.2 to 0.4 mg/kg IV, IM q4-12h

Ethanol

Use Ethylene glycol toxicosis

Dose *Loading dose* 600 mg/kg IV;
     Maintenance dose 100 mg/kg/hour IV infusion in a 7% solution (Pure ethanol contains 754 mg/mL; 190 proof contains 715 mg/mL.)

Famotidine

Uses H_2-receptor blockade

Dose *Dog* 0.5 to 1.0 mg/kg PO, IV q12-24h

Fentanyl

Uses Analgesia

Dose *Dog* 3 to 10 µg/kg IV q30-120min
     or 5 to 10 µg/kg/hr IV infusion
Fentanyl is available as a transdermal patch, which allows transdermal absorption of fentanyl across intact skin. These patches have not been approved for use in animals.

Ferrous sulfate

Use   Iron supplement

Dose   *Dog* 100 to 300 mg PO daily
            Cat   50 to 100 mg PO daily

Flumazenil

Use   Benzodiazepine receptor antagonist

Dose   Empirical at this time 0.1 to 0.5 mg/kg IV, IM, SC

Furosemide

Use   Loop diuretic, pulmonary edema, hypertension, cerebral edema

Emergency dose   1 to 5 mg/kg IV q1-4h PRN

Nonemergency dose   0.5 to 1 mg/kg PO, IM, SC q8-12h

Glyceryl monoacetate

Use   Sodium fluoroacetate toxicosis

Dose   0.55 mg/kg IM q1h to total dose or 2 to 4 mg/kg

Guaifenesin (glyceryl guaiacolate)

Use   Muscle relaxation

Dose   110 mg/kg IV

Haloperidol

Use   Suggested for use in amphetamine toxicosis

Dose   1 mg/kg IV

Heparin

Use   Anticoagulation by activation of antithrombin III; higher doses may also inactivate thrombin and (when combined with AT III) inactivates factors IX, X, XI, XII, and XIII.

Dose   *Microdose* 5 to 10 IU/kg IV, SC q6h
            Minidose   50 to 100 IU/kg IV, SC q6h
            Dose   100 to 250 IU/kg IV, SC q6h

Dosage is usually adjusted to maintain activated PTT at 1.5 to 2.5 times normal.

Hetastarch; *see* Hydroxyethyl starch

Hydralazine

Use   Hypertension

Dose   *Dog*   0.5 to 2.5 mg/kg PO q8-12h
          Cat   2.5 mg PO q12h

Hydrochlorothiazide

Use   Diuretic, pulmonary edema

Dose   2 to 4 mg/kg PO q12-24h

Use   Hypertension

Dose   0.5 to 2.0 mg/kg PO q12-24h

Hydrocortisone sodium succinate

Use   Shock

Dose   10 mg/kg IV

Hydrogen peroxide 3%

Use   Emetic

Dose   1 to 2 mL/kg PO; repeat once in 5 to 10 minutes if vomiting did not occur with first dose.

Hydroxyethyl starch (hetastarch, Hespan)

Use   Colloid volume expander, shock

Dose   20 mL/kg IV

Hypertonic saline (7% to 7.5%)

Use   Shock, rapid volume expansion

Dose   4 mL/kg IV (most effective when combined with a colloid such as dextran 70 or hetastarch)

Insulin (regular, crystalline)

Use   Hyperkalemia

Dose   0.5 to 1 unit/kg IV (with concurrent administration of 2 g of dextrose per unit of insulin) over 30 minutes

Ipecac syrup

Use   Emetic

Dose   *Dog*   1 to 2.5 mL/kg PO (One reference reports that no dog should get more than 15 mL.)
          Cat   1 to 3.3 mL/kg PO

Dose may be repeated once, but if emesis does not occur, ipecac must be recovered by gastric lavage.

Isoproterenol

Use   Shock

Dose   *Dog* 0.04 to 0.08 µg/kg/min IV infusion
Cat 4 to 6 µg total dose IM q30min PRN

Use   Bronchodilator

Dose   *Dog* 0.1 to 0.2 mg IM SC
Cat 4-6 µg total dose IM q30min PRN

Kaolin, pectin

Use   GI protectant, adsorbent for paraquat/diquat poisoning

Dose   1 to 2 mL/kg PO q6-12h

Lactulose

Use   Hyperammonemia, laxative

Dose   *Dog* 5 to 15 mL PO q8-12h
Cat 0.25 to 1 mL PO q8-24h

Leukovorin

Use   Methotrexate toxicity

Dose   *Dog* 3 mg/m^2 IM within 3 hours of methotrexate

Lidocaine

Use   Ventricular dysrhythmias

Dose   *Dog* 1 to 2 mg/kg IV bolus followed by 25 to 75 µg/kg/min IV infusion
Cat 0.25 to 1 mg/kg IV bolus followed by 5 to 40 µg/kg/min IV infusion.

Magnesium chloride

Use   Magnesium supplementation

Dose   1 mEq/kg/day in IV fluids

Use   Life-threatening hypomagnesemia

Dose   0.15 to 0.3 mEq/kg IV slowly over 5 to 15 minutes. (Use commercial parenteral solution only.)

Magnesium hydroxide (milk of magnesia)

Use   Antacid

Dose   *Dog*   5 to 30 mL PO q12-24h
             Cat   5 to 10 mL PO q12-24h, or 2 to 3 mL/kg PO

Use   Cathartic

Dose   *Dog*   10 to 150 mL PO
             Cat   15 to 50 mL PO

Magnesium sulfate

Use   Cathartic

Dose   *Dog*   250 to 500 mg/kg PO
             Cat   200 mg/kg PO

Epsom salt should be mixed with 5 to 10 mL/kg water and administered orally.

Use   Life-threatening hypomagnesemia

Dose   0.15 to 0.3 mEq/kg IV slowly over 5 to 15 minutes. (Use commercial parenteral solution only—not Epsom salt.)

Mannitol

Use   Cerebral edema, acute renal failure or oliguria, rhabdomyolysis

Dose   0.1 to 0.5 g/kg IV (over 5 to 15 minutes) q1-6h PRN

Meperidine

Use   Analgesia

Dose   *Dog*   5 to 10 mg/kg IM, SC q1h PRN
             Cat   2 to 10 mg/kg IM, SC q2h PRN

Meperidine may be given very slowly IV but may cause severe hypotension.

meso-Dimercaptosuccinic acid (succimer, DMSA, Chemet)

Use   Lead, arsenic, and mercury poisoning—acts by chelation

Dose   Unknown. Currently under investigation. It is used in humans at 10 mg/kg q8h either orally or parenterally.

Methionine (DL-methionine)

Use Urinary acidification

Dose *Dog* 200 to 1000 mg PO q8h
Cat 200 to 1000 mg PO daily

Methocarbamol

Use Muscle relaxation for toxicosis (such as metaldehyde, penitrem A)

Dose *Dog* Give slowly to effect; up to 222.2 mg/kg IV as needed.
Cat Give slowly to effect; up to 44.4 mg/kg IV.

Methylene blue

Use Methemoglobinemia

Dose *Dog* 8.8 mg/kg IV slowly, repeat as needed or 3 to 4 mg/kg in 250 mL of saline given IV over 30 minutes Reports of acute toxicity and death have been reported after administration of 10 mg/kg. May form Heinz bodies.
Cat 1.5 mg/kg has been reported to be beneficial to cats with nitrite-induced methemoglobin. Given in the absence of methemoglobinemia, methylene blue may cause Heinz body formation.

Methylprednisolone sodium succinate

Use Brain or spinal cord trauma

Dose 25 to 30 mg/kg IV at entry followed by 12.5 to 15 mg/kg IV at 2 and 6 hours after entry; then 2.5 mg/kg/hour IV continuous infusion for 8 to 42 hours.

4-Methylpyrazole

Use Ethylene glycol toxicosis

Dose *Dog* 20 mg/kg IV, then 15 mg/kg IV at 12 and 24 hours, then 5 mg/kg IV at 36 h
Cat 4-MP is not recommended for cats at this time.

Metoclopramide

Use Antiemetic

Dose *Dog* 0.2 to 0.5 mg/kg PO, SC, IV q8h, or 0.01 to 0.02 mg/kg/hour IV infusion

Metoprolol

Use   Atrial fibrillation, some tachydysrhythmias

Dose *Dog* 0.5 to 1.0 mg/kg PO q8h
        Cat 12.5 to 25 mg PO q12h

An IV dose has been published as 0.04 to 0.06 mg/kg given slowly IV q8h. We have not used this route of administration and would advise caution. IV use of beta-blockers can cause hypotension and decreased cardiac output.

Metronidazole

Use   Antibiotic, antiprotozoal

Dose *Dog* 10 to 30 mg/kg PO q8-12h
        Cat 10 to 25 mg/kg PO q8-12h

Midazolam

Use   Preanesthetic, sedative

Dose *Dog* 0.1 to 0.2 mg/kg IM, SC, IV
        Cat 0.066 to 0.1 mg/kg IV, IM

Misoprostol

Use   Prostaglandin-analog gastric protectant

Dose *Dog* 1 to 5 µg/kg PO q8-12h

Morphine sulfate

Use   Analgesia
Dose *Dog* 0.05 to 1.0 mg/kg IV, SC, IM q1-4h PRN
        Cat 0.05 to 0.1 mg/kg SC, IM q1-4h PRN

Nalbuphine

Use   Analgesia, partial opiate antagonist

Dose *Dog* 0.5 to 1.5 mg/kg IM, IV q1-6h

Nalorphine

Use   Narcotic antagonist

Dose *Dog* 0.1 to 0.4 mg/kg IV; maximum dose, 5 mg total
        Cat 1 mg (total) IV

Naloxone HCl

Use   Narcotic antagonist

Dose *Dog* 0.02 to 0.04 mg/kg IV PRN
        Cat 0.05 to 0.1 mg/kg IV

Use   Shock

Dose   2 mg/kg IV slow infusion

Nandrolone decanoate

Use   Anabolic steroid, bone marrow stimulant

Dose   *Dog* 5 mg/kg/week IM; maximum 200 mg
    Cat 10 to 20 mg/week IM

Neostigmine

Use   Anticholinesterase inhibitor

Dose   *Dog* 0.5 mg/kg PO q8-12h
    1 to 2 mg IM PRN

Nicotinamide

Use   Vacor toxicosis (Vacor is a rodenticide no longer used.)

Dose   500 to 1000 mg IM followed by 200 to 300 mg IM
    q4h. May be continued at 200 mg PO q24h for 2
    weeks after recovery

Nikethamide

Use   CNS stimulant used to counteract CNS-depressant
    drugs

Dose   7.8 to 31.2 mg/kg IV, IM, SC

Nitroglycerin 2% ointment

Use   Cardiogenic pulmonary edema

Dose   *Dog* 1/4- to 1-inch ribbon on bare skin q4-12h
    Cat 1/8- to 1/4-inch ribbon on bare skin q6h

Nitroprusside

Use   Lower blood pressure by decreasing preload, afterload,
    and myocardial work

Dose   *Dog* 0.5 to 10 μg/kg/min IV infusion

Omeprazole

Use   Gastric ulceration

Dose   *Dog* 0.7 mg/kg PO daily

Oral colonic lavage solutions (polyethylene glycol, or PEG, solutions, e.g., GoLYTELY, CoLyte; see p. 369)

Use   Whole bowel irrigation

Dose   22 to 33 mL/kg PO
or 25 to 40 mL/kg PO followed by continuous infusion
(through nasogastric tube) at 0.5 mL/kg/hour.

Oxazepam

Use   Appetite stimulant

Dose   *Cat*   0.2 to 0.5 mg/kg PO q12-24h

Oxymorphone

Use   Analgesia, sedation, anesthesia

Dose   *Dog*   0.02 to 0.1 mg/kg IV q3-6h PRN
0.05 to 0.2 mg/kg IM, SC q2-6h PRN
Cat   0.02 to 0.05 mg/kg IV, SC q2-6h PRN

Oxytriphylline

Use   Bronchodilatation

Dose   *Dog*   4 to 10 mg/kg PO q8h

Pancuronium bromide

Use   Muscle paralysis (for anesthesia or treatment of hyperthermia)

Dose   *Dog*   0.03 mg/kg with methoxyflurane anesthesia
or 0.06 mg/kg IV with halothane anesthesia
Cat   0.05 to 0.1 mg/kg IV. Use lower doses if
inhalation anesthesia is to be used.

PEG solutions (polyethylene glycol solutions)

Use   Whole bowel irrigation

Dose   25 to 40 mL/kg PO followed by continuous oral infusion
of 0.5 mL/kg/hour or 30 to 40 mL/kg PO every 2 hours

D-Penicillamine

Use   Chelator useful in copper or lead toxicity

Dose   *Dog*   COPPER: 10 to 15 mg/kg PO q12h
LEAD: 8 mg/kg PO q6h or 10 to 55 mg/kg PO
q12h

Pentobarbital

Use   Anesthesia, seizure control

Dose   2 to 30 mg/kg IV slowly to effect

Phenobarbital

Use   Seizures

Dose Status epilepticus 2 to 4 mg/kg IV repeated q30min to effect

Maintenance   *Dog*   1 to 8 mg/kg q12h PO, IM, IV

Cat   1 to 2 mg/kg q12h PO, IM, IV

Phenoxybenzamine

Use   Hypertensive crisis

Dose *Dog*   0.2 to 1.5 mg/kg PO q12h

Cat   2.5 to 7.5 mg PO q24h

Phentolamine

Use   Hypertensive crisis

Dose *Dog* 0.02 to 0.10 mg/kg IV

Phenylephrine

Use   Vasopressor

Dose 0.1 to 0.15 mg/kg IV

Phenytoin

Use   Antidysrhythmic

Dose *Dog*   2 to 4 mg/kg IV as needed up to a level of 10 mg/kg total dose.

Cat   Not available

Physostigmine

Use   Muscarinic mushroom toxicity, ivermectin toxicity, anticholinergic overdose

Dose *Dog*   0.06 mg/kg IM or IV over 5 minutes

Potassium bromide

Use   Long-term seizure control

Dose *Dog*   30 to 40 mg/kg PO q24h with food

Potassium chloride

Use   Potassium supplementation

Dose 0.1 to 0.25 mL/kg PO q8h

For IV use, do not exceed 0.5 mEq/kg/hour IV.

Potassium citrate

Use Urine alkalinization

Dose 5 to 7 mg/kg/hour in IV fluids
35 to 50 mg/kg PO q8h

Potassium gluconate

Use Potassium supplementation

Dose 5 to 8 mEq PO q12-24h

Potassium permanganate

Use Strychnine toxicosis

Dose 5 mL/kg in gastric lavage solution

Pralidoxime chloride (2-PAM)

Use Organophosphate toxicosis

Dose 20 to 50 mg/kg IV very slowly (maximum = 500 mg/min)
or SC q12h; start with lower doses. If no response after 3 doses, discontinue.

Prazosin

Use Vasodilatation, hypertension

Dose *Dog* 1 mg/15 kg PO q8-12h

Prednisolone

Use Hypercalcemia

Dose 2 to 3 mg/kg PO, SC q12h
40 mg/m^2 PO q12h

Prednisolone sodium phosphate

Use Shock

Dose 11 mg/kg IV

Prednisolone sodium succinate

Use Shock

Dose 11 to 30 mg/kg IV

Use Cerebral edema (methylprednisolone sodium succinate preferred)

Dose 60 mg/kg IV initially, followed by 30 mg/kg IV 2 and 6 hours after initial dose, followed by tapering dose, over the next 42 hours

Prednisone; *see* Prednisolone

Procainamide

Use Ventricular dysrhythmias

Dose *Dog* 6 to 8 mg/kg IV over 5 minutes followed by 10 to 40 µg/kg/min IV infusion
or 6 to 20 mg/kg IM q4-6h
or 10 to 20 mg/kg PO q6-8h

Propofol

Use Anesthesia

Dose *Dog* 5 to 7 mg/kg IV to effect without preanesthesia; lower doses are required when preanesthetics have been given
Cat 7 mg/kg IV induction; then 0.51 mg/kg/min IV infusion

Propranolol

Use Ventricular dysrhythmias, tachydysrhythmias

Dose Acute   0.02 to 0.06 mg/kg IV over several minutes
Nonacute *Dog* 0.125 to 0.250 mg/kg PO q8-12h
      Cat 2.5 to 5 mg PO q8-12h

Use Hypertension

Dose Use only with concurrent alpha blockade.
0.02 to 0.06 mg/kg IV slowly

Use *Bufo* (toad) poisoning

Dose 1.5 to 5.0 mg/kg IV q20min PRN ECG normalization
This dosage is for Bufo *poisoning ONLY!*

Protamine sulfate

Use Anticoagulant, therapy for heparin overdose

Dose 1 mg of protamine inactivates approximately 100 units of heparin. Administer IV *slowly,* not exceeding 5 mg/min.

Quinidine

Use Ventricular dysrhythmias

Dose *Dog* 6 to 16 mg/kg IM, PO q8-12h
Cat 4 to 8 mg/kg IM, PO q8h

Ranitidine

Use Gastric ulceration, gastritis

Dose *Dog* 1 to 2 mg/kg IV, SC, PO q8-12h
Cat 2.5 mg/kg IV q12h; 3.5 mg/kg PO q12h

Sodium bicarbonate

Use Alkalinization of urine for certain toxicoses

Dose 1 to 2 mEq/kg IV q3-4h; blood pH must be monitored

Use Treatment of metabolic acidosis

Dose Bicarbonate required = $0.3(BW_{kg} \times Base\ deficit)$
Administer $^1/_4$ to $^1/_2$ dose over 1 hour and the remaining over
the next 6 to 12 hours. Monitor blood gases.

Sodium nitrite

Use Confirmed cyanide poisoning

Dose 16 mg/kg IV slowly; repeat in 30 minutes
Sodium nitrite and 25% sodium thiosulfate are given in combination for cyanide poisoning. Cyanide antidote kits may be
found at local human hospitals.

Sodium nitroprusside; *see* Nitroprusside

Sodium polystyrene sulfonate

Use Cation exchange, hyperkalemia

Dose 0.25 to 0.5 g/kg/day PO or as enema

Sodium sulfate (Glauber's salt)

Use Cathartic

Dose *Dog* 250 to 500 mg/kg PO
Cat 200 mg/kg PO
The salt should be mixed with 5 to 10 times as much water for
oral administration.

Sodium thiopental

Use Induction, anesthesia

Dose 3 to 15 mg/kg IV to effect

Sodium thiosulfate

Use   Cyanide poisoning

Dose   *Dog* 1.65 mL/kg 25% sodium thiosulfate IV
Sodium nitrite and 25% sodium thiosulfate are given in combination for cyanide poisoning. Cyanide antidote kits may be found at local human hospitals.

Sorbitol

Use   Cathartic

Dose   4 g/kg PO

Succimer; *see* ***meso*-Dimercaptosuccinic acid**

Succinylcholine

Use   Muscle paralysis with controlled anesthesia

Dose   *Dog* 0.07 mg/kg IV
             Cat 0.06 mg/kg IV

Sucralfate

Use   Gastric or intestinal tract ulceration

Dose   *Dog* 250 to 1000 mg PO q6-8h
             Cat 250 mg PO q6-12h

Terbutaline

Use   Bronchodilatation

Dose   *Dog* 0.05 to 0.1 mg/kg PO q8-12h
             0.01 mg/kg SC q4h
             Cat 0.625 to 1.25 mg PO q8-12h
             0.01 mg/kg SC q4h

Tetramine

Use   Copper hepatopathy

Dose   *Dog* 10 to 15 mg/kg PO q12h

Theophylline

Use   Bronchodilatation

Dose   *Dog* 1 to 2 mg/kg IV or 5 mg/kg IM, PO q6-8h
             Cat 1 to 2 mg/kg IV or 4 mg/kg PO q8h

Thiamine (vitamin B$_1$)

Use   Ethylene glycol toxicosis, thiamine deficiency

Dose 10 to 100 mg/day IM, PO

Use Lead poisoning

Dose 1 to 2 mg/kg IM or 2 mg/kg PO q24h

Tocainide

Use Ventricular dysrhythmias

Dose *Dog* 15 to 30 mg/kg q8-12h

Trimethobenzamide HCl (Tigan)

Use Antiemetic; acts at the chemoreceptor trigger zone (CRTZ)

Dose 3 mg/kg IM q8-12h

Vecuronium

Use Muscle-paralyzing agent

Dose *Dog* 10 to 20 µg/kg IV
Cat 20 to 40 µg/kg in the cat

Vitamin K$_1$

Use Vitamin K–antagonist toxicosis

Dose 1 to 5 mg/kg SC, PO q12-24h for up to 6 weeks
Vitamin K$_1$ has greater bioavailability when given orally than subcutaneously. Therefore it should not be administered by injection unless the patient is vomiting, has received activated charcoal, or has some other complicating factor that precluded oral administration of the drug.

Xylazine

Use Emetic, sedative

Dose *Dog* 1.1 mg/kg IV
1.1 to 2.2 mg/kg IM, SC
Cat 0.44 mg/kg IM, SC

Yohimbine

Use Reversal of xylazine effects, antidote for amitraz intoxication

Dose *Dog* 0.11 mg/kg IV slowly
Cat 0.5 mg/kg IV slowly

Zinc acetate

Use Copper hepatotoxicosis

Dose *Dog* 5 to 10 mg/kg SC q12h

Appendix B
DAILY FLUID REQUIREMENTS

Daily Fluid Requirements for Dogs

Body weight (kg)	Maintenance needs	
	mL/day	mL/hour
1	132	6
2	214	9
3	285	12
4	348	15
5	407	17
6	463	19
7	515	21
8	566	24
9	615	26
10	662	28
11	707	29
12	752	31
13	795	33
14	837	35
15	879	37
16	919	38
17	959	40
18	998	42
19	1037	43
20	1075	45
21	1112	46
22	1149	48
23	1185	49
24	1221	51
25	1256	52
26	1291	54
27	1326	55
28	1360	57
29	1394	58
30	1427	59
35	1590	66
40	1746	73
45	1896	79

Daily Fluid Requirements for Dogs—cont'd

Body weight	Maintenance needs	
(kg)	mL/day	mL/hour
50	2041	85
55	2182	91
60	2319	97
70	2583	108
80	2836	118
90	3080	128
100	3316	138

Data from Haskins SC: *Semin Vet Med Surg (Small Anim)* 3:232, 1988.

Daily Fluid Requirements for Cats

Body weight	Maintenance needs	
(kg)	mL/day	mL/hour
1.0	80	3
1.5	108	5
2.0	135	6
2.5	159	7
3.0	182	8
3.5	205	9
4.0	226	9
4.5	247	10
5.0	268	11

Data from Haskins SC: *Semin Vet Med Surg (Small Anim)* 3:232, 1988.

Appendix C
RECIPES FOR DIALYSATE AND CONTINUOUS DRUG INFUSIONS

Dialysate Recipes

Under aseptic conditions mix:

1. One liter of lactated Ringer's solution, normal saline, or half-strength saline
2. 50% dextrose
   a. For a 1.5% dextrose dialysate solution, add 30 mL/L
   b. For a 2.5% dextrose dialysate solution, add 50 mL/L
   c. For a 4.25% dextrose dialysate solution, add 85 mL/L
3. 1000 units of heparin/L
4. Other medications as required

Warm the dialysate to slightly higher than body temperature (to promote vasodilatation) and administer according to protocol.

Dobutamine drip

Use Inotropic agent, increases cardiac output without much influence on heart rate or blood pressure except at higher doses.

Dose *Dog* 2 to 40 µg/kg/min IV infusion
Cat 2.5 to 15 µg/kg/min IV infusion

Concentration 12.5 mg/mL

Dose (µg/kg/min)	100 mL diluent (D$_5$W)	250 mL diluent	500 mL diluent
2.0	0.96 mL	2.40 mL	4.80 mL
3.0	1.44 mL	3.60 mL	7.20 mL
4.0	1.92 mL	4.80 mL	9.60 mL
5.0	2.40 mL	6.00 mL	12.00 mL
10.0	4.80 mL	12.00 mL	24.00 mL

Remove the amount of diluent listed above and then add that amount of stock dobutamine to the remaining diluent.
Administer at 1 mL/kg/hour
To administer higher doses, combine appropriate columns.
Constant monitoring of blood pressure is advised. Adjust rate according to response.
Tachycardia or cardiac dysrhythmias may be seen at higher doses.
Dobutamine may cause seizures in cats.

Dopamine drip

Use   Inotropic support, blood pressure support

Dose   5 to 20 μg/kg/min IV infusion

Use   Renal vasodilator, acute renal failure

Dose   1 to 3 μg/kg/min IV infusion

Concentration   40 mg/mL (available in 80 mg/mL and 160 mg/mL formulations)

Dose (μg/kg/min)	100 mL diluent (D₅W)	250 mL diluent	500 mL diluent
1.0	0.15 mL	0.38 mL	0.75 mL
2.0	0.30 mL	0.75 mL	1.50 mL
3.0	0.45 mL	1.13 mL	2.25 mL
4.0	0.60 mL	1.50 mL	3.00 mL
5.0	0.75 mL	1.88 mL	3.75 mL
10.0	1.50 mL	3.75 mL	7.50 mL
20.0	3.00 mL	7.50 mL	15.00 mL

The above is only for the 40 mg/mL formulation. Make appropriate adjustments when using other formulations.

Remove the above amount from the volume of diluent (preferably D₅W) and add the volume of stock dopamine from the vial to the container of diluent. Mix well.

The patient must be adequately hydrated before dopamine is administered.

Administer at 1 mL/kg/hour. Dopamine is given "to effect." Urine production should be monitored when dopamine is given at low doses. The rate of administration should be increased or decreased depending on urine production. Normal urine production is approximately 1 mL/kg/hour in the dog and 0.5 mL/kg/hour in the cat.

When dopamine is given to support blood pressure, the blood pressure is to be monitored and the rate of administration adjusted accordingly. The rate of administration must be decreased if tachycardia or cardiac arrhythmias are noted.

Dopamine is incompatible with sodium bicarbonate.

If dopamine leaks perivascularly, the area should be infiltrated with 5 to 10 mg of phentolamine mixed with 10 to 15 mL of saline. If this is not done, severe necrosis and sloughing are possible.

Lidocaine drip

Use Ventricular dysrhythmias

Dose *Dog* 1 to 2 mg/kg IV bolus followed by 25 to 75 µg/kg/min IV infusion

      Cat 0.25 to 1 mg/kg IV bolus followed by 5 to 40 µg/kg/min IV infusion

Concentration 20 mg/mL

Dose (µg/kg/min)	From 500 mL of fluid, remove:	Then add 2% lidocaine
5	7.5 mL	7.5 mL
10	15.0 mL	15.0 mL
20	30.0 mL	30.0 mL
30	45.0 mL	45.0 mL
40	60.0 mL	60.0 mL
50	75.0 mL	75.0 mL
60	90.0 mL	90.0 mL
70	105.0 mL	105.0 mL
75	112.5 mL	112.5 mL
Administer at 1 mL/kg/hour		

Procainamide drip

Use   For treatment of ventricular arrhythmias

Dose   *Dog*   6 to 8 mg/kg IV over 5 minutes followed by 10 to 40 µg/kg/min IV infusion

Concentration   100 mg/mL

Dose (µg/kg/min)	From 500 mL of fluid, remove:	Then add procainamide
10	3.0 mL	3.0 mL
15	4.5 mL	4.5 mL
20	6.0 mL	6.0 mL
30	9.0 mL	9.0 mL
40	12.0 mL	12.0 mL
Administer at 1 mL/kg/hour		

Sodium nitroprusside drip

Use To lower blood pressure by decreasing preload, afterload, and myocardial work.

Dose 0.5 to 10 µg/kg/min

Concentration 25 mg/mL

Dose (µg/kg/min)	100 mL diluent (D₅W)	250 mL diluent
0.5	0.12 mL	0.3 mL
1.0	0.24 mL	0.6 mL
2.5	0.60 mL	1.5 mL
5.0	1.20 mL	3.0 mL
7.5	1.80 mL	4.5 mL
10	2.40 mL	6.0 mL

Remove the amount listed from the diluent and add that amount of sodium nitroprusside solution to the diluent. Sodium nitroprusside decomposes in light and will lose potency if not protected from light. Wrap the diluent and administration set in appropriate light blocker (provided with the sodium nitroprusside in some cases) or wrap in aluminum foil.

Administer the solution at 1 mL/kg/hour. Continuous monitoring of blood pressure is mandatory. Cyanide toxicity may be seen.

Suggested Reading

Chew DJ, DiBartola SP, Crisp MS: Peritoneal dialysis. In DiBartola SP, editor: *Fluid therapy in small animal practice,* Philadelphia, 1992, WB Saunders.

Appendix D
POISON TREATMENT FLOW CHART

Pet's name:_____ Owner's name:_____

Date:_____ Time admitted:_____

Suspected toxin:_____

Treatment:

Secured airway:

Oxygen administered at (flow rate)_____/min

Vein catheterized:

Fluids given:

   Type:_____ Rate:_____

Antidotes given:

1. Product_____ Dose_____ Time_____

2. Product_____ Dose_____ Time_____

3. Product_____ Dose_____ Time_____

4. Product_____ Dose_____ Time_____

5. Product_____ Dose_____ Time_____

6. Product_____ Dose_____ Time_____

Emesis:

(First attempt)

Emesis with_____ Time administered:_____

(Second attempt)

Emesis with_____   Time administered:_____

(Third attempt)

Emesis with_____   Time administered:_____

Lavage:

Gastric or crop lavage with_____   Time:_____

Charcoal:

Activated charcoal with_____   Time:_____

Catharsis:

Catharsis with_____   Time:_____

Bathing:

Bathed with_____   Time:_____

INDEX